Feel Better Fast and Make It Last gives you the latest fascinating and important neuroscience information on how to boost your mood, quiet anxiety, and increase your overall brain health. I highly recommend it.

ANDREW NEWBERG, MD
Thomas Jefferson University; coauthor of *How God Changes Your Brain*

Life is full of challenges for everyone. But contrary to what you may believe, these events need not preclude your ability to be happy and joyful. In *Feel Better Fast and Make It Last*, Dr. Daniel Amen gives us a powerful array of tools to redirect our brains away from despair and grief to a place of happiness, gratitude, and love. This book is truly a precious gift.

DAVID PERLMUTTER, MD
Author of #1 *New York Times* bestseller *Grain Brain* and *The Grain Brain Whole Life Plan*

This book is delightful to read, a guide full of useful information for all of us that will help our brains and help our lives and our habits. All of us who have read it have been helped by it.

ANDREW CAMPBELL, MD
Editor in chief, *Advances in Mind-Body Medicine*

Feel Better Fast and Make It Last is the one book about the brain that you'll want to read this year. I have been working with Dr. Amen for the past 25 years, and this book is his most exciting work yet. Do you want to discover the secrets of quantum change? If you want to transform your life, take the practical steps outlined in this book, which will help you feel better fast and make it last. This book will give you what you need to bring lasting change to your brain. *Feel Better Fast and Make It Last* is your manual for transformed life!

DR. EARL HENSLIN
Clinical psychologist and author of *This Is Your Brain on Joy*

Daniel has taught me (and countless others) the critical role our brain health plays in our careers, families, and overall quality of life. If you truly value the relationships in your life, stop what you're doing and read this book.

TODD DAVIS
FranklinCovey's chief people officer; *Wall Street Journal* bestselling author of *Get Better: 15 Proven Practices to Build Effective Relationships at Work*

This book is your map to an abundant life! Imagine sitting down with one of the smartest, most passionate doctors on the planet and getting a personalized plan for the healthiest version of you. That is the experience of reading *Feel Better Fast and Make It Last.*

To know Dr. Amen is to believe that your life can be all it was meant to be. This book feels like sitting with him in his office and getting his personal plan for your healthiest life.

Healthy people build healthy families. Healthy families create a healthy world. If you want to positively change your life and the lives of generations that will follow you, you must read this book!

JEN ELMQUIST, MA, LMFT
Mental and relational health expert and author of *Relationship Reset*

Our choices determine our results, and our results determine our success. It all begins with choices. But the question is, which choices are right? How can we choose to live with joy, creativity, and prosperity, and free ourselves from depression and panic? With his astonishing new research, Daniel Amen has unlocked the answers. In this book, you'll discover new aspects of who you are and who you can become. Once you understand your own emotions and behaviors, you can replace the negative with a positive future. This book outlines the game plan to your most fascinating and fulfilling life.

SALLY HOGSHEAD
New York Times bestselling author and creator of the Fascination Advantage® personality test

Dr. Daniel Amen keeps writing cutting-edge, easy-to-understand books on what is most important to a healthy and happy brain. This is his best book yet. Dr. Amen shows us how we can all have good brains, overcome life's main stressors, and foster healthy lives. *Feel Better Fast and Make It Last* has motivated me to change my lifestyle, keeping the health of my brain in mind. This book will be on my "must read" list for all my clients—and my family members.

Dr. Amen's *Feel Better Fast and Make It Last* is a get-you-thinking and start-changing book that doesn't make you feel guilty but educates you into wanting to live with your brain as your first priority.

I could not put down *Feel Better Fast and Make It Last*, as it was readable, easy to understand, and related to my life. It shook me up and gave me new habits of asking myself each day, "Is this good or bad for my brain?" and making daily decisions based on "Will this make me feel good now but not later?" Dr. Amen's contribution to brain health is helping us all improve our lives.

SHARON MAY, PhD
Founder of Safe Haven Relationship Center and author of *Safe Haven Marriage*

We've all found ourselves reacting to one event or another—landing in a place we never expected to be. These ground-shaking moments can leave us feeling anxious, sad, angry, scared out of our minds, or worried. We want help, and more importantly, we need it *now*. We don't have to remain stuck in our pain. Dr. Amen's simple, hands-on, and very doable steps can change what seems unchangeable. Why wait, struggle, or hope for tomorrow when you can feel better fast today?

SHERI KEFFER, PhD
Author of *Intimate Deception: Healing the Wounds of Sexual Betrayal*

A SAMPLE OF OTHER BOOKS BY DANIEL AMEN

Memory Rescue, Tyndale, 2017

Stones of Remembrance, Tyndale, 2017

Captain Snout and the Super Power Questions, Zonderkidz, 2017

The Brain Warrior's Way, with Tana Amen, New American Library, 2016

The Brain Warrior's Way Cookbook, with Tana Amen, New American Library, 2016

Time for Bed, Sleepyhead, Zonderkidz, 2016

Change Your Brain, Change Your Life (revised), Harmony Books, 2015, *New York Times* Bestseller

Healing ADD (revised), Berkley, 2013, *New York Times* Bestseller

The Daniel Plan, with Rick Warren, DMin, and Mark Hyman, MD, Zondervan, 2013, #1 *New York Times* Bestseller

Unleash the Power of the Female Brain, Harmony Books, 2013

Use Your Brain to Change Your Age, Crown Archetype, 2012, *New York Times* Bestseller

The Amen Solution, Crown Archetype, 2011, *New York Times* Bestseller

Unchain Your Brain, with David E. Smith, MD, MindWorks, 2010

Change Your Brain, Change Your Body, Harmony Books, 2010, *New York Times* Bestseller

Magnificent Mind at Any Age, Harmony Books, 2008, *New York Times* Bestseller

The Brain in Love, Three Rivers Press, 2007

Making a Good Brain Great, Harmony Books, 2005, Amazon Book of the Year

How to Get Out of Your Own Way, MindWorks, 2005

ADD in Intimate Relationships, MindWorks, 2005

Preventing Alzheimer's, with William R. Shankle, MS, MD, Penguin, 2004

Healing Anxiety and Depression, with Lisa Routh, MD, Putnam, 2003

Healing the Hardware of the Soul, Free Press, 2002

New Skills for Frazzled Parents, MindWorks, 2000

The Most Important Thing in Life I Learned from a Penguin!?, MindWorks, 1995

Unlock Your Brain's Healing Potential to Overcome
Negativity, Anxiety, Anger, Stress, and Trauma

FEEL BETTER
FAST
AND
MAKE IT LAST

DANIEL G. AMEN, MD
#1 *NEW YORK TIMES* BESTSELLING AUTHOR

TYNDALE
MOMENTUM®

The nonfiction imprint of
Tyndale House Publishers, Inc.

Visit Tyndale online at www.tyndale.com.

Visit Tyndale Momentum online at www.tyndalemomentum.com.

Visit Daniel G. Amen, MD, at http://danielamenmd.com.

TYNDALE, *Tyndale Momentum*, and Tyndale's quill logo are registered trademarks of Tyndale House Publishers, Inc. The Tyndale Momentum logo is a trademark of Tyndale House Publishers, Inc. Tyndale Momentum is the nonfiction imprint of Tyndale House Publishers, Inc., Carol Stream, Illinois.

Feel Better Fast and Make It Last: Unlock Your Brain's Healing Potential to Overcome Negativity, Anxiety, Anger, Stress, and Trauma

Designed by Dean H. Renninger

Published in association with the literary agency of WordServe Literary Group, www.wordserveliterary.com.

For information about special discounts for bulk purchases, please contact Tyndale House Publishers at csresponse@tyndale.com, or call 1-800-323-9400.

Library of Congress Cataloging-in-Publication Data

Names: Amen, Daniel G., author.
Title: Feel better fast and make it last : unlock your brain's healing potential to overcome negativity, anxiety, anger, stress, and trauma / Daniel G. Amen, MD #1 New York Times bestselling author.
Description: Carol Stream, Illinois : Tyndale House Publishers, Inc., [2018] | Includes bibliographical references.
Identifiers: LCCN 2018029690 | ISBN 9781496425652 (hc)
Subjects: LCSH: Self-care, Health. | Brain.
Classification: LCC RA776.95 .A464 2018 | DDC 612.8/2--dc23 LC record available at https://lccn.loc.gov/2018029690

ISBN 978-1-4964-3881-2 (International Trade Paper Edition)

Printed in the United States of America

24   23   22   21   20   19   18
7   6   5   4   3   2

MEDICAL DISCLAIMER

The information presented in this book is the result of years of practice experience and clinical research by the author. The information in this book, by necessity, is of a general nature and not a substitute for an evaluation or treatment by a competent medical specialist. If you believe you are in need of medical intervention, please see a medical practitioner as soon as possible. The stories in this book are true. The names and circumstances of the stories have been changed to protect the anonymity of patients.

Contents

Introduction

YOU CAN FEEL BETTER FAST AND MAKE IT LAST: THE BRAIN-XL APPROACH

It is during our darkest moments that we must focus to see the light.
ATTRIBUTED TO ARISTOTLE

Virtually all of us have felt anxious, depressed, traumatized, grief-stricken, or hopeless at some point in life. It's perfectly normal to go through hard times or experience periods when we feel panicked or out of sorts, whether we have a diagnosable condition or not. How we respond to these challenges makes all the difference in how we feel—not just immediately, but in the long run.

All of us want to stop the pain quickly. Unfortunately, many people self-medicate with energy drinks, overeating, alcohol, drugs, risky sexual behavior, angry outbursts, or wasting time on mindless TV, video games, social media, or shopping. Although these substances and behaviors may give us temporary relief from feeling bad, they usually only prolong and exacerbate the problems—or cause other more serious ones, such as energy crashes, obesity, addictions, sexually transmitted diseases, unhappiness, relationship problems, or financial ruin.

I am a psychiatrist, a brain-imaging researcher, and the founder of Amen Clinics, which has one of the highest published success rates in treating people with complex and treatment-resistant mental health issues such as attention deficit hyperactivity disorder (ADHD), anxiety and mood disorders, posttraumatic stress disorder, and more. Thanks to all of this experience, I understand how critical it is for you to know *what will help you feel better right now and later*. In this book I'll be highlighting strategies that will lead you to experience more joy, peace, energy, and resilience, both immediately and in the future.

Plenty of things may help in the short term but will make you feel worse—or cause more problems—in the long term. Here are two stories that illustrate how the right remedies can set you on a healthier, happier course.

CHRIS: HELP FOR A GRIEVING MOM

I met Chris at my Northern California clinic when I was there giving a lecture. She told me that two years earlier she had lost her 12-year-old daughter, Sammie, to bone cancer. Chris had no idea how hard Sammie's death would hit her. Every night she went to bed with Sammie's illness and death playing over and over in her mind. Chris ate more and drank alcohol as a way to cope and quiet her mind, but most mornings she woke up in a panic, and the terror would follow her through her days. She felt so useless and depressed that she had secretly planned on killing herself on the two-year anniversary of Sammie's death.

Just a few weeks before the anniversary, Chris was visiting with a friend of her sister's, whom she described as very fit, with a positive attitude. Chris, who is just five feet one inch tall, weighed a little more than 200 pounds and was walking in a gloom so heavy she thought she'd never smile—and mean it—again. "This friend had a copy of the *Change Your Brain, Change Your Body Daily Journal*," Chris explained. "Flipping through it, I thought, *Okay, I like this. It makes sense to me. I have to start looking for the brighter side of life.* After all, my choices at that point were to take my life, drink myself to death, or end up in rehab. And I was way too proud to go to rehab." Chris went home and downloaded my book *Change Your Brain, Change Your Body* and read it cover to cover in one night. "I can still remember how I felt in the moment when I read . . . that alcohol stops you from feeling 'empathy and compassion for others.' I knew I needed to get my feelings of empathy and compassion back for my other children and husband. I needed to find a way to be happy and whole again for their sakes and my own.

"I went hard-core into the plan," Chris said. "In fact, I did a 28-day cleanse. I tossed out all the alcohol, ate no processed food, and began taking fish oil and vitamin D." Chris felt better nearly immediately. "Within eight days I didn't care if I never dropped a pound again. I was free! Because I was eating food that actually nourished my cells, the food and alcohol cravings stopped. I got rid of all the diet drinks and colas. I slept through the night for the first time in four years, and I didn't wake up in a panic." After 10 weeks she had lost 24 pounds and was running four days a week. After five months she was down 35 pounds and had lost eight inches off her waist.

Her skin was brighter, and she felt like a completely new woman. Of course she will never forget her daughter, but there is no way that Sammie would have wanted her mother to be in such pain. Now Chris believes that Sammie would be proud of her.

The best time to start healing from a crisis is before it starts. Giving yourself the excuse to eat bad food, drink alcohol, or smoke pot to deal with the pain only prolongs it. Never let a crisis be your excuse to hurt yourself.

If you're like me, when you hurt, you want to feel better now, fast, pronto! During my psychiatric training I had a wonderful supervisor, Dr. Jack McDermott, who was a world leader in psychiatry. I loved his mentorship on how to help children, teens, adults, and families who were hurting. In his professional evaluation of me at the end of the year, he wrote, "Dr. Amen is a bright, competent, and caring physician, who will make a wonderful psychiatrist; but he needs to be more patient. He wants people to get better fast." Then and now, I don't see wanting people to get better quickly as a problem. That is what people who are in pain want. No one wants to be patient. No one wants a prolonged process. They want to feel better fast, and they want that feeling to last.

LEIZA: REVERSING DEPRESSION AND MEMORY PROBLEMS

Leiza, an attractive woman with flaming red hair, was 50 years old when she first came to our Atlanta clinic. She had seen one of my public television programs and brought her teenage son to us for ADHD because he had not responded to treatment. She also decided to be scanned because, as she said, "I'm very scattered, always late, and my memory is poor. . . . My father and his mother had dementia, and I don't want it. . . . I really feel like I am in the early stages of dementia. . . . I am tired of being depressed and beating myself up." She had been an actor and then a stay-at-home mother for 20 years. As her children were becoming more independent, she wanted to act again, but she didn't believe she could. She told one of her friends, "I could never go back to work. I can't remember anything. I can't focus. I can't make any decisions."

The two years before Leiza came to see us were the most challenging in her life. She had felt a lot of anxiety while taking care of her son's learning disabilities, her daughter's depression, and her father's dementia, and in dealing with the death of her mother-in-law. With the chronic stress, Leiza noticed more problems with her memory. She would make appointments and then forget to show up, despite having put the appointment on her calendar. Six months before her appointment with us, she was diagnosed with ADHD and put on Adderall, but she didn't think it helped her.

As part of our workup of Leiza, we did a brain imaging study called SPECT (single photon emission computed tomography), which looks at blood flow and activity—essentially, how the brain works. Her SPECT scan showed severe decreased blood flow across her whole brain, which was very concerning given the family history of Alzheimer's disease. Our research, and that of others, has shown that Alzheimer's disease and other forms of dementia start in the brain decades before people have any symptoms. Leiza was already symptomatic, and her brain showed that she was headed for the same fate as her father and grandmother.

Leiza's scan was the wake-up call she needed to get serious about rehabilitating her brain *now* if she wanted to feel better fast and avoid eventually being a burden to her children. She was motivated to do everything we recommended, including taking supplements and doing a treatment called hyperbaric oxygen therapy (HBOT; see appendix A, page 292), which boosts blood flow to the brain. Within several months she noticed significant improvement in her mood, focus, and memory. She started to audition for television and landed a lead role in a TV pilot as the FBI director. She told me none of it would have been possible without rehabilitating and caring for her brain. Her follow-up scan two years later showed remarkable improvement, which is something we have seen repeatedly over the past three decades. Your brain can be better and you can feel better—and we can prove it!

How to Read SPECT Scans

Throughout this book you'll see a number of SPECT scans from Amen Clinics patients.

We will include four images; they show the brain first from underneath and then, moving clockwise, from the right side, the top, and the left side. For detailed information about how the SPECT scan works and who should get one, see "When Should You Think about Getting a Functional Imaging Study, Such as SPECT?" on page 271.

HEALTHY SPECT SCAN

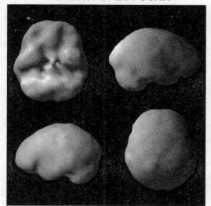

Full, even, symmetrical activity

LEIZA'S SPECT SCAN

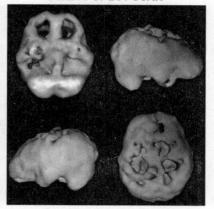

Holes indicate areas of severe decreased blood flow.

LEIZA'S AFTER TREATMENT SPECT SCAN

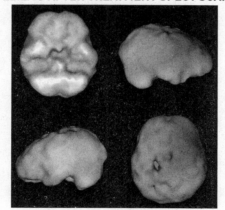

Marked overall improvement

THE MISSING STRATEGY TO FEELING BETTER FAST

One of the most important secrets to our success at Amen Clinics is that we focus first on understanding, healing, and optimizing the physical functioning of the brain (hardware), and second on properly programming it (software). Both always work together, and if you ignore one while only working on the other, you will have a harder time consistently feeling better.

Unfortunately, the vast majority of professionals who are trained to help people who are struggling with how they feel receive little to no training on how to heal and optimize the brain, which limits their success. I recently lectured to 5,000 mental health professionals and asked them how many had received *any* training on how to optimize the physical functioning of the brain during their education; fewer than one percent raised their hands.

Physicians have been trying to drug the brain into submission since the 1950s. The outcomes have been poor because doctors too often ignore the necessity of first putting the brain into a healing environment by addressing issues such as sleep, toxins, diet, exercise, and supplementation. Dr. Thomas Insel, former director of the National Institute of Mental Health, wrote, "The unfortunate reality is that current medications help too few people to get better and very few people to get well."[1] In contrast with antibiotics, which can cure infections, none of the medications for the mind cure anything. They only provide a temporary bandage that comes off when the psychotropic medications are stopped, causing symptoms to recur. In addition, many of these medications are insidious; once you start on them, they change your brain chemistry so you need them in order to feel normal. There is a better way. *Feel Better Fast and Make It Last* is the manual that helps you unlock your brain's healing potential to quickly overcome negativity, anxiety, anger, stress, grief, and trauma.

Honestly, I, too, undervalued brain health for nearly a decade as a young psychiatrist until our group at Amen Clinics found a practical way to look at the brain. Before we started our brain imaging work in 1991, I had been trained and board-certified as a child-and-adolescent psychiatrist and general psychiatrist and was busy seeing children, teens, adults, and older adults with a wide variety of issues connected with mental health, including depression, bipolar disorder, autism, violence, marital conflict, school failure, and ADHD. During that time, I was flying blind and not thinking much about the actual physical functioning of my patients' brains. Researchers at academic centers told us that brain imaging tools were not ready for clinical practice—maybe someday in the future.

I loved being a psychiatrist, but I knew we were missing important puzzle pieces. Psychiatry was, and unfortunately remains, a soft, ambiguous science, with many competing theories about what causes the troubles our patients experience. In medical school and during my psychiatric residency and child-and-adolescent psychiatry fellowship, I was taught that while we really didn't know what caused psychiatric illnesses, they were likely the result of a combination of factors, including

- Genetics—but no one knew exactly which genes were the real troublemakers;
- Abnormal brain chemistry—which gave us many medications to try, but they only worked some of the time;
- Toxic parenting or painful childhood experiences—but some people thrived even though they were raised in abusive environments, while others withered;
- Negative thinking patterns—but correcting the erroneous thought patterns helped some people and not others.

The lack of neuroimaging led to a "brainless" psychiatry, which kept my profession steeped in outdated theories and perpetuated stigma for our patients. I often wondered why all other medical specialists looked at the organs they treated—cardiologists, for example, scanned the heart, gastro-enterologists scoped the gut, and orthopedists imaged bones and joints—while psychiatrists were expected to guess at what was wrong by talking to patients. *And we were dealing with the most complicated organ of all—the human brain!* Our patients are every bit as sick as those with heart disease, osteoporosis, or cancer. Depression, bipolar disorder, addictions, and schizophrenia are all potentially lethal disorders, and even issues such as chronic stress, anxiety, and ADHD can affect all aspects of our lives.

IMAGING CHANGED EVERYTHING

In 1991, everything changed for me. My lack of respect for the brain vanished almost instantly when I started looking at the brains of my patients with a nuclear medicine study called SPECT, mentioned in Leiza's story on page xvi. It is different from CT or MRI scans, which look at the brain's anatomy or structure. SPECT looks at brain function, which is helpful because functional problems almost always precede structural problems. SPECT is a leading indicator of trouble, pointing to issues years before they manifest, while CT and MRI are lagging indicators of trouble that reveal abnormalities later in illnesses. SPECT basically answers a key question about each area of the brain: Is it healthy, underactive, or overactive? Based on what we see, we can stimulate the underactive areas or calm the overactive ones with supplements, medicines, electrical therapies, or other treatments, all of which optimize the brain. We can also help patients ensure that the healthy areas of their brains stay healthy.

Almost immediately after starting to look at scans, I became excited about the possibilities of SPECT to help my patients, my family, and myself. The scans helped me be a better doctor, as I could observe the brain function of my patients. I could see if their brains were healthy, which meant the issues they were facing were more likely to be psychological, social, or spiritual rather than biological in nature. I could see if there was physical trauma from concussions or head injuries, causing trouble to specific areas of the brain, or if there was evidence of toxic exposure from drug or alcohol abuse (addicts rarely admit to how much they are using, but it is hard to stay in denial when looking at a damaged brain) or other toxins, such as mercury, lead, or mold. I also could see if my patients' brains worked too hard, which is associated with anxiety disorders and obsessive-compulsive tendencies.

I was so excited about imaging that I scanned many people in my own family, including my 60-year-old mother, who had one of the healthiest SPECT scans I had seen. Her scan reflected her life. As a mother of seven children and grandmother and great-grandmother of 44, she has always been everyone's best friend. At the time of this writing, she has been married to my father for 68 years, and she is consistently loving, attached, focused, and successful in every way, including being the club golf champion and a top golfer for more than 50 years. After scanning my mom, I scanned myself, and my results were not so good. I had played football in high school and gotten sick with meningitis as a young soldier, plus I had a lot of bad brain habits, such as not sleeping more than four hours a night, struggling with being overweight, eating junk food, and being chronically stressed at home and at work. Seeing my mom's scan and then my own, I fell in love with my brain and vowed to make it better. I also developed what I call brain envy. I come from a very competitive family and was highly irritated that my 60-year-old mother had a better-looking brain than I did at 37. Much of my life after that moment has been about making my brain better and teaching others what I learned about how to do it. When my brain was rescanned 20 years later, it was much healthier.

Now, close to 30 years after we started to look at the brain at Amen Clinics, we have built the world's largest database of nearly 150,000 brain SPECT scans on patients from 120 countries. Our work has clearly taught us that unhealthy brain function is associated with a higher incidence of

- Sadness
- Anxiety
- Fear
- Panic
- Brain fog

- Poor focus
- Addictions
- Domestic violence
- Incarceration
- Loneliness

- Suicidal behaviors
- Violence
- School failure

- Divorce
- Dementia

By contrast, healthy brain function is correlated with improved

- Happiness
- Joy
- Energy
- Resilience
- Focus
- Longevity

- Relationships
- School performance
- Business success
- Wealth management
- Creativity

This is what feeling better looks like. As your brain becomes healthier, you will experience fewer of the problems on the first list and more of the rewards on the second. And as these positive personal characteristics take hold, you'll experience constructive changes in your attitude, your ability to respond to challenges, and your sense of purpose.

THE BRAIN-XL APPROACH

Using the mnemonic, or memory aid, BRAIN-XL as our framework, I'll introduce you to the latest research, as well as our clinical experience, to help you feel better fast and make it last. First, I want to acquaint you with the four aspects of health, which I often share with my patients: biological, psychological, social, and spiritual. They all work together, and we need to be aware of each one as we take steps to feel better. If there's a root biological cause for our problems, such as a genetic inheritance or the lasting effects of a head injury, we need to deal with that first. But we also need to be aware of psychological aspects, like negative thought patterns or an early childhood trauma, as well as the way our social interactions and connections can affect us. And finally, our health can have a spiritual component. When we have a strong sense of purpose—of living for something larger than ourselves—we find inspiration that can go a long way to helping us feel better. As we work through the BRAIN-XL acronym, we'll touch on all of these areas.

I chose BRAIN-XL because improving your brain health is the core strategy of the program, and XL has many terrific meanings, including *excel*, *extra large*, *extra load*, *extended life*, and *extra love*. Of course, no one feels joyful all the time, but with an understanding of how your physical brain, mental processes, social attachments, and spiritual connection work and some strategies that will enhance their functioning, you are more likely to love your life and feel better every day. Here is what BRAIN-XL stands for:

B Is for Brain

Chapter 1: Use Your Brain to Rescue Your Mind and Body. Whenever you feel sad, mad, nervous, or out of control, it is critical to have emotional-rescue techniques. This chapter will introduce you to six powerful practices to help you feel better fast.

Chapter 2: The Missing Strategy. The secret to feeling better fast now and for a lifetime is to immediately work on optimizing the physical functioning of your brain. This chapter summarizes my latest thinking on how to help you have the best brain possible, as quickly as possible.

Chapter 3: Control Yourself. Are you impulsive, distracted, and disorganized . . . or thoughtful, focused, and organized? The part of your brain that determines which of these descriptions fits you is the *prefrontal cortex*, or *PFC*, in the front third of your brain. Neuroscientists call it the "executive" part of the brain because it acts like your own internal chief executive officer or boss. This chapter will help you strengthen your PFC to make great decisions and avoid ones that can ruin your life.

Chapter 4: Change Is Easy—If You Know How to Do It. Your brain likes to do what it has always done, even when that is not in your best interest. Getting stuck in unhelpful behaviors, holding grudges, and engaging in unproductive worrying all cause immense suffering. There is an area deep in the frontal lobes called the *anterior cingulate gyrus*, the brain's gear shifter, which allows you to move from thought to thought or idea to idea. When this part of the brain is healthy, you are flexible and adaptable, and you can easily shift your attention and learn from your mistakes. When it is overactive, you can get stuck on negative thoughts (obsessions) or behaviors (addictions), say no even when saying yes may be good for you, and notice what is wrong a lot more often than you notice what is right. This chapter will help you optimize this part of the brain to turn your ruts into superhighways of success.

R Is for Rational Mind

Chapter 5: Master Your Rational Mind. Once the physical functioning of your brain is healthy, it is critical to know how to strengthen your rational mind.

This chapter will help you develop the mental discipline necessary for feeling better fast, including eliminating the ANTs (automatic negative thoughts), quieting your mind, focusing on gratitude, and even welcoming failure.

A Is for Attachments

Chapter 6: Healing Connections. Our attachments bring us the greatest joys and the most painful sorrows. When relationships are stressed or break apart, people become unhappy and vulnerable to acting in counterproductive ways. In a computer analogy, social attachments are like network connections. The way the brain is functioning is often the missing piece in understanding healthy or difficult relationships, trauma, and grief. This chapter explores how to use your brain to improve any relationship, helping you to feel better fast. Knowing this information can help you save your job, your marriage, your friendships, or your relationships with your children—or all four.

Chapter 7: Overcoming Trauma and Grief. Emotional trauma can get stuck in the brain, causing your emotional circuits to overfire—sometimes for years. This chapter explores healthy ways to eliminate the hurts that haunt you.

I Is for Inspiration

Chapter 8: Create Immediate and Lasting Joy. True inspiration comes from knowing why you are on the planet and grasping the meaning and purpose underlying what you do. Knowing and acting on your "why" is critical to living each day with joy. Purposeful people are happier and healthier, and they live longer. This chapter shows you how to protect your brain's pleasure centers to live with passion and purpose and avoid addictions and depression. This knowledge can help you feel joyful every day.

N Is for Nourishment

Chapter 9: The Feel Better Fast Diet. Your brain needs a constant source of energy to run your life. Think of it as the battery that powers your life. This chapter explains which foods you need (and which you should toss) to immediately boost your focus, memory, and mood.

Chapter 10: Advanced and Brain-Type Nutraceuticals. This chapter gives you a personalized, targeted approach to getting the nutrients your brain and body need. It provides detailed descriptions of the nutraceuticals I think everyone should take, together with ones targeted to specific brain types.

X Is for the X Factor

Chapter 11: Think Different. In any given situation, the X factor is the variable that has the most significant impact on the outcome. That perfectly describes the brain imaging work we've been blessed to do at Amen Clinics. It changed everything we do. By looking at the brain in people who had complex problems or were treatment resistant, we gained new insights that often made the difference between success and failure, healing and maintaining illness, even life and death. This chapter reveals the top 10 lessons we and our patients have learned from our experience with brain SPECT imaging. It also lists the circumstances in which you or a loved one should consider a scan.

L Is for Love

Chapter 12: Love Is Your Secret Weapon. Doing the right thing is the ultimate act of love for yourself and others. Here you will learn about the science of epigenetics and how caring for your brain and body can impact generations to come. That really makes the good feelings last a long time.

IS IT REALLY POSSIBLE TO FEEL BETTER FAST?

Many people, mental health professionals included, think therapy needs to be long, hard, and painful. They believe that if you start medication for anxiety or depression, you're making a lifelong commitment. Certainly some people will need help longer than others, but in my experience, many people can feel better fast if they engage in the right behaviors and strategies, which include knowing about and optimizing their brains.

Think about it: You know you can make yourself feel worse almost immediately by dwelling on the worst possible outcome of a situation, spending time with highly toxic people, or sabotaging each of your senses with dreadful sounds, smells, tastes, touches, or sights. You can just as easily make yourself feel better through simple choices like practicing gratitude, surrounding yourself with caring people, and using many other techniques that I will demonstrate throughout the book.

: 15 MINUTES **Keep an eye out for the stopwatch:** You will find it next to strategies that work quickly to help you feel better. The stopwatch will indicate the amount of time, up to 60 minutes, you need to devote to that strategy for it to begin to work. Although there are many helpful and valuable strategies in the coming pages, I am highlighting the fast-acting ones so that you can choose them when you need the most immediate relief.

The truth is, we live in an impatient society. When people seek help for mental health issues, the most common number of therapy sessions they receive is one. Either they find benefit from getting their worries off their chests and learning simple strategies—or they conclude therapy won't be helpful for them. Even when they commit to ongoing therapy, the average number of sessions a patient attends is six or seven, regardless of the psychotherapist's theoretical orientation.[2]

Almost everyone wants to feel better fast, and research suggests it is possible. Studies since the 1980s have shown the value of single-session therapies (SSTs). In one study, a single session of hypnosis significantly decreased anxiety and depressive symptoms after coronary artery bypass surgery.[3] In another, Australian researchers found that 60 percent of children and teens with mental health issues showed improvement after 18 months from just one session of therapy.[4] On page 190, I share the story of a man who was suffering from crushing grief and was helped by just one session with famed psychiatrist and Holocaust survivor Viktor Frankl. The components of SSTs are helping people tap into their strengths, offering simple solutions, and providing support—three strategies that I will also provide throughout the book.

Helping people change their feelings and behaviors and optimize their lives has been my passion as a psychiatrist for the past four decades. Amen Clinics partnered with Professor BJ Fogg, director of the Persuasive Tech Lab at Stanford University, and his sister, Linda Fogg-Phillips, to help our patients with behavior change. They teach that only three things change behavior in the long run:

1. An epiphany
2. A change in the environment (what and who surrounds you)
3. Taking baby steps[5]

When Leiza saw her troubled SPECT scan, it was a wake-up call for her to get healthy, as it is for so many of our patients. When I read a study by my friend Dr. Cyrus Raji[6] on what I call the dinosaur syndrome (as your weight goes up, the size and function of your brain go down—with a big body and a little brain, you're likely to become extinct), I had an epiphany and found the discipline to lose 25 pounds. But you don't have to wait for an epiphany to change your behavior. You don't need to have a heart attack or get cancer in order to get serious about your health. Most people can change their environment (friends, workplace, church) or the people they surround

FEEL BETTER FAST NOW BUT NOT LATER	FEEL BETTER FAST NOW AND LATER

themselves with, and all of us can make small changes that, over time, create amazing results.

High motivation helps you do hard things. But if your motivation is medium or even low, you can still change for the better. In fact, the Foggs encourage starting with baby steps, or what they call "Tiny Habits."[7] These are easy changes that will boost your sense of accomplishment and competence and, over time, evolve into bigger changes. At the end of each chapter, look for a list of Tiny Habits that you can incorporate each week, one or more at a time. Each one is tied to a habitual activity you do every day—like getting out of bed, brushing your teeth, answering the phone, or driving your car—which serves as a prompt to remind you to take action. The Tiny Habits format is "When I do x (or when x happens), I will do y." Then when you do y, celebrate to reinforce the new behavior and good feeling. Celebrations can be as simple as a fist pump or saying an "Atta boy" or "Atta girl" to yourself. Remember, small daily improvements are the key to spectacular long-term results.

Here's one you can start right now that will make a huge and lasting change: Whenever you come to a decision point in your day, ask yourself, "Is the decision I'm about to make good for my brain or bad for it?" If you consistently make decisions that serve your brain's health—and you'll learn more about how to do that in each chapter of this book—you are well on your way to feeling better fast in a way that will make it last.

PART 1

B IS FOR BRAIN

Amen Clinics are virtually unique in our focus on the brain as the source of many of our patients' problems. We always begin by addressing the brain's physical function and then move on to how it is programmed. It's absolutely necessary to do both. Sadly, many people forget the brain—or try to tame it with drugs, a temporary fix that will wear off sooner or later, causing symptoms to return. These next four chapters will give you brain-based strategies to gain control over anxiety, worry, sadness, stress, and anger.

In chapter 1 we'll look at quick, practical strategies that will help you feel better fast and pave the way for longer-term change, whether you're trying to rescue a bad day or dealing with an issue such as chronic anxiety or depression. Think of this as a tool-box you can put to immediate use. Then in chapters 2 through 4, we'll consider the brain's hardware, looking at specific areas of the brain that control different aspects of our mental processes. I'll give you lots of ideas for how you can help your brain function better.

CHAPTER 1

USE YOUR BRAIN TO RESCUE YOUR MIND AND BODY

QUICK TECHNIQUES WHEN LIFE FEELS OUT OF CONTROL

Climbing above one's difficulties always takes carefully considered action. There is always a way out, but it's easier to move effectively with the help of an experienced guide.

SIR EDMUND HILLARY, THE FIRST CONFIRMED MOUNTAIN CLIMBER TO SUMMIT MOUNT EVEREST

It was 6:30 in the morning in the busy emergency room at the Walter Reed Army Medical Center in Washington, DC. I was just putting on my white lab coat as I walked through the doors to the unit. It was my third day as an intern, and the emergency room would be my home for the next month. Down the hall from me, a woman was screaming. Curious, I went to see what was going on.

Beth, a 40-year-old patient, was lying on a gurney with a swollen right leg. She was in obvious pain and screamed whenever anyone touched her leg. Bruce, a brand-new psychiatry intern like me, and Wendy, the internal medicine chief resident, were trying to start an IV in Beth's foot. She was anxious, scared, uncooperative, and hyperventilating. A blood clot in her calf was causing this tremendous swelling. The IV was necessary so Beth could be sent to the X-ray department for a scan that would show exactly where the clot was, allowing surgeons to operate and remove it. With each stick of the IV needle to her swollen foot, Beth's screams became louder. Wendy was obviously frustrated and irritated, and sweat started to roll down her temples.

"Calm down!" she snapped at the patient.

Beth looked scared and confused. There was a lot of tension in the room.

Wendy paged the surgeon on call. She paced during the several minutes it took for him to get back to her. When the phone rang, Wendy quickly answered it, saying, "I need you to come to the ER right away. I need you to do a 'cut down' on a patient's foot. It looks like she has a blood clot in her leg, and we need to start an IV before sending her to X-ray. Her foot is swollen, and she's being difficult!"

Wendy listened for a few moments and then said, "What do you mean you can't come for an hour? This has got to be done right away. I'll do it myself." She cursed as she slammed down the phone.

Hearing this, Beth looked even more panicked.

Being new, I didn't want to say anything, especially because I had heard of Wendy's reputation for harassing interns, but I hated to see Beth in pain. *This is going to be an interesting day*, I thought to myself. I took a deep breath.

"Wendy, can I try to start the IV?" I asked softly.

She glared at me, and with a tone that was both sarcastic and condescending, she said, "Your name is Amen, right? I've been starting IVs for five years. What makes you think you're so special? But if you want to try and look stupid, hotshot, go for it." She rudely tossed the IV set at me and left the room. I motioned to Bruce to shut the door.

The first thing I did was walk around the gurney to Beth's head and establish eye contact with her. I gave her a gentle smile. Wendy had been yelling at Beth from the other end of the gurney, at her feet.

"Hi, Beth, I'm Dr. Amen. I need you to slow down your breathing. When you breathe too quickly, all of the blood vessels constrict, making it impossible for us to find a vein. Breathe with me." I slowed my own breathing, thinking that Wendy was going to kill me when I finished.

"Do you mind if I help you relax?" I asked. "I know some tricks."

"Okay," Beth said nervously.

"Look at that spot on the ceiling," I said, pointing to a spot overhead. "I want you to focus on it and ignore everything else in the room . . . I'm going to count to 10, and as I do, let your eyes feel very heavy. Only focus on the spot and the sound of my voice. 1 . . . 2 . . . 3 . . . let your eyes feel very heavy . . . 4 . . . 5 . . . let your eyes feel heavier still . . . 6 . . . 7 . . . 8 . . . your eyes are feeling very heavy and want to close . . . 9 . . . 10 . . . let your eyes close, and keep them closed.

"Very good," I said as Beth closed her eyes. "I want you to breathe very slowly, very deeply, and only pay attention to the sound of my voice. Let your whole body relax, from the top of your head all the way down to the bottoms of your feet. Let your whole body feel warm, heavy, and very relaxed. Now

I want you to forget about the hospital and imagine yourself in the most beautiful park you can imagine. See the park—the grass, the hillside, a gentle brook, beautiful trees. Hear the sounds in the park—the brook flowing, the birds singing, a light breeze rustling the leaves in the trees. Smell and taste the freshness in the air. Feel the sensations in the park—the light breeze on your skin, the warmth of the sun."

All of the tension in the room had evaporated. Wendy popped her head in the room, but Bruce put his index finger to his lips and motioned for her to leave. She rolled her eyes and quietly shut the door.

"Now I want you to imagine a beautiful pool in the middle of the park," I continued. "It is filled with special, warm healing water. In your mind, sit on the edge of the pool and dangle your feet in it. Feel the warm water surround your feet. You are doing really great."

Beth had gone into a deep trance.

I went on. "Now I know this might sound strange, but many people can actually make their blood vessels pop up if they direct their attention to them. With your feet in the pool, allow the blood vessels in your feet to pop up so that I can put an IV in one and you can get the help you need, still allowing your mind to stay in the park and feel very relaxed."

In medical school, I took a monthlong elective in hypnosis. I had watched a film of an Indian psychiatrist who put a patient in a hypnotic trance and had her dilate a vein in her hand. The doctor stuck a needle through the vein and then removed it, causing blood to flow out of both sides of the vein. Next, at the doctor's suggestion, the patient stopped the bleeding, first on one side of the vein and then the other. It was one of the most amazing feats of self-control I had ever seen. Beth's situation reminded me of the film. In truth, I had no expectation that she would actually be able to dilate the vein in her foot.

To my great surprise, the moment I made the suggestion, a vein clearly appeared on top of Beth's swollen foot. I gently slipped the needle into the vein and attached it to the bag of IV fluid. Bruce's eyes widened. He couldn't believe what he had just seen.

"Beth," I said softly, "you can stay in this deep relaxed state as long as you need. You can go back to the park anytime you want."

Bruce and I wheeled Beth to X-ray.

When I returned to the unit an hour later, Wendy gave me a hostile look, but I smiled inside.

With the right plan, you can feel better fast and make it last, even when you are in the midst of an emotional or physical crisis. That is why I have provided the following emergency rescue plan, which includes the techniques I used to help calm Beth—hypnosis, progressive muscle relaxation, and guided imagery—among others. Before we get to the plan, it is critical to understand how your brain and body work in a crisis, especially as it relates to your emergency alarm system—the fight-or-flight response.

THE FIGHT-OR-FLIGHT STRESS RESPONSE

The fight-or-flight response is hardwired into our bodies to help us survive. It is mobilized into action whenever a stress appears, such as what happened to Beth in the emergency room. Harvard physiology professor Walter Cannon first described the fight-or-flight response in 1915. He said it was the body's reaction to an acute stress, harmful event, or threat to survival, such as experiencing an earthquake or being robbed—or having the chief resident scream at you while she is poking you with a needle. Acute stress activates the sympathetic nervous system, which prepares you to either put up a fight or flee a dangerous situation. The fight-or-flight response is triggered by

1. the amygdala, an almond-shaped structure in the temporal lobes that is part of the limbic or emotional brain, which sends a signal to

2. the hypothalamus and pituitary gland to secrete adrenocorticotropic hormone (ACTH), which signals

3. the adrenal glands, on the top of the kidneys, to flood the body with cortisol, adrenaline, and other chemicals to rocket you into action.

The graphic on pages 8–9 illustrates what happens in our bodies when this response is set off.

The fight-or-flight response is part of a larger system in the body called the autonomic nervous system (ANS). It is called "autonomic" because its processes are largely automatic, unconscious, and out of our control, unless we train it otherwise (more on that coming up). It contains two branches that counterbalance each other: the sympathetic and parasympathetic nervous systems. Both regulate heart rate, digestion, breathing rate, pupil response, muscle tension, urination, and sexual arousal. The sympathetic nervous system (SNS) is involved in activating the fight-or-flight response, while the parasympathetic nervous system (PNS) helps to reset and calm our bodies.

Our very survival depends upon the fight-or-flight response, as it helps move us to action when there is a threat. But when stress becomes chronic, such as if you live in a war zone, grow up in an unpredictable alcoholic home, are sexually molested over time, or wet your bed and wake up every morning in a panic, your sympathetic nervous system becomes overactive. When that happens, you are more likely to suffer from anxiety, depression, panic attacks, headaches, cold hands and feet, breathing difficulties, high blood sugar, high blood pressure, digestive problems, immune system issues, erectile dysfunction, and problems with attention and focus.

In his groundbreaking book *Why Zebras Don't Get Ulcers*, Stanford University biologist Robert Sapolsky pointed out that for animals such as zebras, stress is generally episodic (e.g., running away from a lion) and their nervous systems evolved to rapidly reset. By contrast, for humans, stress is often chronic (e.g., daily traffic, a difficult marriage, job or money worries). Sapolsky argued that many wild animals are less susceptible than humans to chronic stress-related illnesses such as ulcers, hypertension, depression, and memory problems.[1] He did write, however, that chronic stress occurs in some primates (Dr. Sapolsky studies baboons), specifically individuals on the lower end of the social dominance hierarchy.

In humans, one big stress (such as being robbed, raped, or in a fire) or multiple smaller stressors (such as fighting with your spouse or children on a regular basis) can turn on a chronic fight-or-flight state in the body, leading to mental stress and physical illness. But you can learn to quiet your SNS and activate the PNS, which will lead you to feel calmer, happier, and less stressed. Improving the PNS is associated with lower blood pressure, more stable blood sugar, and better energy, immunity, and sleep.

THE FEEL BETTER FAST RESPONSE

After I finished my psychiatric training in 1987, I was stationed at Fort Irwin in California's Mojave Desert. Halfway between Los Angeles and Las Vegas, Fort Irwin was also known as the National Training Center—the place where our soldiers were taught to fight the Russians (and later others) in the desert. At the time, I was the only psychiatrist for 4,000 soldiers and a similar number of their family members. It was considered an isolated assignment. There were problems with domestic violence, drug abuse (especially amphetamine abuse), depression, and stress-related ailments from living in the middle of nowhere. I dealt with many people who suffered from headaches, anxiety attacks, insomnia, and excessive muscle tension.

THE FIGHT-OR-FLIGHT RESPONSE

Threat: an attack, harmful event, or threat to survival

Brain: processes the signals, beginning first in the amygdala and then in the hypothalamus

ACTH

ACTH: pituitary gland secretes adrenocorticotropic hormone

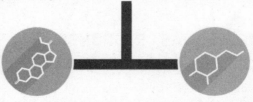

Cortisol released

Adrenaline released

PHYSICAL EFFECTS

Heart beats faster
and harder

Bladder relaxes

Pupils dilate for better
tunnel vision, but there is a
loss of peripheral vision

Erections are inhibited
(other things to
think about)

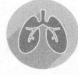

Air passages open and rapid
shallow breathing increases

Blood pressure increases

Production of tears
and saliva decreases

Digestion slows

Hearing diminishes

Muscles become tense;
trembling may occur.
Muscles around hair
follicles constrict, causing
goose bumps

Blood vessels shunt blood
to upper arms and upper
legs (fight or flee) and
away from hands and feet,
which get colder

Veins in skin constrict
(colder hands and feet) to
send more blood to major
muscle groups (to fight or
flee), causing the "chill"
sometimes associated
with fear

Blood sugar level
increases for energy

Brain has trouble focusing on
small tasks; it's thinking only
of dealing with the threat

Immune system
shuts down

Shortly after arriving at Fort Irwin, I went through the cabinets in the community mental health clinic, which was housed in a World War II Quonset hut, to see what helpful tools had been left behind by my predecessors. To my delight, I found an old biofeedback temperature trainer. Biofeedback is based on the idea that if you get immediate feedback on the physiological processes in your body, such as hand temperature, breathing, or heart rate, you can learn to change them through mental exercise. I had attended one biofeedback lecture during my psychiatric training, so I dusted off the old machine and started using it with patients who had migraine headaches. My staff and I taught them how to warm their hands using only their imaginations. Hand warming triggered an immediate parasympathetic relaxation response, which significantly decreased their migraine pain. It was fascinating to see how patients could raise their hand temperature with their minds, sometimes by as much as 15 to 20 degrees. Temperature training taught patients how to participate in their own healing process.

A few months after arriving at Fort Irwin, I wrote a request to our hospital commander, asking him to buy $30,000 worth of the latest computerized biofeedback equipment for our soldiers, including 10 days of training for me in San Francisco. While he laughed at me at first, eventually I got approval simply because he needed to spend his whole budget by the end of the year.

The biofeedback training was the most stimulating and intense learning experience I'd had as a physician. I learned how to help people relax their muscles, warm their hands (much faster than with the old equipment), calm sweat-gland activity, lower blood pressure, slow their own heart rates, breathe in ways that promoted relaxation, and even change their own brain wave patterns.

When I returned to Fort Irwin, my patients loved biofeedback because it helped them feel better fast. I loved it for the same reason and spent time each day doing it myself. I became masterful at breathing with my diaphragm, and I could slow my heart rate and even warm my own hands more than 15 degrees whenever I felt stressed. I had struggled with anxiety for most of my early life, which came in part from having an older brother who beat me up regularly when I was young, and in part from wetting my bed at night until about age nine. Waking up every morning in a panic, not knowing if the sheets would be wet or dry, changed my nervous system to be on alert and expect bad things to happen. Using these tools to calm myself was a wonderful relief.

Based on my work with hypnosis, biofeedback, and quickly enhancing brain function, here are six simple techniques that use your brain to control your mind and body, helping you to feel better fast.

Technique #1: Use hypnosis, guided imagery, and progressive muscle relaxation to enter a deep, relaxed state.

Many people associate hypnosis with loss of control or stage tricks. But doctors know it to be a serious science, revealing the brain's ability to heal medical and psychiatric conditions. "Hypnosis is the oldest Western form of psychotherapy, but it's been tarred with the brush of dangling watches and purple capes," said psychiatrist David Spiegel, MD, the son of a famous hypnotist and associate chair of psychiatry and behavioral sciences at Stanford University School of Medicine. "In fact, it's a very powerful means of changing the way we use our minds to control perception and our bodies. . . . The power of hypnosis to immediately change your brain is real."[2]

Using hypnosis, guided imagery, or progressive muscle relaxation (PMR) increases parasympathetic tone and can quickly decrease the fight-or-flight response in a wide variety of conditions, as it did for Beth. These techniques have been found to have many benefits, including lowering anxiety, sadness, and tension in parents of children with cancer;[3] pain and fatigue in those receiving chemotherapy;[4] stress in those with multiple sclerosis;[5] anxiety and depression;[6] migraine frequency;[7] tension headaches;[8] craving and withdrawal symptoms in people quitting smoking;[9] poststroke anxiety (a result of listening to a PMR CD five times a week);[10] and phantom limb pain.[11] They can also improve quality of life in the elderly[12] and dialysis patients,[13] fatigue in the elderly, and sexual function in postmenopausal women.[14]

Learning hypnosis, guided imagery, and progressive muscle relaxation is simple; there are many online audios that can guide you. We have several on our Brain Fit Life site (www.brainfitlife.com). You can certainly do it yourself. Below are the instructions I give my patients to help them go into a deep relaxed state. The skill builds over time, so it is important to practice this exercise to gain mastery. Set aside two 15-minute periods a day and go through the following five steps.

15 MINUTES SELF-HYPNOSIS, GUIDED IMAGERY, AND PROGRESSIVE MUSCLE RELAXATION: A HEALING PRACTICE

1. Sit in a comfortable chair with your feet on the floor and your hands in your lap. Pick a spot on the opposite wall that is a little bit above your eye level. Stare at the spot. As you do, slowly count to 20. Notice that your eyelids soon begin to feel heavy, as if they want to close. Let them. In fact, even if they don't feel as if they want to close, slowly lower them as you get to 20.

2. Take a deep breath, as deep as you can, and very slowly exhale. Repeat the deep breath and slow exhale three times. With each in-breath, imagine taking in peace and calmness, and with each out-breath, blow out all the tension—all the things getting in the way of your relaxing. By this time, you'll notice a calm come over you.

3. Squeeze the muscles in your eyelids, closing your eyes as tightly as you can. Then slowly let the muscles in your eyelids relax. Imagine that relaxation slowly spreading, like a warm, penetrating oil, from the muscles in your eyelids to the muscles in your face—down your neck, into your shoulders and arms, into your chest, and throughout the rest of your body. The muscles will take the cue from your eyelids and relax progressively all the way down to the bottoms of your feet.

4. When all the tension has left your body, imagine yourself at the top of an escalator. Step on the escalator and ride down, counting backward from 10. By the time you reach the bottom, you'll be very relaxed.

5. Enjoy the tranquility for several moments. Then get back on the escalator riding up, counting to 10 as you go. When you get to 10, open your eyes, feeling relaxed, refreshed, and wide awake.

To make these steps easy to remember, think of the following words:

- Focus (focus on the spot)
- Breathe (slow, deep breaths)
- Relax (progressive muscle relaxation)
- Down (ride down the escalator)
- Up (ride up the escalator and open your eyes)

If you have trouble remembering these steps, you may want to record them as you read them aloud and then do the exercise as you listen to the audio.

Allow yourself plenty of time to do this. Some people become so relaxed that they fall asleep for several minutes. If that happens, don't worry. It's a good sign—you're really relaxed!

:20 ADD VISUAL IMAGERY TO ENVISION A BETTER LIFE
MINUTES When you've practiced this technique a few times, add the following steps:

Choose a haven—a place where you feel comfortable and that you can imagine with all your senses. I usually "go" to the beach. I can see the ocean, feel the sand between my toes and the warm sun and breeze on my skin, smell the salt air and taste it faintly on my tongue, and hear the seagulls, the waves, and children playing. Your haven can be any real or imaginary place where you'd like to spend time.

After you reach the bottom of the escalator, use all your senses to imagine yourself in your special haven. Stay for several minutes. This is where the fun starts and where your mind becomes ripe for change.

Begin to experience yourself—not as you currently are, but as you *want* to be. Plan on spending at least 20 minutes a day on this refueling, life-changing exercise. You'll be amazed at the results.

During each session, choose one goal to work on. Stay with that goal until you can imagine yourself reaching it, going through each of the steps required to attain it. If your goal is to own your own business, for example, use all your senses to imagine yourself in that business. See the office or shop. Interact with your customers. Smell the environment around you. Feel your desk. Sip a cup of coffee in your chair, savoring the taste and aroma. Experience your dream. Make it real in your imagination, thereby beginning to make it real in your life. Or, if your goal is to improve your relationship with your spouse, friend, or children, imagine the relationship as you want it to be, in as much detail as you can. The way to improve your expectations is to first imagine the situation as you want it to be instead of imagining the worst, as you likely have been doing.

IT EVEN WORKS AT HOME

Years ago, on the Fourth of July, we had a party at our house. As the fireworks started outdoors, our then-eight-year-old daughter, Chloe, was creating her own fireworks in our kitchen. My wife, Tana, had created a new dessert for the party, a combination of coconut and almond butter. Chloe decided to heat it up. When she took it out of the microwave, she tested it with her finger—and that's when the screaming started. It was very hot, and the concoction stuck to her finger. She first tried to shake it off, then wiped it off with a towel and stuck her finger in her mouth. Next, she put her hand in ice water, then aloe gel, and then ice cubes. The pain and frustration escalated as she unraveled, and the automatic negative thoughts (ANTs; see chapter 5) started to take over. "I'm so stupid," she said. "Why did I do that?" Her mother gave her ibuprofen for the pain and started putting her to bed, but Chloe was not calming down.

The negative thoughts were now coming in droves. "I can't do this. It's too much. I can't take it. I'm so stupid. I can't believe I did it. I wish I could go back and do it over."

Tana tried to distract Chloe by reading to her, but it didn't work. She then prayed with her, but Chloe couldn't focus. Nothing worked, so Tana walked into my office and said I needed to help.

I sat on Chloe's bed and assessed the situation. As I had done for many patients in the hospital, I used a simple hypnotic trance to calm her. Using the outline above, I had her focus on a spot on the wall, close her eyes, start to relax her body, and slow her breathing. I then asked her to imagine walking down a flight of stairs as I counted backward from 10. Next I had her imagine going to a special park that she imagined with all of her senses, where it was safe and she was with her mother and friends. I had her imagine going into a warm pool. The water had special healing powers that soothed and helped her finger, taking away the pain. The water also helped to calm her thoughts and her body. She did not need to be so hard on herself. We all make mistakes. Being angry only made the pain worse.

Chloe became visibly more relaxed and started to drift off to sleep. The park and special healing pool was a place she could go back to anytime she was upset or needed to calm down. Then she fell asleep. Quietly, we left her room, wondering how she would do. We did not see her until the next morning, and even though she had a small blister on her finger, she said it didn't hurt and all was well. "Everyone makes mistakes," she said. "I guess that was one of mine. I won't do it again." This technique is very powerful—with adults and with children, too.

Technique #2: Master diaphragmatic breathing.

In the chapter's opening story, the first thing I did with Beth was help her to slow her breathing, so she could get more oxygen to her brain. Diaphragmatic breathing is a core biofeedback technique to help you feel better fast. It is simple to teach and, once practiced, simple to implement and maintain. Like brain activity, breathing is essential to life and involved in everything you do. Breathing delivers oxygen from the atmosphere into your lungs, where your bloodstream picks it up and takes it to all of the cells in your body so that they can function properly. Breathing also allows you to eliminate waste products, such as carbon dioxide, which can cause feelings of disorientation and panic. Brain cells are particularly sensitive to oxygen; within four minutes of being deprived of it, they start to die. Slight changes in oxygen content in the brain can alter the way you feel and behave.

When someone gets upset, angry, or anxious, their breathing becomes shallow and fast (see the "Breathing Anatomy" diagram below). This causes the oxygen in an angry person's blood to decrease, while toxic carbon dioxide increases. Subsequently, the oxygen/carbon dioxide balance is upset, causing irritability, impulsiveness, confusion, and bad decision-making.

Learning how to direct and control your breathing has several immediate benefits. It calms the amygdala (part of the emotional brain), counteracts the fight-or-flight response, relaxes muscles, warms hands, and regulates the heart's rhythms. I often teach patients to become experts at breathing slowly, deeply, and from their bellies. If you watch a baby or a puppy, you will notice that they breathe almost solely with their bellies—the most efficient way to breathe.

Expanding your belly when you inhale flattens the diaphragm, pulling the lungs downward and increasing the amount of air available to your lungs and body. Pulling your belly in when you exhale causes the diaphragm to push the air out of your lungs, allowing for a more fully exhaled breath, which once again encourages deep breathing. In biofeedback, patients are taught to breathe with their bellies by watching their breathing pattern on the computer screen. In 20 to 30 minutes, most people can learn how to change their breathing patterns, which relaxes them and gives them better control over how they feel and behave.

BREATHING ANATOMY

INHALATION   EXHALATION

Oxygen Intake   Carbon Dioxide

Lungs

Diaphragm

Diaphragm pulls downward, helping lungs expand with oxygen

Diaphragm returns upward, forcing lungs to expel carbon dioxide

The diaphragm, a bell-shaped muscle, separates the chest cavity from the abdomen. Many people never flatten the diaphragm when they inhale, and thus with each breath they have less access to their own lung capacity and have to work harder. By moving your belly out when you inhale, you flatten the diaphragm, significantly increase lung capacity, and calm all body systems.

BREATHING DURING ANGER

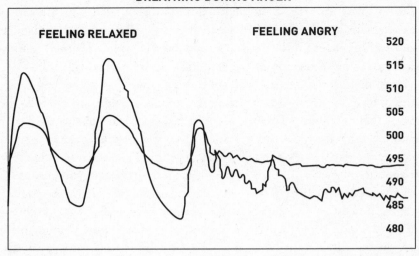

The large waveform is a measurement of abdominal or belly breathing, by a strain gauge attached around the belly; the smaller waveform is a measurement of chest breathing, by a strain gauge attached around the upper chest. At rest, this person breathes mostly with his belly (a good pattern), but when he thinks about an angry situation his breathing pattern deteriorates, markedly decreasing the oxygen to his brain (common to anger outbursts). No wonder people who have anger outbursts often seem irrational!

Controlled diaphragmatic breathing has been shown to improve focus and lower anxiety, stress, negative feelings, and cortisol;[15] decrease depression[16] and asthma;[17] reduce obesity in children,[18] pain,[19] blood pressure,[20] motion sickness,[21] and seizure frequency;[22] and boost the quality of life in heart failure patients.[23]

Technique #3: Become expert at warming your hands with your mind.

Take a moment to focus on your hands, feeling their energy and temperature. When you intentionally learn how to warm your hands with your brain by directing your thoughts to warming images (such as holding your palms up in front of a fire), your body goes into a relaxed state. Scientific research has shown that using this technique can be helpful for anxiety,[24] migraine headaches in both children[25] and adults,[26] blood pressure,[27] and irritable bowel syndrome (IBS).[28] New evidence shows that when you hold something warm, such as a warm hand, you are more trusting and giving, and you feel closer to others. Cold hands have the opposite effect.

Researchers studied college students to assess how hand temperature

Breathing Techniques to Help You Calm Down Fast

:05 *Breathing Technique #1:* While few people have access
MINUTES to sophisticated biofeedback equipment, these simple techniques can be effective for everyone. Try the following exercise right now: Lie on your back and place a small book on your belly. When you inhale, make the book rise by expanding your belly; when you exhale, pull your belly in, which will lower the book. Shifting the energy of breathing lower in your body—from your upper chest into your abdomen—will help you feel more relaxed and in better control of yourself almost instantaneously. Practice this for five minutes every day until it feels natural. You can use this breathing technique to gain greater focus and control over your temper. It is easy to learn, and it can also help with sleep and anxiety issues.

:02-03 *Breathing Technique #2:* Whenever you feel anxious,
MINUTES mad, or tense, take a deep breath, hold it for one or two seconds, and then slowly exhale for about five seconds. Then take another deep breath, as deep as you can, hold it for one to two seconds, and again slowly exhale. Do this about 10 times, and odds are that you will start to feel very relaxed, if not a little sleepy. I have used this technique myself for 30 years whenever I feel anxious, angry, or stressed, or when I have trouble falling asleep. It sounds so simple, but breathing is essential to life. When we slow down and become more efficient with our breathing, most things seem better.

affects emotions.[29] They found that holding warm things may actually make people view others more favorably and may also make them more generous. In one study, a tester met each of the 41 participants in the lobby of the building where the tests were being conducted. In the elevator on the way up, the tester casually asked the participant to hold his cup of coffee while he recorded some information on his clipboard. The participant did not know that this request was part of the experiment. Half the participants were asked to hold a cup of warm coffee, and half were asked to hold a cup of iced coffee. Once in the testing room, participants were given a packet of information on an unknown person and then asked to evaluate the person's personality using a questionnaire. Participants who had held the warm coffee were much more likely to score the unknown person as warmer than those who had held the iced coffee.

In a second study by the same researchers, participants were asked to hold either a hot or a cold therapeutic pad. Participants thought their role was to evaluate the product. After the "test," they were offered a reward for themselves or a treat for a friend. The people who had held the warm pad were more likely to choose the treat for a friend. Dr. John Bargh, coauthor of the study, said, "It appears that the effect of physical temperature is not just on how we see others, it affects our own behavior as well. Physical warmth can make us see others as warmer people, but also cause us to be warmer—more generous and trusting—as well." Coauthor Dr. Lawrence Williams said, "At a board meeting, for instance, being willing to reach out and touch another human being, to share their hand, those experiences do matter although we may not always be aware of them."[30] These studies are striking because we know that when our hands are cold, we are more likely to be anxious and fearful, traits that decrease intimacy and closeness to others.

Bring Warmth to Intimate Relationships

: 🔲 To develop heartfelt closeness, when you hold your
MINUTES partner's hand, imagine warm, loving energy going from your hand to his or hers. With each exhalation send warm, intentional thoughts of love and gratitude. Do this just a few times a day, and soon you will begin to notice a positive difference in your relationship.

Visualizing warmth, especially in your hands, is another tool to help you feel better fast and counteract the fight-or-flight response. I've found that teaching patients to warm their hands calms down their bodies and minds just as effectively as prescription drugs. Hand warming elicits an immediate relaxation response. We know this because biofeedback instruments allow us to measure hand temperature and then teach people how to warm their hands. Interestingly, children are better at this than adults because kids readily believe they have power over their bodies, whereas adults do not.

When my daughter Breanne was eight years old, she could increase her hand temperature by up to 20 degrees. She was so good at it, I brought her along with me when I did a biofeedback lecture to physicians at a Northern California hospital. In front of 30 physicians, I had her demonstrate her amazing skill. However, for the first three minutes her hands did nothing but get ice cold, because she felt such performance anxiety. In those few minutes I was horrified, feeling like a terrible father who was exploiting his daughter to be important in front of his colleagues. Then I whispered in her ear that she should close her eyes, take a deep breath, and imagine her hands in the warm sand at the beach (the image that worked best for her). Over the next seven minutes, her hands warmed 18 degrees. The doctors were amazed, she was so happy with herself, and I was relieved that I had not scarred her for life.

How can you warm your hands with your mind? You do it with diaphragmatic breathing and the visualization that works for you. For some, like Breanne, it's imagining putting your hands in warm sand at the beach. For others, it's thinking about holding a loved one's hand or touching their warm skin. For still others, it's visualizing holding a warm, furry kitten or puppy.

:03–04 *Hand-Warming Technique.* Close your eyes and hold out your
MINUTES hands, palms down, and visualize a campfire in front of you. Focus. Think heat. You can hear the fire crackle, smell the aroma of fresh-cut wood burning, see the sparks float up into the sky. Now feel the soothing heat as it penetrates the surface of your skin and goes deep to warm your hands. Picture this as you breathe deeply, and count slowly to 20. Did you feel an increase in warmth? Relaxation? Did you find you started to hold your hands closer as if there were actually a fire in front of you? Practice this technique for a few minutes every day, and you'll find you get to the relaxation response more easily and faster over time. Find the hand-warming images that work for you, and you will reset your nervous system to be more relaxed and counteract your stress response. You can buy temperature sensors online (under brand names Biodots, Stress Cards, and Stress Sheets) to get feedback on your progress.

13 Hand-Warming Images

1. Holding someone's warm hand or touching their warm skin
2. Visualizing (in great detail) someone you appreciate
3. Putting your hands in warm sand at the beach
4. Taking a hot bath or shower
5. Sitting in a sauna
6. Cuddling a baby
7. Cuddling a warm, furry puppy or kitten
8. Holding a warm cup of tea or sugar-free cocoa
9. Holding your hands in front of a fire
10. Wearing warm gloves
11. Being wrapped in a warm towel
12. Getting a massage with warm oil
13. Holding a hot potato while wearing warm gloves

Technique #4: Pray and/or practice meditation (especially Loving-Kindness Meditation).

Focusing on your breathing, a beautiful outdoor scene, or Scripture for just five to ten minutes a day is a simple yet powerful way to improve your life. Prayer and meditation have been found to calm stress; improve focus, mood, and memory; and enhance prefrontal cortex function to help you make better decisions. What's more, meditation benefits your heart and blood pressure, digestion, and immune system, as well as improving executive function and emotional control and reducing feelings of anxiety, depression, and irritability.[31]

There are many effective techniques, including reading, memorizing, or meditating on Scripture; writing out a personal prayer; reading classic spiritual writings; or focusing on gratitude. One of my personal favorite forms of meditation is called Loving-Kindness Meditation (LKM), which is intended to develop feelings of goodwill and warmth toward others. It has been found to quickly increase positive emotions and decrease negative ones,[32] decrease pain[33] and migraine headaches,[34] reduce symptoms of posttraumatic stress disorder[35] and social prejudice,[36] increase gray matter in the emotional processing areas of the brain,[37] and boost social connectedness.[38] Here's how to start to practice:

: 🔟 *Loving-Kindness Meditation.* Sit in a comfortable and relaxed posi-
MINUTES tion and close your eyes. Take two or three deep breaths, taking twice
as long to exhale as inhale. Let any worries or concerns drift away, and feel
your breath moving through the area around your heart. As you sit, quietly
or silently repeat the following or similar phrases:

May I be safe and secure.
May I be healthy and strong.
May I be happy and purposeful.
May I be at peace.

Let the intentions expressed in these phrases sink in as you repeat them.
Allow the feelings to grow deeper.

After a few repetitions, direct the phrases to someone you feel grateful for
or someone who has helped you:

May you be safe and secure.
May you be healthy and strong.
May you be happy and purposeful.
May you be at peace.

Next, visualize someone you feel neutral about. Choose among people
you neither like nor dislike, and repeat the phrases.

Now visualize someone you don't like or with whom you are having a hard
time, and repeat the phrases with that person in mind. Kids who are being
teased or bullied at school often feel quite empowered when they send love
to the people who are making them miserable.

Finally, direct the phrases more broadly: *May everyone be safe and secure.*
You can do this for up to 30 minutes; it is up to you.

Technique #5: Create your emotional rescue playlist.

Music can soothe, inspire, improve your mood, and help you focus. It is important in every known culture on earth, with ancient roots extending back thousands of years.[39] After evaluating more than 800 people, researchers have found
that people listen to music to regulate their energy and mood, to achieve self-
awareness, and to improve social bonds. Music provides social cement—think
of work and war songs, lullabies, and national anthems.[40] In his powerful book
The Secret Language of the Heart, Barry Goldstein reviewed the neuroscientific
properties of music. He suggested that music stimulates emotional circuits in

the brain[41] and releases oxytocin, the "cuddle hormone," which can enhance bonding, trust, and relationships.[42] He wrote, "Listening to music can create peak emotions, which increase the amount of dopamine, a specific neurotransmitter that is produced in the brain and helps control the brain's reward and pleasure centers. . . . Music was used to assist patients with severe brain injuries in recalling personal memories. The music helped the patients to reconnect to memories they previously could not access."[43] Be aware, however, that music you strongly like or dislike may impair your focus.[44]

Based on the concept of entrainment, which means your brain picks up the rhythm of your environment, you can manipulate your mind with the music you choose. In a fascinating study, research subjects rated Mozart's Sonata for Two Pianos (K. 448) and Beethoven's Moonlight Sonata as happy and sad, respectively.[45] Listening to happy music (Mozart's piece) increased activity in the brain's left hemisphere, associated with happiness and motivation, and decreased activity in the right hemisphere, often associated with anxiety and negativity. Beethoven's piece did the opposite. According to research published in the *Journal of Positive Psychology*, you can improve your mood and boost your overall happiness in just two weeks, simply by having the intention of being happier and by listening to specific mood-boosting music, such as Aaron Copland's *Rodeo*, for 12 minutes a day.[46] Having only the intention to be happier was not as effective. Listening to happy instrumental music (versus music with lyrics) was more powerful in activating the limbic or emotional circuits of the brain.[47]

Create your own emotional rescue playlist to boost your mood quickly. Research shows it can be effective to start with musical pieces you love. If you're not sure where to start, try some of these pieces, which have been shown through research to boost mood.

RESEARCH-BASED FEEL BETTER FAST MUSIC

:03-25
MINUTES
　　　　　Without lyrics (words can be distracting[48]):

Sonata for Two Pianos in D Major, third movement (K. 448) – Mozart (~ 6 min.)
"Clair de Lune" – Debussy (~ 5 min.)
"Adagio for Strings" – Samuel Barber (~ 8 min.)
Piano Sonata no. 17 in D Minor ("The Tempest") – Beethoven (~ 25 min.)
"First Breath after Coma" – Explosions in the Sky (9:33 min.)
"Adagio for Strings" – Tiësto (9:34 min. original; 7:23 min. album version)

"Fanfare for the Common Man" – Aaron Copland (~ 4 min.)
"Weightless" – Marconi Union (8:09 min.)
"Flotus" – Flying Lotus (3:27 min.)
"Lost in Thought" – Jon Hopkins (6:16 min.)
"The Soundmaker" – Rodrigo y Gabriela (4:54 min.)
"See" – Tycho (5:18 min.)
"Spectre" – Tycho (3:47 min.)

Add nature sounds (your own recordings or downloads of favorites) to boost mood and focus.[49]

:02-05
MINUTES
With lyrics:[50]

"Good Vibrations" – The Beach Boys (3:16 min.)
"Don't Stop Me Now" – Queen (3:36 min.)
"Uptown Girl" – Billy Joel (3:23 min.)
"Dancing Queen" – ABBA (3:45 min.)
"Eye of the Tiger" – Survivor (4:11 min.)
"I'm a Believer" – The Monkees (2:46 min.)
"Girls Just Want to Have Fun" – Cyndi Lauper (4:25 min.)
"Livin' on a Prayer" – Bon Jovi (4:09 min.)
"I Will Survive" – Gloria Gaynor (3:11 min.)
"Walking on Sunshine" – Katrina and the Waves (3:48 min.)

Brain-enhancing music specifically composed by Barry Goldstein to enhance creativity, mood, memory, gratitude, energy, focus, motivation, and inspiration can be found at www.mybrainfitlife.com. Treat your brain and listen often.

Technique #6: Flood your five senses with positivity.

The brain senses the world. If you can change the inputs, you can often quickly change how you feel.

:03-25 *Hearing*—Music can help to optimize your state of being, as we
MINUTES have just seen.

:20-60 *Touch*—Positive touch is powerful. Getting a hug, a massage,
MINUTES acupuncture, or acupressure or spending time in a sauna can
improve mood.

- Massage has been shown to improve pain, mood, and anxiety in fibromyalgia patients;[51] mood and pain in cancer patients;[52] and mood after open-heart surgery.[53] It has also been shown to improve mood and behavior in students with ADHD.[54] (30–60 min.)
- Acupuncture and acupressure can help with premenstrual syndrome (PMS),[55] depression,[56] anxiety and anger,[57] and pain.[58] (60 min.)
- Saunas have been shown to enhance mood after just one session,[59] increase endorphins (feel-good chemicals),[60] and decrease the risk of Alzheimer's disease.[61] (20 min.)

TINY HABITS THAT CAN HELP YOU FEEL BETTER FAST—AND LEAD TO BIG CHANGES

:02–20 MINUTES Each of these habits takes just a few minutes. They are anchored to something you do (or think or feel) so that they are more likely to become automatic. Once you do the behaviors you want, find a way to make yourself feel good about them— draw a happy face, pump your fist, or do whatever feels natural. Emotion helps the brain to remember.

1. Whenever I feel anxious or stressed, I will take three deep belly breaths and imagine a safe haven or place that relaxes me.

2. When I hold my partner's or child's hand, I will think of warmth radiating between our hands.

3. When I start to feel irritated, I will look at some photos of nature.

4. When I feel upset, I will put on the playlist I developed to feel happy.

5. Before I go to bed, I will pray or do a short Loving-Kindness Meditation.

:05 *Smell*—Certain scents are known to have positive effects on how
MINUTES we feel, especially lavender oil (for anxiety,[62] mood,[63] sleep,[64] and
migraine headaches[65]), rose oil,[66] and chamomile.[67]

:05 *Sight*—Soothing images can impact your mood. Images of nature[68]
MINUTES and fractals (never-ending patterns)[69] can soothe stress. In one study,
people who looked at real plants or posters of plants experienced less
stress while waiting for medical procedures.[70]

:05 *Taste*—Flavoring food with cinnamon, saffron, mint, sage, or
MINUTES nutmeg has been shown to enhance mood.[71]

Find fun ways to put this all together to change your state of mind: Take
a sauna while listening to "Good Vibrations" and watching scenes of the
ocean, all with the scent of lavender or rose oil in the air and while sipping
on a cinnamon almond-milk cappuccino.

These six techniques are effective ways to help you feel better fast when
you're anxious or upset. Come back to them anytime you need to regain
control over your mind and body.

SIX BRAIN-BASED TECHNIQUES TO REGAIN CONTROL OVER YOUR MIND AND BODY

1. Use hypnosis, guided imagery, and progressive muscle relaxation
   to go into a deep, relaxed state.

2. Master diaphragmatic breathing.

3. Become expert at warming your hands with your mind.

4. Pray and/or practice meditation (especially Loving-Kindness
   Meditation).

5. Create your emotional rescue playlist.

6. Flood your five senses with positivity.

You can listen to hypnosis audios, breathing games, and meditations at
www.brainfitlife.com.

CHAPTER 2

THE MISSING STRATEGY

BOOSTING BRAIN HEALTH CAN MAKE YOU FEEL GREAT NOW AND FOR A LIFETIME

The chief function of the body is to carry the brain around.
THOMAS EDISON

RAIN: THE RIGHT TREATMENT FOR A TROUBLED CHILD

At 2:10 one morning in June 2010, life changed forever for Trish, a California mom of three. She received a call from Child Protective Services asking if she was interested in picking up her 10-month-old niece, Rain, who had been taken into custody after being exposed to domestic violence. Trish had never met the child before and discovered that Rain was quiet, malnourished, and almost catatonic. Trish thought at first that she could be autistic, but once around Trish's teenage children, Rain started to come out of her shell. At 18 months Rain went to her first preschool, but within two months she had been kicked out of three schools. She was described as impulsively mean, even though at times she could be very empathetic, especially to animals. At this young age, Rain head-butted, kicked, hit, pinched, and punched. She had to stay with a nanny until she went to kindergarten.

Rain was suspended from school the first month for violent behavior. This continued into first grade. After many painful meetings with the school, it was decided to place Rain in a school that deals with behaviorally disordered children. She went to a level 1 school, which lasted 90 days. She was then transferred to a level 2 school for children with more severe behavioral issues, which only lasted 30 days, and finally to the most restrictive type of school, level 3, which still couldn't help her control her tantrums. The school system totally failed Rain. The principal told Trish the school would only keep Rain if she were put on psychiatric medication, which Trish refused to do because she thought they didn't really know what was going on with her child.

"We tried and tried and tried to get her help and failed miserably. Nothing is worse than not being able to help your child, especially not understanding *why* she suffered," Trish told me. "We wondered, *What are we doing wrong as parents?* We had three kids in college, so our track record was pretty good. We simply did not know what to do besides pray. So, we prayed—a lot!"

Yet another new school suspended Rain within two months for destruction of property and fighting with other kids. At age seven, she was now being placed in a private school with a locked campus. Trish had just started to work as the director of the call center at Amen Clinics.

"I was ready to quit my job. I was called to the school every day, like clockwork, for 10 consecutive days. As a parent I was simply exhausted and out of hope. But I did have an advantage: I worked at Amen Clinics. Although we see kids all day, it just had not sunk in that this could be a 'mental health' issue. So we scanned her brain."

Rain's scan was very abnormal. She had a pattern we call the "ring of fire," with excessive activity in her whole brain, especially her anterior cingulate gyrus, meaning she would get stuck on negative thoughts and behaviors. The child's brain was working way too hard, giving her little control over her own behavior. It was easy to call her a bad girl until you looked at her brain. We put Rain on supplements to calm her brain, had her see a neurofeedback therapist, and changed her diet, eliminating gluten and dairy.

RAIN BEFORE

RAIN AND TRISH AFTER

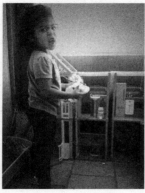
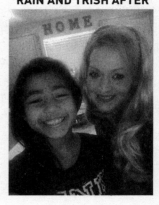

**NORMAL "ACTIVE" BRAIN
SPECT SCAN**

**RAIN'S
SPECT SCAN**

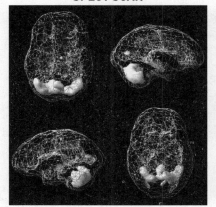
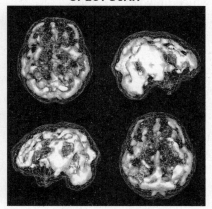

Most active areas in cerebellum
at back of brain

Ring of fire pattern:
overall increased activity

In the first 30 days Rain had fewer issues. Within 60 days the school had stopped calling. Trish thought, *Is this really happening?* After about 90 days, Rain said for the first time ever, "Mom, I like school." Trish cried tears of joy. What's even more amazing is that Rain, now eight years old, is in second grade, but she reads, writes, and tests in science and math at the sixth-grade level. She is in a new school, which wanted to move her ahead two grades. She was never academically tested prior to second grade because she was so overfocused that she was unable to cooperate or pay attention. Trish told me, "She won 'writer of the year' and 'most empathic peer.' My child, who wanted to burn down the school, is finally not fighting her own brain. My daughter smiles, laughs, reads, and has not been kicked out of school or put her hands on another child since getting the help she needed."

HELPING YOUR BRAIN IS THE MISSING STRATEGY

Too often, when people feel sad, nervous, panicky, grief-stricken, or unhappy, they engage in behaviors that hurt their brains, and thus their lives. And well-meaning professionals often prescribe medications without ever looking at the brain. Whenever you have negative or out-of-control feelings, the secret to feeling better fast is to engage in behaviors that serve the physical health of your brain, rather than hurt it.

Over the years, I have been able to simplify brain health into these three steps:

1. Develop brain envy.
2. Avoid anything that hurts your brain.
3. Engage in regular brain-healthy habits.

Strategy #1: Develop brain envy.

Anyone who has read my books is familiar with a concept I call *brain envy*. To truly be your best, you need to love and care for the three-pound supercomputer between your ears. And it helps to have a healthy envy of the people around you who respect and take care of their brains, as it acts as a powerful motivator to emulate their behavior. Yet very few people really care about their brains, likely because they cannot see them. You can see the wrinkles in your skin, the fat around your belly, the flab on your arms, or the graying hair around your temples, and you can do something about any of those things if they make you unhappy. But because very few people ever look at their brains with imaging studies like SPECT, many just don't pay attention to them. As a result, they don't care about them, which is why parents allow children to hit soccer balls with their heads, play tackle football, or do dangerous gymnastic or cheerleading routines—and why they feed their kids unhealthy food. It is also why you may text while driving, drink too much alcohol, smoke pot, eat low-quality fast food on the run, allow automatic negative thoughts (ANTs) to infest your mind, or not make sleep a priority.

Once you truly love your brain, everything in your life changes because you have a heightened sense of urgency to care for it, just as you would care for a new $300,000 Ferrari. Would you ever pour sugar or salt into the gas tank? Would you run the car until it couldn't go anymore without maintenance? Of course not! But isn't your brain worth so much more? Of course it is. Your brain needs you to love and care for it, or it will never be able to fully take care of you.

When you develop brain envy and truly love your brain, it becomes easier to focus on the right habits to keep it healthy over time. You're also more likely to make these changes with a great attitude. Doing the right things for your brain is self-reinforcing. Gradually you realize that you don't feel deprived. Rather, you start to feel bad when you do the wrong things because you realize you are hurting the most important part of you, the part that runs everything in your life. That is the epitome of self-destructive behavior. Ultimately, as we will see in chapter 12, taking care of our brains is about loving ourselves and others.

To drive this point home, let's contrast ten statements I hear from my patients who have brain envy with the assertions I hear from those who have brain apathy.

BRAIN ENVY STATEMENTS	BRAIN APATHY STATEMENTS
I love my brain.	I never think about my brain.
Every day, I make the best decisions I can.	Everything in moderation. (This opens the door to illness because it becomes your excuse to keep doing the wrong thing.)
I am aware of the pitfalls around me.	Don't take things so seriously.
I try to do the best for my brain every day, including holidays.	It's the weekend. I should live a little.
I focus on getting good sleep.	Sleep is not a priority. I'm just too busy.
I only buy healthy food for my family.	My kids won't eat anything healthy. I buy them what they want, so at least they'll eat something.
I get my important health numbers tested every year.	I haven't had a checkup in years.
I won't let my kids play sports where they could hit their heads.	I allow my kids to make their own decisions about sports.
I have dementia in my family. I am going to do everything I can to avoid it.	I have dementia in my family. It's genetic, so there's nothing I can do about it.
I keep my weight at a healthy level, to protect my brain.	Everyone's overweight. What's the big deal?
I gave up sugar to save my brain.	I'd rather get Alzheimer's disease than give up sugar.

It should be obvious which column will give you better overall brain health.

How can you make brain envy actionable in your life? Use the Tiny Habit you learned in the introduction: *Whenever you come to a decision point in your day, ask yourself, "Is the decision I'm about to make good for my brain or bad for it?"* In the rest of this chapter and the chapters to come, we'll take a look at many specific behaviors and choices that will positively affect your brain, so you'll be fully equipped to answer this question. But you may already know more than you think you do. Consider these three examples:

- You just had a fight with your spouse. Should you

   1. respond in anger and tell him or her just what is on your mind?
   2. have a donut to calm your nerves?
   3. grab an apple and a few nuts, and take a walk to calm down and consider what you can do to make the situation better?

Which of these options will help your brain work better?

- Your stock portfolio went down after a stock market sell-off. Should you

  1. stay up all night to figure out your next best move?
  2. make sure you get seven hours of sleep so you are well rested and can make good decisions about your stocks the next day?
  3. smoke a joint to relax?

Which of these options will help you make better decisions?

- Your boss just told you she was unhappy with your performance. Should you

  1. skip lunch, put your head down, and work harder?
  2. complain to your coworkers about how unreasonable your boss is over a beer and nachos after work?
  3. take a walk to clear your head, return, and ask your boss for feedback on how you can improve?

Which of these choices will help your brain help you improve your life?

If you practice brain envy and make a habit of asking, "Is this decision good for my brain or bad for it?" at the moment of choice, and then make the best decision for the health of your brain, it will help you feel better fast in a way that will be long lasting.

Love your brain by asking yourself at the moment of every choice, "Is this good for my brain or bad for it?"

Strategy #2: Avoid anything that hurts your brain.

One of the world's richest men, famed business investor and CEO of Berkshire Hathaway Warren Buffett, has two rules of investing:

Rule #1: Never lose money.

Rule #2: Never forget rule #1.

In the same way, the most important rules of brain health are

Rule #1: Never lose brain cells.

Rule #2: Never forget rule #1.

Losing brain cells is much harder to recover from than any financial loss. Just ask anyone who has had a serious brain injury or stroke. When I was in medical school, we were taught that people were born with all of the brain cells they would ever have, and once those were gone, that was it. While we now know that is not completely true, only certain small areas of the brain make new cells every day. That's why you should do everything you can to avoid losing the brain cells you have.

In my book *Memory Rescue: Supercharge Your Brain, Reverse Memory Loss, and Remember What Matters Most*, I developed the mnemonic BRIGHT MINDS to help you remember the 11 major factors that steal brain cells and lead to cognitive impairment. You can prevent or treat almost all of these risk factors, and even the ones that you can't, such as having a family history of dementia, can be ameliorated with the right strategies. Here is a brief summary of the BRIGHT MINDS risk factors. The risks marked with an asterisk (*) are things that might make you feel better temporarily but will hurt you in the long run.

B – Blood flow: Circulation is essential to life. It is the conduit for transporting nutrients to, and toxins away from, your cells. Low blood flow shrinks the brain and kills its cells. In fact, low blood flow on brain imaging is the number one predictor of future Alzheimer's disease. What's more, if you have blood flow problems anywhere, you likely have them throughout your body.

Blood Flow Risks That Drain Your Brain

- Excessive caffeine*
- Nicotine*
- Dehydration
- Hypertension
- Any cardiovascular disease
- Erectile dysfunction
- Oxygen deprivation (such as near drowning)
- Too little exercise*

R – Retirement/Aging: The risk of brain dysfunction increases with age. When you stop learning or connecting with others, your brain starts dying.

Retirement/Aging Risks That Drain Your Brain

- Loneliness or social isolation
- Being in a job that does not require new learning
- Retirement without new learning endeavors

I – Inflammation: Chronic inflammation is like a low-level fire in your body that destroys your organs. Here's a list of inflammation promoters.

Inflammation Risks That Drain Your Brain

- Leaky gut
- Gum disease
- Low omega-3 fatty acids
- High omega-6 fatty acids
- High C-reactive protein (CRP)
- Fast and processed food, pro-inflammatory diet*

G – Genetics: Your inheritance matters, but your lifestyle matters more. As we will see, genetic risk is not a death sentence; it should be a wake-up call to get serious about brain health.

Genetic Risks That Drain Your Brain

- Family member with cognitive impairment, dementia, Parkinson's disease, or a mental health issue
- Apolipoprotein E (*APOE*) e4 gene (one or two copies raise your risk for cognitive problems)

H – Head trauma: Your brain is soft, about the consistency of soft butter, and it is housed in a very hard skull with multiple sharp, bony ridges. Head injuries, such as concussions, even mild ones, can kill brain cells and cause significant, lasting cognitive problems. Even one concussion triples the risk of suicide.[1]

Head Trauma Risks That Drain Your Brain

- History of one or more head injuries with or without loss of consciousness
- Playing contact sports,* even without a concussion
- Activities that increase the risk of brain trauma, such as texting while driving,* trying to carry too many packages at one time, or going up on any roof (don't unless it's absolutely safe)

T – Toxins: Toxins are a major cause of brain dysfunction. Your brain is the most metabolically active organ in your body, which makes it more vulnerable to damage from a long list of toxins. Personal care products are particularly dangerous, because what goes on your body goes in and becomes your body.

Toxin Risks That Drain Your Brain

- Nicotine (smoking cigarettes, chewing tobacco, vaping)*
- Drug abuse, including marijuana,* which increases the risk of psychosis in teenagers,[2] decreases motivation and school performance, and decreases overall blood flow to the brain, especially in areas vulnerable to Alzheimer's disease[3]
- Moderate to heavy alcohol use*
- Many legal drugs, such as benzodiazepines, sleeping medications, and chronic pain medications*
- Pesticide exposure in air or food, recently shown to decrease serotonin and dopamine in the brain[4]
- Environmental toxins, such as mold, carbon monoxide, or air or water pollution
- Personal care products (such as shampoos and deodorants) made with parabens, phthalates, or PEGs*
- Artificial food additives, dyes, and preservatives
- Drinking* or eating* out of plastic containers
- Heavy metals, such as lead or mercury
- Cancer chemotherapy
- General anesthesia (use local or spinal anesthesia whenever possible)
- Health issues with the organs of detoxification—liver, kidneys, skin, or gut
- Handling cash register receipts (plastic coating can get through your skin)

M – Mental health: Untreated problems ranging from chronic stress and anxiety to bipolar disorder and addictions are associated with cognitive impairment and early death.

Mental Health Risks That Drain Your Brain

- Chronic stress
- Depression
- Anxiety disorders
- Attention deficit hyperactivity disorder (ADHD)
- Posttraumatic stress disorder (PTSD)
- Bipolar disorder
- Schizophrenia
- Addictions (drugs, alcohol, sex)*
- Gadget addiction*
- Negative thinking

I – Immunity/Infection issues: These are common but often unrecognized causes of brain dysfunction.

Immunity/Infection Risks That Drain Your Brain

- Chronic fatigue syndrome
- Autoimmune diseases, such as rheumatoid arthritis, multiple sclerosis, and lupus
- Untreated infections, such as Lyme disease, syphilis, and herpes
- Hiking* where you may be bitten by a tick
- Low vitamin D level

N – Neurohormone deficiencies: When your hormone levels are unbalanced, your brain is too.

Neurohormone Deficiencies That Drain Your Brain

- Low or high thyroid
- Low testosterone (males and females)
- Low estrogen and progesterone (females)
- Low DHEA
- High cortisol levels
- Hormone disruptors, such as BPA, phthalates, parabens, and pesticides
- Protein* from animals raised with hormones or antibiotics that can disrupt your hormones
- Sugar,* which disrupts hormones

D – Diabesity: The term describes a combination of being diabetic or pre-diabetic and being overweight or obese. The standard American diet is a major cause of diabesity, which contributes to chronically high blood sugar levels. These hurt blood vessels and cause inflammation and hormone disruption as well as the storage of toxins—all of which damage the brain.

Diabesity Risks That Drain Your Brain

- Diabetes or prediabetes
- High fasting blood sugar or HbA1c (hemoglobin A1c)
- Being overweight or obese
- Standard American diet* of processed foods, sugar, and unhealthy fats
- Drinking fruit juice* (high in sugar)

S – Sleep issues: All sleep problems are a major cause of brain dysfunction, but especially chronic insomnia and sleep apnea. When you sleep, your brain cleanses itself of debris. Without proper sleep, trash builds up, harming the brain.

Sleep Issues That Drain Your Brain

- Chronic insomnia
- Chronic use of sleep medication*
- Sleep apnea
- Drinking/eating caffeinated drinks or food after 2 p.m.*
- Sleeping in a warm room
- Light or noise at night
- Gadgets* that wake you up
- Irregular sleep schedule
- Anger or upset before bed

Whatever you want in life, it is easier to achieve when your brain works right. It is important to have the right attitude as you make these changes. You don't avoid things in order to deprive yourself. You avoid things that hurt your brain because it is the ultimate act of love—for yourself and others.

"But How Can I Have Any Fun?"

For the past 13 years, Dr. Jesse Payne and I have taught a high school course we created called "Brain Thrive by 25" that teaches teens how to love and care for their brains. It has now been taught in 42 states and 7 countries. Independent research in 16 schools found it decreased drug, alcohol, and tobacco use as well as depression, and improved self-esteem. Whenever we teach the section of the course on things to avoid to have a healthy brain, invariably a teenage boy—rarely a girl—will raise his hand and ask, "But how can I have any fun?"

Whenever we get this question, we play a game with the teens called "Who has more fun? The teen with the good brain or the one with the bad brain?" I recently gave a lecture to 7,000 high school students and their parents at the Congress of Future Physicians. These were high-performing teens who wanted to become physicians. I played this game with them and asked the crowd, "Who gets into the college of his choice . . . the teen with the good brain or the one with the bad brain?"

In unison, they screamed, "The teen with the good brain."

I then asked, "Who gets the girl and gets to keep her because he doesn't act like a jerk . . . the guy with the good brain or the one with the bad brain?"

The girls in the arena roared with approval, "The guy with the good brain."

I then wondered, "Who gets the best jobs and keeps them . . . the woman with the good brain or the one with the bad brain?"

"The woman with the good brain" was the answer that came back to me.

"Who makes the most money . . . the person with the good brain or the one with the bad brain?" I asked.

"The person with the good brain," they agreed.

"Who is the best parent . . . the dad or mom with the good brain or the one with the bad brain?"

"The dad or mom with the good brain," they shouted.

And finally, I said, "Who takes the coolest vacations, drives the coolest cars, and has the most meaning and purpose in their lives?"

"The ones with the good brains," they roared.

Then I told them about one of my celebrity friends whom I had helped to quit smoking pot 12 weeks earlier. The week before the lecture, I texted her this question: "Are you having more fun with your good habits or with the bad ones?"

She texted me right back, "Ha! Good! By a billion!"

Strategy #3: Engage in regular brain-healthy habits.

Now that you know what risk factors to avoid, it is critical that you develop discipline around building the best daily habits. I'll discuss them in the context of our BRIGHT MINDS program, starting with several overarching habits you will want to adopt.

General Strategies

- Worry—a little. According to research, people whose motto is "Don't worry; be happy" die the earliest from accidents or preventable illnesses. Some anxiety is good. Obviously too much is bad, but so is too little.
- Make yourself less vulnerable to poor decisions. Ultimately, the quality of your decisions determines the health of your brain and body. Be

sure to have clear goals, get seven hours of sleep every night, and keep your blood sugar on an even keel by eating protein and fat at every meal. Low blood sugar levels are associated with poor decisions.

- Identify your daily motivation. In chapter 8 I'll introduce what I call the "One-Page Miracle," which you can look at every day for inspiration and focus.
- Select a healthy peer group. You become like the people with whom you spend time, and being with healthy people is a good way to develop brain envy.

FEEL BETTER FAST NOW AND LATER TIP: *Find the healthiest person you can stand and then spend as much time around him or her as possible.*

B - Simple Brain-Healthy Habits to Improve Brain Blood Flow

:05-60
MINUTES

- At least twice a week, engage in regular exercise and healthy sports that require coordination and complex moves (dancing, table tennis, tennis, martial arts without head contact, golf, tai chi, qigong, yoga)
- Focus on staying hydrated—drink five to eight glasses of water a day
- Drink decaffeinated green tea
- Have a small piece of sugar-free dark chocolate
- Spice up your food with cayenne pepper and rosemary (for more detailed information on brain-healthy foods, see chapter 9)
- Eat beets
- Eat green leafy vegetables to boost vitamin E and blood flow
- Eat pumpkin seeds to boost dopamine and increase focus
- Take supplements: ginkgo biloba and vinpocetine (see chapter 10 for a discussion on nutraceuticals)

FEEL BETTER FAST NOW AND LATER TIP: *Eat a beet salad, sprinkled with pumpkin seeds, and small pieces of dark chocolate with a cup of green tea.*

R - Simple Antiaging Brain-Healthy Habits

:05-60
MINUTES

- Start a daily practice of learning something new
- Take up a musical instrument as a new learning strategy
- Listen to upbeat, happy music to boost your brain
- Join a singing group[5]

- Learn new dance steps to help keep the brain young[6]
- Use cloves, a potent antioxidant, in cooking
- Eat shrimp to boost acetylcholine, the neurotransmitter of memory
- Stay connected, seek social support, volunteer
- Take supplements: acetyl-L-carnitine (to improve mitochondrial energy), huperzine A (to boost acetylcholine), and the herbs rhodiola and ashwagandha (to increase overall energy)

FEEL BETTER FAST NOW AND LATER TIP: *Listen to stimulating music or sing. Make a playlist of the songs that make you feel amazing (see chapter 1, pages 22–23).*

I - Simple Brain-Healthy Habits to Decrease Inflammation

:05-30
MINUTES

- Get your CRP level tested (blood test)
- Test your Omega-3 Index (blood test); the goal is to get above 8
- Eat more toxin- and pollutant-free fish or take fish oil supplements
- Eat more omega-3 rich foods, such as nuts, seeds, avocados, and green leafy vegetables
- Increase consumption of probiotic foods or supplements
- Floss your teeth daily and care for your gums

FEEL BETTER FAST NOW AND LATER TIP: *Eat more omega-3 rich foods, such as clean fish, avocados, and walnuts.*

G - Simple Brain-Healthy Habits to Improve Your Genetics

:05-30
MINUTES

- If you have dementia in your family, be serious about brain health as soon as possible and go in early for memory screening
- Test your *APOE* gene type; if you have the *APOE* e4 gene, avoid contact sports and other head trauma risks
- Eat foods with turmeric or take the supplement curcumin
- Eat organic blueberries
- Cook with sage
- Take supplements: CoQ10, vitamin D, sage, curcumin, and green tea extracts

FEEL BETTER FAST NOW AND LATER TIP: *Defrost a cup of frozen organic blueberries to have as a snack. My daughter Chloe calls them God's candy.*

H - Simple Brain-Healthy Habits to Decrease Head Trauma Issues

:05-60
MINUTES

- Always wear your seat belt when you drive or ride in a vehicle
- Wear a helmet when skiing, biking, etc.
- Slow down and be careful when going downstairs; hold the handrail
- If you have had a head trauma, check your hormones and optimize any that are low
- Use peppermint (the herb) to help with healing
- Consider hyperbaric oxygen therapy (HBOT; see appendix A). My colleagues and I published a study on soldiers who had suffered brain injuries.[7] We saw increased blood flow to their brains after the first session and lasting improvements to blood flow, mood, and processing speed after 40 sessions. Improved sleep was one of the most consistent findings with HBOT.
- Take supplements: omega-3 fatty acids and multivitamins

FEEL BETTER FAST NOW AND LATER TIP: *Talk to your doctor about HBOT treatments.*

T - Simple Brain-Healthy Habits to Detoxify Your Brain and Body

- Buy organic
- Breathe, drink, and eat clean (air, water, and food)
- When pumping gas, avoid breathing in fumes
- Limit alcohol to two servings a week
- Support the four organs of detoxification
  - Kidneys—drink more water
  - Liver—eat detoxifying vegetables, such as cabbage, cauliflower, and brussels sprouts
  - Gut—eat more fiber
  - Skin—work up a sweat with exercise or use a sauna
- Use apps, such as Think Dirty or Healthy Living (EWG.org), to scan your personal care products and eliminate as many toxic ingredients as possible
- Get your home tested for mold if it has been flooded or had any water damage
- Take supplements: N-acetyl-cysteine (NAC, for your liver) and fiber

FEEL BETTER FAST NOW AND LATER TIP: *Take a sauna bath—the more often, the better.*[8]

M - Simple Brain-Healthy Habits to Improve Your Mental Health

:05-60
MINUTES

- Practice stress management techniques, such as those described in chapter 1
- When you awaken in the morning, say to yourself, *Today is going to be a great day!*
- Every day, write down three things you are grateful for
- If you have trouble with focus, consider a high-protein, lower-carbohydrate diet
- Eat up to eight servings of fruits and vegetables a day; a linear correlation shows that this will increase your level of happiness. Tomatoes have been shown to help mood.
- Learn to meditate, especially the Loving-Kindness Meditation (see chapter 1, page 21), which has been shown to increase energy to the brain
- Go for a walk in nature (or at least outdoors)
- Use brighter lights, especially full spectrum bulbs that have ultraviolet radiation similar to the sun's[9]
- If natural interventions are not effective, work with a local therapist or psychiatrist
- Kill the ANTs (automatic negative thoughts; see chapter 5, pages 99–100): Whenever you feel mad, sad, nervous, or out of control, write down your negative thoughts and learn to talk back to them
- Take supplements: s-adenosyl-methionine (SAMe), saffron, and omega-3s to support mood; 5-hydroxytryptophan (5-HTP) if you are a worrier

FEEL BETTER FAST NOW AND LATER TIP: *When your mood is low, take a walk in nature while drinking vegetable juice.*

I - Simple Brain-Healthy Habits to Improve Your Immunity

- If you are struggling with brain fog or memory issues, consider being tested for exposure to infectious diseases
- Do an elimination diet for a month to see if you have food allergies, which can damage your immune system
- Eat immunity-enhancing foods, such as onions, mushrooms, and garlic
- Watch a comedy or go to a comedy club to boost energy[10] and immunity

- Take supplements: vitamin D (know and optimize your level), aged garlic, and vitamin C

FEEL BETTER FAST NOW AND LATER TIP: *Eat a stir-fry with onions, garlic, mushrooms, and a protein; skip the rice.*

N - Simple Brain-Healthy Habits to Improve Your Neurohormones

- Have your hormones tested on a regular basis
- Add fiber to eliminate unhealthy forms of estrogen
- For women: Optimize estrogen for brain health
- Consider hormone replacement when necessary
- Take supplements: zinc (to help boost testosterone) and ashwagandha (to reduce cortisol and support the thyroid)

FEEL BETTER FAST NOW AND LATER TIP: *Lift weights and eliminate sugar to help raise your testosterone level.*

D - Simple Brain-Healthy Habits to Decrease Your Risk of Diabesity and Improve Your Weight and Blood Sugar

- Maintain a healthy weight; lose weight slowly if you are overweight (develop lifelong habits)
- Eat a brain-healthy diet (see chapter 9, page 203)
    - Anti-inflammatory and colorful foods
    - Low-glycemic, high-fiber carbs
    - Protein and fat at each meal (to stabilize blood sugar and cravings)
    - Healing spices
- Know your body mass index (BMI) now and check it monthly
- Flavor dishes with cinnamon and nutmeg
- Chew sugar-free gum to boost oxygen and blood flow to your brain[11]
- Take supplements: chromium picolinate and alpha-lipoic acid (to decrease cravings and support healthy blood sugar levels)

FEEL BETTER FAST NOW AND LATER TIP: *Sniff a cinnamon stick or peppermint.*

S - Simple Brain-Healthy Habits to Improve Your Sleep

- If you snore, get assessed for sleep apnea
- Put blue-light blockers on your gadgets

- Turn off gadgets or keep them away from your head at night
- Cool your home a bit before bedtime
- Darken your bedroom
- Maintain a regular sleep schedule
- Listen to a hypnosis sleep audio
- Take supplements: melatonin and magnesium; 5-HTP (if worrying keeps you up)

FEEL BETTER FAST NOW AND LATER TIP: *At bedtime, put the scent of lavender nearby and listen to a hypnosis sleep audio.*

I've given you a lot of strategies here, but I want you to come away feeling empowered, not overwhelmed. You can make so many small daily decisions to improve your brain health. They are within your reach! Start with just a few and add from there.

Meanwhile, keep that key question in mind as you go through each day: *Is this good for my brain, or bad for it?* Choosing what's good for your brain is the way to feel better fast.

THREE KEY BRAIN HEALTH STRATEGIES

1. Develop brain envy.

2. Avoid anything that hurts your brain.

3. Engage in regular brain-healthy habits to create a strong foundation for success. For now, pick one new BRIGHT MINDS habit a week to plant into your life.

Never forget:

Rule #1 of brain health is **Never lose brain cells.**

Rule #2 of brain health is **Never forget rule #1.**

The health of your brain is foundational to feeling better fast—now and later. Love and take care of your brain, so you can love your life.

TINY HABITS THAT CAN HELP YOU FEEL BETTER FAST—AND LEAD TO BIG CHANGES

30 SECONDS -:20 MINUTES Each of these habits takes just a few minutes. They are anchored to something you do (or think or feel) so that they are more likely to become automatic. Once you do the behaviors you want, find a way to make yourself feel good about them— draw a happy face, pump your fist, or do whatever feels natural. Emotion helps the brain to remember.

1. When I have used the bathroom, I will drink a glass of water (blood flow).

2. After I hang up my car keys, I will learn a new chord on my instrument (retirement/new learning).

3. When I finish brushing my teeth before bed, I will floss (inflammation).

4. After I open the refrigerator, I will grab a handful of organic blueberries (genetics).

5. When I go downstairs, I will hold the handrail (head trauma).

6. When I pump gas, I will stand away from the nozzle so I don't breathe fumes (toxins).

7. When I am feeling sad, I will take a walk in nature (mental health).

8. When I prepare vegetables for dinner, I will add garlic and onions to the mix (immunity).

9. When I go to the salad bar, I will get a half cup of beans (neurohormones).

10. When I eat dinner, I will add one colorful vegetable to my plate (diabesity).

11. After I get into bed, I will listen to a hypnosis sleep audio (sleep).

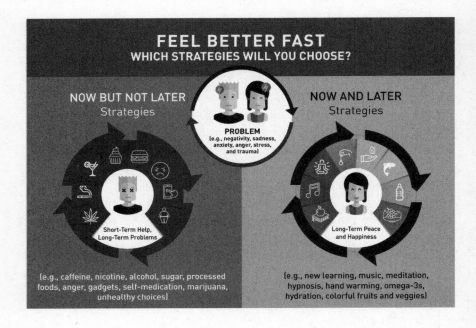

CHAPTER 3

CONTROL YOURSELF

BOOST THE BRAIN'S EXECUTIVE CENTER TO MAKE GREAT DECISIONS AND AVOID ONES THAT RUIN YOUR LIFE

The best car safety device is a rearview mirror with a cop in it.
BRITISH COMEDIAN DUDLEY MOORE

The prefrontal cortex (PFC), the front third of the brain, is the cop in your head that helps you decide between right and wrong and determine whether an action is beneficial. It assists you in directing your behavior toward your goals and braking when it starts to get out of control. The PFC is the leader in you and is arguably the most important part of your brain when it comes to making the decisions that will help you feel better fast and make it last.

Neuroscientists call the PFC the executive part of the brain because it functions as the chief executive officer of your life. When it is healthy, this boss in your head is goal-oriented, focused, organized, thoughtful, and simultaneously present- and future-oriented; exhibits good judgment; learns from mistakes; and is able to control your impulses. When this part of the brain is hurt, for whatever reason, it is as if the leader in your head has gone on vacation (*when the cat's away, the mice will play*), and you are more likely to act in impulsive, ineffective, irresponsible, or abusive ways. This not only hurts you but can hurt others as well. Healing the PFC can therefore help you and those around you—colleagues, employees, your kids—feel better fast. In this chapter, we'll explore how the PFC develops and how to protect and strengthen it.

The PFC is proportionally larger in humans than it is in any other animal by far. It represents 30 percent of a human's brain, 11 percent of a chimpanzee's brain, 7 percent of a dog's brain, 3 percent of a cat's brain (which is why cats need nine lives), and one percent of a mouse's brain. The PFC is the part of your brain that makes you human. It is involved in the following executive functions:

- Focus
- Forethought
- Planning
- Judgment
- Decision-making
- Organization
- Follow-through
- Empathy
- Learning from mistakes
- Problem-solving
- Expressive language
- Impulse control
- Saying no to behaviors inconsistent with goals
- Conscientiousness—e.g., consistently showing up when you say you will

THE PREFRONTAL CORTEX

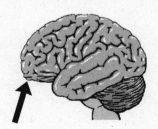

Pinocchio's Jiminy Cricket embodies the role of the PFC. Near the opening of the movie, the Blue Fairy dubs Jiminy "Pinocchio's conscience, lord high keeper of the knowledge of right and wrong, counselor in moments of high temptation, and guide along the straight and narrow path." Jiminy's job is to help Pinocchio work toward his goal of becoming a real boy. When Jiminy is away from Pinocchio, the wooden boy nearly loses his life from a series of bad decisions. Similarly, not having a healthy PFC costs many people their success in life and, in some cases, their very lives. The PFC supervises you. It is the small voice in your head or the angel on your shoulder encouraging you to do the right thing and to reach the goals that are most important to you. When your PFC is hurt or its activity level is low (as it often is in people who have attention deficit hyperactivity disorder, or ADHD), your impulses—the devil on the other shoulder whispering in your ear to do the wrong thing that feels right in the moment—are more likely to win. Before we look at the differences between a healthy and a troubled PFC, here is a quick overview of how this brain region develops.

THE BRAIN'S LATE BLOOMER

Brain development is a fascinating construction tale, where genes and environment work together to make us who we are. At times during pregnancy, the fetus's brain produces 250,000 new cells per minute. Babies are born with 100 billion neurons; however, only a relatively small number of those neurons are connected. About three-quarters of the brain develops outside the womb, in response to our environment and experience. Nature and nurture always work together. Brain development is especially rapid during the first few years of life. By age three, a toddler's brain has formed close to 1,000 trillion connections—about twice as many connections as adults have. Between the ages of 3 and 10 is a time of rapid social, intellectual, emotional, and physical development. Brain activity in this age group is more than twice that of adults, and although new synaptic connections continue to be formed throughout life, never again will the brain be as capable of easily mastering new skills or adapting to setbacks.

The abundance of connections helps explain why it is generally easier for children to learn languages and music. Young children are able to learn just about any language and how to play musical instruments more easily than adults, even though adults often have more motivation. With age, the number of connections decreases, which helps to explain why it becomes harder to pick up an instrument, acquire languages, lose native accents, and even roll our *r*'s!

On the next page is a graph of activity in the prefrontal cortex across the lifespan, based on more than 70,000 scans we've done at Amen Clinics. You can see that, on average, a child's PFC is very active. In this case, that does not mean better function but is more akin to unbridled activity. However, over time the activity begins to settle down and work more efficiently for two main reasons: pruning and myelination.

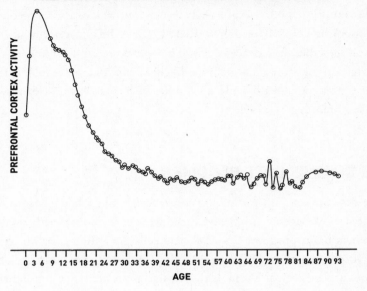

PREFRONTAL CORTEX ACTIVITY OVER THE LIFE SPAN

In the first years of life, the brain has an abundance of cells, connections, and possibilities. As we age, our brains begin the pruning process, eliminating connections that are unnecessary, incorrect, or not being stimulated, in order to strengthen and enhance the connections that are being used. Pruning helps the brain become more efficient, similar to the effect of pruning on plants, but it's crucial that the right things get pruned. As you can see in the graph ("Prefrontal Cortex Activity over the Life Span" above), at around age seven, PFC activity begins to decrease at a rapid rate. That's because the brain has begun to prune extraneous connections. The brain is one of the best examples of the "use it or lose it" principle. Connections that are used repeatedly in the early years become permanent, while those that are not used are pruned. This is why it's important for children to be raised in an enriched environment. It allows them to keep more of the tracks in their brains since the brain strengthens what is used and eliminates the unstimulated connections. Experience, opportunity, and stress all influence how much pruning takes place.

At the same time pruning is occurring, brain cells are being wrapped with a white fatty substance called myelin that works like insulation on copper wires. Myelination helps nerve cells work 10 to 100 times faster. A myelinated cell is much more efficient, which is another reason why the PFC becomes less active from about the age of 7 to 25 (seen on the graph) as myelination progresses.

Myelination starts in the back of the brain and over time works its way to the front. In infants, the cerebellum (coordination center) and occipital lobes (vision) develop first, which support balance, coordination, speech, vision, and motor movements. During this time, young ones are learning how to crawl, walk, and talk. The parietal lobes, at the top back part of the brain, develop more in the elementary school years. They're involved with throwing and catching balls and the ability to read and solve math problems. During the teenage years, the limbic or emotional brain becomes much more active. The limbic system is involved with feelings, bonding, and friendships. The PFC is the last part of the brain to develop, and it continues during late adolescence and into the mid- to late twenties. Healthy myelination of the PFC is also associated with intelligence, attention, processing speed, reaction time, musical ability, and working memory.

UNMYELINATED VS. MYELINATED NEURON

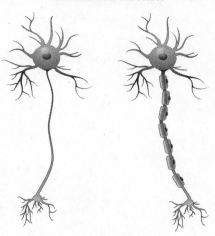

Anything that disrupts myelin formation can delay or damage brain development. Here are the main culprits:

- Smoking
- Alcohol
- Drug use
- Depression
- ADHD
- Brain trauma
- Toxins or infections
- Inflammation
- Poor diet

- Low omega-3 levels
- Low vitamins B12, C, or D
- Low zinc
- Low total cholesterol
- Low-fat diet (myelin is 80 percent fat)
- Excessive stress
- Limited exercise
- Less-than-optimal sleep

Even though we think of 18-year-olds as adults, their brain development is far from finished. Myelin continues to be deposited in the PFC until age 25 or 26, making the executive part of the brain work at a higher, more efficient level. Were you more mature at 25 than at 18? I sure was. It is ironic that the car insurance industry knew about maturity and brain development long before society did. When do car insurance rates change? At age 25.

Why? Because that is when people display better driving judgment and are statistically less likely to get into accidents, which means they cost insurance companies less money.

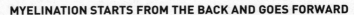

MYELINATION STARTS FROM THE BACK AND GOES FORWARD

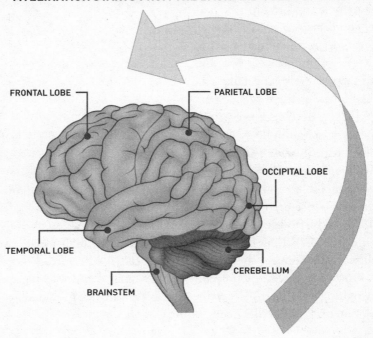

It is critical for more people to be aware that brain development continues into early adulthood. In addiction medicine, it is common for therapists to say a teen's development becomes arrested at the age he or she started to use drugs. If a teen starts abusing alcohol, drugs, or both at age 15 and doesn't stop until he is 30, emotionally, as a 30-year-old, he will seem about the same as a 15-year-old. Teenage and early adult smoking and drug or alcohol abuse, as well as brain injuries from contact sports, all have the potential to disrupt brain development—in some cases permanently.

One of neurologist Sigmund Freud's concepts that has proved useful is that human personality is made up of the id, the ego, and the superego. The id is our child mind that wants what it wants when it wants it; the ego is our healthy adult mind; and the superego is the parent inside our heads telling us what we should and should not do. Effective CEOs have healthy egos. If their superegos are too strong, they are likely to be punitive micromanagers who hold on to hurts. If their ids are in control (which means their PFCs are less active), they may be chasing the secretary around the office. They're not working effectively but are letting the child within run things.

To keep the PFC healthy, you have to stop poisoning the brain. Frequent happy hours will not help to build a healthy ego or PFC. I have never understood why business events are typically filled with alcohol. After all, the business of life is about brain function. If you're constantly diminishing brain function, over time your life is less likely to be what you want it to be.

THE ROLE OF THE PFC

A helpful analogy for understanding the PFC is to imagine yourself at the top of a mountain road in the Colorado Rockies. It's winter, and you're in a high-performance sports car, such as a Lamborghini, Porsche, or Ferrari. Your goal is to get to the bottom of the mountain safely, while enjoying the ride along the way. To navigate the miles of steep, winding roads and hairpin turns, effective brakes are a must. When the brakes are worn or damaged, you are much more likely to get into a serious accident. Brakes help the car and driver adjust to whatever situation presents itself—wind, rain, snow, ice, and other drivers who may be sleep-deprived or may have had too much to drink. A healthy PFC serves the same function as the car's brakes, allowing you to safely navigate life, adjusting to whatever situations arise. This brain region is especially critical during the stressful or scary turns in life. When the PFC is hurt or too low in activity, the brakes are weak, and all sorts of problems arise. For one, you are more likely to figuratively skid off the road you intended to be on. And when the PFC works too hard, as it often does in obsessive-compulsive disorder (OCD), the brakes are always on, stopping any progress down the mountain or in your life.

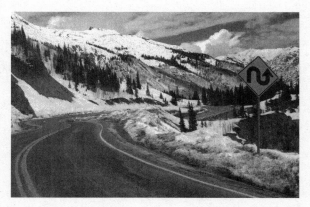

You need brakes when driving on a dangerous Colorado mountain road.

Problems with the PFC

When the PFC is hurt or damaged for whatever reason, people often struggle with

- Short attention span
- Distractibility
- Poor planning
- Lack of perseverance
- Impulsivity
- Erratic decision-making
- Chronic lateness and poor time management
- Disorganization
- Procrastination
- Difficulty being in touch with their emotions
- Trouble expressing feelings
- Poor judgment
- Lack of empathy
- Trouble learning from experience
- Saying yes too often
- Lack of conscientiousness

With these issues, there is also a higher incidence of

- School failure
- Divorce
- Job failure
- Legal issues
- Speeding tickets
- Incarceration
- Financial problems
- Mental health issues, especially ADHD and addictions

As you can see, protecting your PFC means protecting your ability to feel good now and later.

The brain is a sneaky organ. We all have weird, crazy, stupid, sexual, violent thoughts that no one should ever hear. The PFC protects us from allowing those senseless thoughts to escape our mouths or stops our fingers from pressing the send button on an inappropriate or unhelpful e-mail, text, or tweet.

Several years ago, while attending a medical conference, I was sitting in the back of the room with a friend I'll call Joelle. As I mentioned in *Memory Rescue*, Joelle had been in a car accident a few years earlier. She had been stopped at a traffic light when a pickup truck going 70 miles per hour plowed into the back of her BMW. The driver's-side airbag deployed, but the violent impact of the rear-end collision and the airbag crashing against Joelle's head slammed her soft, gelatin-like brain against the front part of her skull, ripping blood vessels and bruising and damaging her PFC. From the time of the accident, Joelle's reactions were unfiltered, and she was much more likely to say anything that came into her mind. Often it was funny, but sometimes it could be very hurtful. Before the medical conference session started, two obese women sitting in front of us were discussing their weight. One woman said to the other, "I don't know why I'm overweight; I just eat like a bird."

Joelle looked at me and said, loud enough for everyone around us to hear, "Yeah, like a condor." My face immediately turned red, and I looked at Joelle in complete embarrassment. Horrified, she put her hand to her mouth and said, "Oh no, did that get out?"

"Yes." I nodded.

"I'm so sorry," she said as the women moved away from us.

While I was writing this chapter, one of my friends got an inappropriate text from a consultant employed by her investment firm. They had worked together for more than a year without incident. But one evening when the consultant had too much to drink, he texted her, "Please send sexy pics." Shocked, my friend ended the consultancy. The man lost a high-paying job because his PFC went on temporary leave. *When the cat's away . . .*

I once had lunch with a close friend who was having marital problems. I knew Chuck had ADHD, which is associated with low PFC function, and was struggling at home in his relationships with his wife and children. As usual, Chuck was telling me about the turmoil in his life. All of a sudden his affect changed, his eyes brightened, his tone became more excited, and in a hushed voice he told me about a woman he had recently met on an airplane. She was pretty, smart, and interesting, and she seemed to like him a lot. She had even come to his office for a visit. As he started to go on, I interrupted him.

"Chuck, do you like attorneys?"

"What do you mean?" he said, looking surprised.

"Play it out," I said. "You're having marital problems, you meet this attractive woman who seems interested in you, and she's been to your office. The next step, if it hasn't happened already, is you are going to have an affair. Your wife will likely find out, and she will never forgive you. She'll file for divorce. You'll spend a lot of money on attorneys and hate yourself for putting your family through your betrayal. Then, a year from now, you will have lost half your net worth and be visiting your children on the weekends. Plus, they will be upset that you betrayed them, too."

"Wow," Chuck said, looking deflated. "I never thought about it like that."

"That is what your prefrontal cortex does for you," I said. "It plays things out."

Chuck later told me that he never called the woman back. *The cat was back.*

Thoughtfulness, Consideration, and Love

A fascinating lesson from our brain imaging work is that when I help my patients' brains function better, especially the PFC, they are significantly more thoughtful, considerate, and loving.

Bryan called himself "the anger broker of the San Fernando Valley." He came to see me after he got out of the hospital following a serious suicide attempt. Two weeks earlier his wife had served him with divorce papers; that night he locked himself in a closed garage with his car running. When the paramedics broke in to rescue him, he screamed obscenities at them. And when I first met Bryan, he was condescending and hostile to my office staff and then to me. I listened patiently for the first hour, then told him that if he wanted me to help him, he had to get scanned. I was not going to put up with his abuse for long and had no intention of allowing him to abuse our staff, so we had to get him the best help quickly. While Bryan was being scanned, he even complained about Mike, our amazing scan technologist, which was a first.

Bryan's PFC was clearly damaged, including on the left side, which tends to be the happier side of the brain. Damage to the left PFC is often associated with depression, irritability, and aggression. We put him on our BRIGHT MINDS brain rehabilitation program (see chapter 2, pages 39–44), which included supplements, HBOT (hyperbaric oxygen therapy), and dietary changes, and after three months the differences in both his behavior and his scan were stunning. He literally became one of the nicest people I've known. He still brings our staff gifts and talks to them with gratitude and love. When your brain works right—especially the PFC—you work right.

BRYAN'S INITIAL SPECT SCAN

AFTER TREATMENT SPECT SCAN

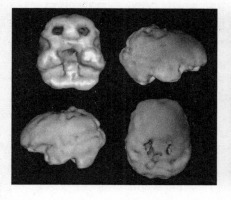

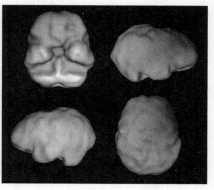

Low PFC activity

Overall improvement

Conscientiousness and Longevity

One of the executive functions of a healthy PFC is conscientiousness, and its payoff can be a longer life. We know this thanks to the remarkable work of Dr. Lewis Terman, a Stanford University psychologist who studied 1,548 bright children who were roughly 10 years old in 1921 when Terman's research began. Now, more than 90 years later, the long-term study has produced a treasure trove of insights linking healthy brain function to longevity.[1]

On the positive side, thoughtful planning, hard work, perseverance, and accomplishing goals were all associated with longevity in the study. Prudent, persistent achievers who had stable families and social support (all signs of a healthy brain) also lived longer. And those who did the best on long-life measures had habits, routines, and social networks that encouraged exercise. Clearly, your social relationships have an impact on your health, and associating with others who are healthy is one way to improve your own well-being.

On the negative side, participants who were most disappointed with their achievements died the youngest. In fact, a lack of success and dependability in one's career (a common sign of a low-functioning PFC) was linked with a huge increase in mortality. How one reacted to a loss also affected longevity: If the loss led to drinking, depression, anxiety, or catastrophizing (exacerbating poor brain function), an early death was often the result; but if instead the loss led to renewed zest for life after a period of grief (thanks to employing brain-healthy recovery skills), the result was a five-year longevity boost beyond the average.

In one of the more intriguing findings, the study showed that people with a carefree outlook underestimated risks and tended to die early from accidents and preventable illnesses. While this finding has often been taken to mean that pessimists outlive optimists, the truth is that optimists who work hard and are more careful tend to live longer than average. It's only the optimists who don't worry, plan, or think about the consequences of their actions who wind up dying sooner. Worry, as it turns out, is a necessary function for staying healthy if it means that you care and think about the future. My clinical experience backs up this observation. A moderate level of anxiety is a good thing. Of course, too much anxiety is not good, but not having enough is connected with taking unreasonable risks that can harm health and safety.

Leadership

The brain is involved in everything we do, including how we think, feel, act, and get along with others. Leadership is all about people—managing and guiding their brains, minds, thoughts, actions, and behavior. Yet in graduate schools of business, where people train to be leaders, there is very little formal education about the brain.

In his groundbreaking book *Emotional Intelligence*, Daniel Goleman listed five traits leaders should have; all five involve your PFC. First is *self-awareness*. Unless you, as a leader, understand yourself, it will be hard for you to understand others. Next is *self-regulation*, which is knowing how to manage your own internal state, your impulses, and your resources. Third is *motivation*, which involves handling and controlling your emotional tendencies and which, in turn, guides and facilitates interactions with people (a combination of your emotional brain and PFC). Then there is *empathy*, which is the awareness of other people's needs and concerns. Finally comes *social skills*, which help leaders adapt to the various environments they find themselves in. Other leaders have discussed perseverance; integrity (listening to the angel on your shoulder); and cautious, thoughtful risk-taking—all characteristic of a healthy PFC—as traits that have helped them succeed.

Self-regulation—being able to manage your impulses—is critical to leading others and yourself. Leaders who lack good impulse control may get hit with a sexual harassment suit or make decisions that put their businesses at risk. The PFC also learns from mistakes—which is a key leadership trait since leaders make a lot of mistakes. Many of the world's best leaders are proud of their mistakes because they learned critical lessons from them. If you make a mistake and you learn from it, you will be a better leader. If you make a mistake but deny it, and instead of looking at it you just put it in a corner somewhere in your mind, odds are you're going to repeat it.

PROTECT YOUR PFC

Understanding and optimizing PFC development is critical to raising healthy humans, which is why protecting it needs to be one of society's main priorities. In particular, the PFC needs to be protected from head trauma, toxins (such as alcohol and marijuana), gadget addiction, lack of sleep, low-quality diets, and chronic stress. (For more risk factors to avoid, see chapter 2, pages 33–37.)

Stop the Insanity of Children Hitting Their Heads against Helmets and Soccer Balls

The US Soccer Federation recently banned children under the age of 11 from hitting soccer balls with their heads (it's actually called "heading"). This is clear progress, as the PFC sits right behind the forehead and is easily damaged by repetitive blows to the head. However, when I heard about the ban, I wondered, *Don't they like kids who are 11 to 25? Why 11, when we know the PFC is not finished developing until 25 in females, and a bit later in males?* Society changes slowly, often to its detriment.

Flying soccer balls are a real menace. It is estimated that a ball that's been kicked hard can impact a player's head with a force of 175 pounds! Children or teens meet that missile with their skulls, slamming their PFCs against the sharp, bony ridges of the skull's frontal bones. Does that sound like a good idea when we all need our PFCs for the rest of our lives so that we can be good workers, parents, and grandparents? Here's the story of one young man who made a smarter choice.

WILL: TOO MANY HEAD WHACKS

Will, age 16, played soccer at an advanced level. He was so good, he even played in Europe for a year. But after he sustained his fourth concussion from being kicked in the head, he had to take off a whole year from school. He was irritable, moody, and easily distracted, and he started making poor decisions. His parents were very concerned when they brought him to the clinic. His SPECT scan showed significant damage to his PFC, in the front of his brain, and damage to his occipital lobes in the back. The brain is housed in a closed space. If it gets hit on one side, it slams against the other side, causing what is called a coup-contrecoup injury (see illustration on page 60).

Even though Will desperately wanted to continue playing the game he loved, he decided to stop. He told me, "I love soccer, but I know I'll love my future wife and children more. I have to do a better job of protecting my brain." Using the rehabilitation protocol we developed at Amen Clinics, Will did much better over time and returned to school. His mood, irritability, and decision-making dramatically improved.

WILL'S SPECT SCAN

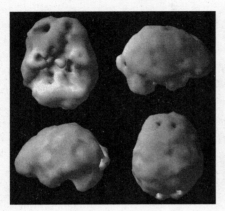

The holes indicate damage to the front and back of his brain.

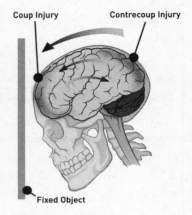

Other common PFC-damaging activities include football, cheerleading, hockey, horseback riding, and trail biking, among others. According to a new study on more than 13,000 teens, 20 percent reported a concussion at some point in their lives.[2] One of the most important lessons I've learned from looking at nearly 150,000 scans is that mild traumatic brain injury can ruin people's lives. Concussions that affect the PFC can permanently decrease a person's executive function unless it is fully rehabilitated. It is vitally important to make protecting our children's and young adults' PFCs a priority.

SIX STRATEGIES TO STRENGTHEN YOUR INTERNAL CEO

Consider the metaphor of the elephant and the rider. The PFC is the rider—the thoughtful part of your brain that attempts to direct your life. The limbic system, where your pleasure centers are housed, is the elephant—the powerful, emotional part of you that drives your impulses and desires. As long as the elephant wants to go where the rider directs him, things work fine. But when the elephant wants to go in a different direction, who is going to win that tug-of-war? Most bets are on the elephant. Cravings (elephant) are often controlled by the PFC (rider) when things are going well, but if the elephant is spooked or becomes nervous or afraid, it can take control. (Think of a food binge.) Keeping the rider healthy, strong, and strategic is critical to staying in control of your life.

How do we integrate the rider and the elephant so that our PFCs and limbic brains, our goals and desires, and our thoughts and behaviors are more in sync? We do it by being purposeful with our goals and strengthening our PFCs through continual training. Here are six strategies to strengthen your executive function, which is instrumental in helping you make good decisions, overcome anxiety, negativity, anger, and stress—and feel better fast.

Strategy #1: Learn to say no to yourself.

Experiments starting in the 1960s reveal how critical a healthy PFC is, even at an early age. These studies have focused on the concept of delayed gratification—being able to wait for a reward. One trial that psychologist Walter Mischel used involved preschoolers and marshmallows. The children were told that they could either eat the marshmallow in front of them immediately or wait for a few minutes and get two. Some kids were unable to wait and ate the marshmallow straight off, while others used tactics like clapping their hands or turning their backs on the one marshmallow to resist. After following the children for 14 years, Mischel found that those who had waited—delaying gratification—had higher self-esteem, better coping skills for stress and frustration, higher academic performance (with SAT scores that were significantly higher, on average), and greater social skills than the children who had been unable to wait.[3] (There are reenactments of this landmark work on YouTube; search for "marshmallow test.")

Similarly, a more recent test with raisins predicted how 20-month-old toddlers—some of whom had been born prematurely, making them more likely to have PFC issues—would perform at the age of eight.[4] The toddlers were tested on how long they could wait before picking up raisins that had been placed under an opaque plastic cup. They were given several training sessions and then asked to wait until they were told that 60 seconds had passed before they retrieved the raisins. Kids who had been born prematurely were more likely to eat the raisins before the full minute elapsed, and those who couldn't control their behavior were likelier to struggle in school seven years later. Unless they learn how to delay gratification or someone helps them rehab their brains, it's also likely that those kids will continue to struggle for the rest of their lives.

The PFC is like a muscle: You have to use it so you don't lose its power to help you exercise patience and make good decisions. Fortunately, you can learn how—there's even proof in Mischel's follow-up studies. He asked adults to demonstrate delayed gratification to the preschoolers, using several tactics to keep themselves from eating the lone marshmallow. When the kids were put to the test again and had to resist their impulses, those who had previously grabbed the single marshmallow used the strategies they had just seen the adults practice, successfully "earning" two marshmallows through their patience. Later, the same kids performed similarly to the ones who had a natural ability to delay gratification.[5]

Kids can learn to develop their PFCs—and you can too. In fact, it's during childhood that the majority of us learn how to exercise our PFCs. We ask our parents if we can do things that aren't good for us, such as riding a bike without a helmet or eating a lot of sweets, and when their answer is no, we learn how to say no to ourselves. But if you grew up with absent parents, you might not have learned the self-control to say no. Or if one or both of your parents struggled with drugs or alcohol, you might have learned instead to give in to your impulses. You might even have lost your ability to say no because of your own addiction.

Saying no to yourself is like being a loving parent—to yourself. Giving in to your bad behavior, whether it's eating too much junk food or channel surfing instead of exercising, can ruin your health and lead to premature death. But if you practice saying no, effectively strengthening your willpower and your PFC, you will find it easier to continue to do so over time. By exercising your PFC, you are making and strengthening nerve cell connections in a process known as long-term potentiation (LTP). Your brain makes new connections when you learn something new. Initially the connections are weak, but with practice—saying no to marijuana, candy, alcohol, lashing out at others, gambling, or using your smartphone incessantly—the PFC circuits in your brain are strengthened, or potentiated. When that happens, behaviors become almost automatic—your brain makes it easier to continue doing the right thing! Conversely, if you are ruled by your impulses, your willpower weakens, which makes it more likely that you will continue to be impulsive.

:03-05 One strategy that can help you say no is to use distraction whenever you feel tempted to do something that's outside your goals.
MINUTES
Create a list of activities that will distract you from giving in to the craving or behavior—things as simple as taking 10 deep breaths, humming to yourself, going for a brief walk, closing your eyes and focusing on your goals, or even

playing the game Tetris on your smartphone. Research has shown that just three minutes of Tetris decreased cravings for food, drugs, cigarettes, alcohol, and coffee, as well as gaming and engaging in sex,[6] and the benefits lasted for the seven days of the study.

Strategy #2: Practice saying no to others.

Tony Blair, the former prime minister of Great Britain, said, "The art of leadership is saying no, not saying yes. It is very easy to say yes." Warren Buffett once said, "The difference between successful people and really successful people is that really successful people say no to almost everything."[7] My father, who was chairman of the board of a $4 billion grocery business, always used to say no. I found it irritating when I was a child, but later I realized the wisdom of it. Saying no is like having effective brakes. In our fast-paced, distraction-filled society, our brakes are becoming weaker and weaker, and we say yes at a dizzying pace to the texts, tweets, posts, and e-mails that distract us from our purpose. Learning to say no to the mundane is essential to being able to accomplish greatness in your life. If you want high-performance results, you must be careful to spend your time wisely and only pursue the most meaningful activities, no matter what others want you to do. Steve Jobs said, "People think focus means saying yes to the thing you've got to focus on. But that's not what it means at all. It means saying no to the hundred other good ideas that there are."[8]

:01-30 Many of my patients with ADHD, who have low PFC activity,
MINUTES
don't think before they act and often overcommit themselves by saying yes to too many things. I have them practice saying these words in front of the mirror: "I have to think about it." Whenever a friend or someone at church asks you to do something, say, "I have to think about it," then go home and ask yourself if the request fits in with the goals you have for your life. Odds are, the trouble that has occurred in your life is not from saying no, but from saying yes to things that were not fully thought through.

Time is such a precious commodity today, with the constant bombardment of distractions. Learning to say no can help save your brain and your life. If the answer to a request to spend your time is not an enthusiastic yes, the answer should probably be no.

Strategy #3: Strengthen your decision-making skills.

The best way to reduce stress in your life is to stop screwing up.
ROY BAUMEISTER, PhD

Making good decisions over and over for a lifetime often adds up to good health and success. And when you have made lots and lots of bad decisions, the end result can be struggles with your health and with success in life. You don't have to be perfect and get every decision right, but the more healthy decisions you make, the better you are likely to look, feel, and act. A bonus is that improving self-control in one area of your life means improving it in other areas. If you start walking every day, for example, you are also likely to start eating better.

Use the following strategies to improve the functioning of your PFC, which in turn will boost the quality of your decisions:

- *Be clear about your goals.* Define them (see the One-Page Miracle, pages 190–193) and review them every day.

- *Decide on a few simple brain health rules ahead of time.* It's easier to stay the course when you have a plan. When you're eating out, for example, you might decide to skip bread and alcohol before your meal (both lower PFC function and can negatively impact your decisions). Thinking ahead can also help you avoid putting yourself in vulnerable situations. If you are planning to attend a party where you know there could be heavy drinking, ask for a wine spritzer and top it up with club soda when it gets low. Be sure to have an exit strategy, too.

- *HALT poor judgment.* In addiction medicine, we often use the acronym HALT in relapse prevention. Do not let yourself get too **hungry** (low blood sugar is associated with low blood flow to the PFC and more bad decisions), **angry** (anger lowers PFC function), **lonely** (being disconnected from others increases bad decisions), or **tired** (a lack of sleep is associated with low PFC function). All of these factors impair decision-making skills.

- *Cut out sugar and artificial sweeteners.* They often trigger cravings and poor decisions.

- :03-05 *Start a journal.* Writing things down is an invaluable way to
  MINUTES stay focused and on track. Recording what you eat is a well-known technique for boosting weight loss—doubling it in one Kaiser Permanente Center for Health Research study.[9] Journaling helps reinforce the habits you want to strengthen until they become second nature. Within a matter of months, you can strengthen the brain circuits that will help you stay healthy for life. How can journaling do all this? The secret is in how you use your journal. If you notice you are struggling with food

CONTROL YOURSELF ✳ 65

cravings or gambling, for example, a journal can help you pinpoint where you might have gone off track—if you skipped a meal, were under intense stress, or spent time with unhealthy people. Being able to recognize your vulnerable times allows you to develop strategies to overcome them. Note down your temptations and look for any patterns—time of day, amount of sleep or food, stress level, and more. Your mistakes are your best teachers, particularly if you let yourself explore them without judging yourself. Knowing what triggers your good decisions and your poor ones can help you become more self-aware.

Strategy #4: Protect myelination and stop letting children hit things with their heads.

There are many healthy, enjoyable sports that will not compromise your child's brain health and future. Tennis, table tennis (my personal favorite), all forms of swimming, running, golf, and dance are wonderful ways to exercise a growing body. Encourage your children to protect their PFCs and their future.

Strategy #5: To feel better fast, you have to go slow.

Slow down, you move too fast.
SIMON AND GARFUNKEL, "THE 59TH STREET BRIDGE SONG (FEELIN' GROOVY)"

In our fast-paced society, it is often the person who can slow down, think about his or her goals, and act accordingly who ends up feeling better fast now and later. Whenever you feel out of sorts, take 10 slow, deep belly breaths, identify your goal in your current situation, and choose the best option for now and later. This simple, thoughtful strategy activates your PFC to calm your emotional brain. It helps you make better decisions and can even alleviate anxiety.[10]

Behaviors you want to change must be practiced slowly, deliberately, and repeatedly so that when you need them, you can implement them immediately. As with learning any new skill, it takes time for the brain to develop new circuits. Be slow and patient when learning anything new.

Strategy #6: Take supplements to sharpen your focus and PFC.

Supplements can help to support focus and executive function. These include rhodiola, green tea extract, L-theanine, ashwagandha, panax ginseng, ginkgo biloba, and phosphatidylserine. See chapter 10 for more information on each, including dosage considerations.

NICK: A PFC PICK-ME-UP FOR A MIXED MARTIAL ARTIST

Nick, 25, was an MMA fighter who was brought to the clinic by his mother because he had been arrested after a drunken bar fight and now had started to express suicidal thoughts. I met him when I gave a lecture at the clinic. During the question-and-answer period, he told me I wouldn't like his profession as an MMA fighter. I smiled and said I liked him but wished he wouldn't put his brain at risk of damage. Later that evening I reviewed Nick's scan with him. It showed low PFC and temporal lobe activity. I asked him if he wanted to do an experiment the next day.

I had just finished one of our studies on professional football players. Amen Clinics did the first and largest brain imaging and rehabilitation study on active and former NFL players. We saw high levels of damage on SPECT scans, especially to the PFC, temporal lobes, and cerebellum (which controls motor and thought coordination). This was not a surprise, as anyone who made it to the NFL in all likelihood had already played football for anywhere from 8 to 12 years and had been hit in the head thousands of times during games and practices. The exciting news from our study was that when we worked to rehabilitate their brains through diet, exercise, and the principles in this book, 80 percent of our players showed improvement, especially in blood flow to the PFC, temporal lobes, and cerebellum, and in memory, mood, motivation, and sleep. Our rehabilitation program also included a sophisticated combination of nutritional supplements (a high-level multivitamin, high-dose omega-3 fatty acids, and nutrients that supported brain function through a number of different mechanisms, including ginkgo, rhodiola, ashwagandha, ginseng, and phosphatidylserine).

I told Nick I knew the supplements worked, but I didn't know how quickly. I said, "How about you come at 8 a.m. tomorrow, I will give them to you, and then we will scan you two and a half hours later at 10:30 a.m." Nick was excited to see if the supplements could help, and they did (see the before and after scans opposite). The second scan revealed a marked increase of blood flow to his whole brain, especially the PFC and temporal lobes. This did not mean he was cured after one dose of supplements; it meant that his brain had the potential to respond if he consistently put it in a healing environment and gave it the nutritional support it needed.

Nick's story is encouraging. If an MMA fighter with a history of brain trauma could see rapid improvement in PFC activity, you can see change too. Strengthen your PFC and you'll make better decisions and feel better fast.

**NICK'S BEFORE AND AFTER SPECT SCANS
(TWO AND A HALF HOURS AFTER TAKING SUPPLEMENTS)**

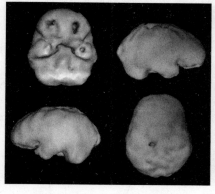

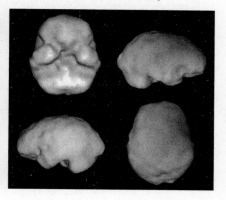

Low PFC and temporal lobe activity　　　Improved PFC and temporal lobe activity

SIX KEY STRATEGIES TO STRENGTHEN YOUR INTERNAL CEO

1. Learn to say no to yourself.

2. Practice saying no to others.

3. Strengthen your decision-making skills:
   - Be clear about your goals.
   - Decide on a few simple brain health rules ahead of time.
   - HALT poor judgment—don't allow yourself to get too hungry, angry, lonely, or tired.
   - Cut out sugar and artificial sweeteners.
   - Start a journal.

4. Protect myelination and stop letting children hit things with their heads.

5. To feel better fast, you have to go slow.

6. Take supplements to sharpen your focus and PFC.

TINY HABITS THAT CAN HELP YOU FEEL BETTER FAST—AND LEAD TO BIG CHANGES

:02-20
MINUTES

Each of these habits takes just a few minutes. They are anchored to something you do (or think or feel) so that they are more likely to become automatic. Once you do the behaviors you want, find a way to make yourself feel good about them—draw a happy face, pump your fist, or do whatever feels natural. Emotion helps the brain to remember.

1. When I am tempted by something that is bad for my brain (like candy or cigarettes), I will hum to myself for a few minutes until the temptation passes.

2. After I open my refrigerator, I will throw out one food that is bad for my brain.

3. When a friend or someone at church asks me to take on a new task, I will say, "I have to think about it."

4. When I go to a party, I will ask for a wine spritzer and top it up with club soda so I'm sure I don't drink too much.

5. When I slip up on my goals, I will note it down in my journal.

6. When my child asks if he or she can play a contact sport like football or soccer, I will say, "No, I want to protect your brain from harm."

7. When I feel out of sorts, I will take 10 deep breaths and focus on my goals.

8. When I eat breakfast, I will take a supplement to improve my brain.

CHAPTER 4

CHANGE IS EASY—IF YOU KNOW HOW TO DO IT

TURN YOUR RUTS INTO SUPERHIGHWAYS OF SUCCESS

People don't change when they see the light,
only when they feel the heat.
PASTOR RICK WARREN

Change is easy—if you know how to do it. But it is hard if you keep doing things that reinforce negative behavior circuits in the brain. If you were an anxious child, for example, anxiety built specific connecting highways (neural networks) in your brain. Odds are you still feel anxious as an adult unless you did something to rewire them. If you deal with pressure by drinking alcohol or lashing out at those around you, you are likely to continue that behavior whenever you feel stressed—unless you develop a new model of doing things.

Once the brain learns how to do something, it becomes wired to do it automatically and reflexively through a process called neuroplasticity. New learning and change take strategy, effort, and resources, which is why we often get stuck. I find this to be true in my own life and bet you do too. Depending on what you've taught your brain to do, this neuroplasticity can help you develop and maintain good habits, or it can cause you to get stuck in ruts that steal portions of your life. An example of the former: When a waiter brings bread to my table at a restaurant, I now automatically request that it be taken away. An example of the latter: For years, my e-mail and smartphone controlled me.

When neurons fire together, they wire together, through a process called long-term potentiation (LTP), and habits and responses become an ingrained part of your life. LTP occurs when the brain learns something new, whether it's good or bad, and causes networks of brain cells to make new connections. Early in the learning process the connections are weak, but over time, as behaviors are repeated, the networks become stronger, making the behaviors more likely to become automatic, reflexive, or habitual. At this point, the networks are said to be "potentiated."

With the brain, what you practice and reinforce becomes your reality. One of my patients, Hank, learned that alcohol powerfully calmed his anxiety, and he couldn't break the wiring underlying his addiction until the pain of losing his family short-circuited the connections. After repeated explosions at home, Hank's children's brains learned they could not trust that they would be safe and became hypervigilant, always watching for the next bad thing to happen. Fear became potentiated in their brains. The stronger the emotion, the more powerful the wiring or connections in the behavior. Some fears or habits will develop after repeated mild-to-moderate exposures, but others will develop after just one exposure if it is intense enough, such as after physical abuse, a fire, robbery, or rape.

Kindling is an important process to understand as it relates to the brain and change. When a scientist passes a low-volt electrical current through a nerve cell, initially nothing happens, but as the voltage is raised to a certain threshold, the cell will begin to fire. If the electrical intensity remains high enough for a long enough period of time, the cell will become kindled, meaning it is more sensitive. The voltage can then be lowered, and it will still cause nerve cell firing. Every time an emotional explosion happened at home, Hank's kids experienced intense nerve cell firing in the limbic or emotional centers of their brains. Over time, as the trauma continued, it took less and less drama to trigger anxious feelings. Even years later, small things, such as an awkward look from a store clerk, could trigger big emotional reactions in the now-grown children.

Your brain has roughly 100 billion brain cells, or neurons. Throughout the day they are either at rest or firing to spark your thoughts, behaviors, and emotions. The activity becomes more intense in high-stress situations, such as the one described above. If you experience enough anxious moments as a child, your neurons may fire faster even at rest, making you feel on edge. As an adult, your neurons are still on guard, ready to fire with little provocation, like a hairpin trigger. Your son drops a plate, and the crashing noise makes you flip out. Someone raises his voice to make a point, and you start feeling panicky. You see someone intoxicated at a party, and you quickly leave, even though you wanted to stay. Because the resting state of your brain is elevated, which we have seen in our brain imaging work on posttraumatic stress disorder, you may be more inclined to drink alcohol, take painkillers, or overeat as a way to soothe your brain. Now your brain has become stuck in a rut, which the *Oxford Dictionary*, in one definition, describes as "a habit or pattern of behaviour that has become dull and unproductive but is hard to change."[1]

Whatever behaviors formed or you allowed into your life, productive or not, are the ones that are likely to continue. *This is why it is critical to assess your automatic behaviors and ask yourself if they are helping or hurting you.*

> *Be very careful of the behaviors you allow into*
> *your life. They may end up hijacking it.*

The exciting news is that you can change unwanted behaviors. Practicing good behaviors, such as getting seven to eight hours of sleep a night, exercising, and saying no to constantly checking your gadgets, strengthens the willpower circuits in the brain. Alternatively, giving in to negative behaviors, such as emotional explosions, mindlessly eating cookies at work, guzzling sodas, consuming excessive amounts of alcohol, procrastinating, or giving in to the urge to look at Internet pornography, strengthens those particular circuits. Whatever behaviors you engage in are the ones you are likely to continue doing. If you allow yourself to yell at your children or be rude to your spouse or coworkers, you are much more likely to do it again and again.

No one wants to be controlled by things that were done to them or by their own past negative choices. To feel better fast, you need to learn to make deliberate choices that will create new pathways in your brain. In this chapter, we'll explore more about how ruts and negative behaviors develop in the brain and how you can quickly develop more positive habits, while becoming more adaptable and flexible. When you repeatedly engage in positive behaviors, you build the superhighways of success that help you reflexively do the things you want to do. I'll show you how you can use your brain to change your habits.

WHY WE GET STUCK IN RUTS: HABITS AND THE BRAIN

Along with long-term potentiation and kindling, it is important to know about two areas of the brain that are involved with mental flexibility and habit formation: the *anterior cingulate gyrus*, which I think of as the brain's gear shifter, and the *basal ganglia*, where habits are formed and sustained.

INSIDE VIEW OF THE BRAIN

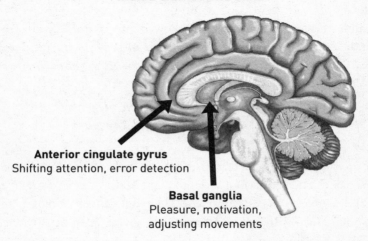

Anterior cingulate gyrus
Shifting attention, error detection

Basal ganglia
Pleasure, motivation,
adjusting movements

The Brain's Gear Shifter

There's an area deep in the frontal lobes called the anterior cingulate gyrus, or ACG, which allows us to shift our attention, go from thought to thought, move from idea to idea, see options, go with the flow, and cooperate, which involves getting outside ourselves to help others. The ACG is also involved in error detection. If you come home and see the front door wide open, for example, even though you know you locked it, it triggers an appropriate danger reaction in your mind.

When the ACG is healthy, we tend to be flexible, adaptable, and cooperative, learn from our mistakes, and effectively notice when things are wrong. When it is underactive, often due to head trauma or exposure to damaging toxins, we tend to be quiet and withdrawn. Alternatively, when the ACG is overactive, often due to low levels of the calming neurotransmitter serotonin, we tend to get stuck on negative thoughts (obsessions) or negative behaviors (compulsions/addictions) and be uncooperative. Serotonin-enhancing strategies, such as taking medicine that increases the availability of serotonin (SSRIs, or selective serotonin reuptake inhibitors), have been used for decades to treat anxiety, depression, and obsessive-compulsive disorder (OCD).

Practically speaking, getting stuck has many different potential manifestations, including worrying, holding grudges, and becoming upset if things don't go your way. On the surface, people with high ACG activity may appear selfish ("My way or the highway"), but from a neuroscience standpoint, they're not selfish; they're rigid. Inflexibility causes them to automatically say no even when saying yes may be their best choice. They have trouble seeing options and tend to be argumentative and oppositional. Plus, they tend to see too many errors—in themselves, their spouses, kids, coworkers, and organizations, such as schools, government, and churches.

In doing research on our extensive brain imaging/clinical database, we discovered that patients who have OCD or posttraumatic stress disorder (PTSD) show increased activity in the ACG. In both disorders, people get stuck on negative feelings, thoughts, and behaviors (see "When the Gear Shifter and Enabler Are Over- or Underactive" on page 74). Knowing this information gives us the clue that strategies to boost serotonin could help increase cognitive flexibility to enable change. Research suggests that is indeed true[2]—more on this below (see Strategy #1, pages 76–77).

The Brain's Enabler

Deep in the brain are two large structures called the basal ganglia (BG). Among other roles, they are involved with integrating thoughts, emotions, and movement, which is why we jump when we get excited or freeze when we become scared. The BG also help to shift and smooth motor behavior and may be involved in habit formation, according to studies. When they are overactive, our research and that of others suggests, people struggle with generalized anxiety, dislike uncertainty, and avoid conflict.[3] With increased BG activity we also see repetitive behaviors, such as tics, nail biting, and teeth grinding, as well as compulsions, such as hand washing and checking locks. When the BG are underactive, people tend to have low motivation, poor handwriting, and trouble feeling pleasure. They are also more vulnerable to attentional problems and movement disorders, such as Parkinson's disease.

When the Gear Shifter and Enabler Are Over- or Underactive

BRAIN AREA
ANTERIOR CINGULATE GYRUS

FUNCTION
- Shifts attention
- Increases cognitive flexibility
- Encourages adaptability
- Moves from idea to idea
- Sees options
- Goes with the flow
- Cooperates with others
- Detects errors

UNDERACTIVE SYMPTOMS
- Low motivation
- Low energy
- Low movement
- Decreased speech

OVERACTIVE SYMPTOMS
- Dislikes change
- Has trouble shifting attention
- Has difficulty seeing options
- Holds own opinions, doesn't listen to others
- Gets locked into a course of action, even though it may not be beneficial
- Says no automatically without thinking first
- Needs things done a certain way
- Engages in compulsive behaviors, such as excessive hand washing, checking locks, counting, or spelling, and experiences anxiety if these are not done
- Is oppositional
- Is argumentative
- Gets upset when things don't go as expected
- Obsessive-compulsive disorder (OCD)
- Posttraumatic stress disorder (PTSD)

BRAIN AREA
BASAL GANGLIA

FUNCTION
- Integrates feeling and movement
- Shifts and steadies fine motor movements
- Suppresses unwanted motor behaviors
- Helps to set the body's anxiety level
- Involved in habit formation
- Generates motivation and drive
- Mediates pleasure/ecstasy

UNDERACTIVE SYMPTOMS
- Low motivation
- Poor handwriting
- Tremors
- Parkinson's disease
- Fine motor problems

OVERACTIVE SYMPTOMS
- Generalized anxiety
- Uncertainty about the future or ambiguity[4]
- Predicts the worst
- Avoids conflict[5]

WHAT DO RUTS LOOK LIKE IN YOUR LIFE?

Getting stuck in a rut can take many forms, including addictions, depression, impulse-control issues, bad habits, staying in difficult or abusive relationships, or maintaining outdated business processes. Worry, holding grudges, obsessive thinking, compulsive behaviors, persistent anger, rude behavior, and being oppositional or argumentative can also be caused by ruts in the brain.

Check the questions that apply to you.

☐ Do you dislike change?
☐ Do you tend to get stuck in loops of thinking?
☐ Do you struggle with repetitive, negative thoughts?
☐ Do you have difficulty seeing options in stressful situations?
☐ Do you tend to hold on to your own opinions and not listen to others?
☐ Do you get locked into a course of action, even though it may not be good for you?
☐ Do you tend to automatically say no without thinking?
☐ Do you get upset if you are surprised or if things don't go the way you expect they should?
☐ Do you struggle with compulsive behaviors, such as hand washing, checking locks, counting, or spelling?
☐ Do you tend to be oppositional or argumentative?
☐ Have you been diagnosed with OCD or PTSD?

The more questions you checked, the more likely you have an ACG that is working too hard. Where do you feel stuck in your life?

☐ Personal habits
☐ Relationships
☐ Health
☐ Work
☐ Money

Think about your day and the automatic behaviors you engage in without much thought, such as

- Using your cell phone or other gadgets
- Brushing your teeth
- Making coffee or tea
- Eating breakfast, healthy or not

- Being polite or curt to your kids or partner
- Reading the news
- Answering e-mail
- Exercising
- Showering
- Driving to work
- Texting with family or friends
- Snacking
- Eating lunch by yourself or with coworkers
- Eating dinner
- Having dessert
- Engaging in bedtime rituals

Ask yourself if the way you accomplish each of your behaviors is helping or hurting you. Do you lunch on salad and soup or wolf down fast food? Do you take regular breaks from e-mail and texting or spend endless hours on one or both? Do you listen to soothing music while driving or tailgate whenever you get behind the wheel?

Have you tried to change habits that have not been helpful but failed miserably over time? That happens to most people because they do not understand the brain. As we have seen, it is in your brain where you become adaptable, flexible, and able to change, or it is in your brain where you get stuck in a rut.

NINE STRATEGIES TO QUICKLY TURN YOUR RUTS INTO SUPERHIGHWAYS OF SUCCESS

Scientists have studied how the brain *can* facilitate change, whether it is to lose weight, beat an addiction, stay off your computer, be more successful at work, change personal habits, or revise business processes. Based on this research, together with our clinical experience at Amen Clinics, here are nine simple brain-based habits to promote change.

Strategy #1: Naturally boost serotonin.

:05-60 When serotonin levels are low, the ACG and BG tend to be more
MINUTES active, which can inhibit change and also contribute to mental inflexibility and getting stuck on negative thoughts or behaviors. Increasing serotonin can help calm these areas of the brain.[6] This can be done with four simple strategies:[7]

- Physical exercise increases the ability of tryptophan, the amino acid precursor of serotonin, to enter the brain. Walking, running, swimming, or playing table tennis will help you feel happier and more mentally flexible. Exercise alone has been found to treat depression, with effectiveness similar to an SSRI antidepressant.[8] Whenever you feel stuck in a rut, get moving.

- Bright light exposure has been shown to increase serotonin and is a natural treatment for seasonal depression and premenstrual tension syndrome, as well as depression in pregnant women.[9] Depression and inflexibility are more common in winter and in places where sunlight is lacking. To improve your mood and increase cognitive flexibility and learning, get more sun or use bright light LED therapy,[10] which is a standard treatment for seasonal depression.

- Eating foods that contain tryptophan can increase serotonin levels. Whenever you feel stuck in a rut, combine tryptophan-containing foods, such as eggs, turkey, seafood, chickpeas, nuts, and seeds, with healthy carbohydrates, such as sweet potatoes and quinoa, to elicit a short-term insulin response that drives tryptophan into the brain. Dark chocolate also increases serotonin.[11]

- Nutritional supplements can also raise brain levels of serotonin. My favorite ones are L-tryptophan, 5-hydroxytryptophan (5-HTP), and saffron.[12] See chapter 10 for more information on these.

Strategy #2: Define what you want and why.

: 15 - 30
MINUTES
To help you make better behavioral choices, your BG and ACG need your prefrontal cortex to step in and take charge. For this to occur, it helps if you clarify which behaviors you want to change. Your brain makes happen what it sees. What patterns are making you feel worse by contributing to your anxiety, anger, stress, or worry? What ruts would you like to turn into superhighways of success, leaving you feeling better? Write them out. Create a vivid and believable "Future of Success" in detail. How will you feel in one, five, and ten years if you consistently engage in the new behavior? You could write, "I'll feel amazing, healthy, energetic, cognitively better than I have ever been, in control." Next, envision a vivid and believable "Future of Failure" in detail. How will you feel in one, five, and ten years if you do not stop this negative behavior? What will your life look like going forward? You might write, "I'll feel embarrassed, lose my family, have a smaller brain, suffer from early disease and death!"

Define what you want, and then ask yourself if your behavior is getting you what you want. If not, be clear with yourself that every time you engage in the wrong behavior, it is strengthening your brain to do the wrong thing. Whenever you do the right thing, it is beginning to strengthen those circuits instead. Practice does not make perfect; it makes the brain do what you practice. Perfect practice makes perfect.

Strategy #3: Assess your readiness for change.

Remember this joke? "How many psychiatrists does it take to change a light bulb? One, but the light bulb really has to want to change."

Likewise, your consent and motivation are critical elements of change. Are you ready to eliminate the ruts in your life? One of my favorite techniques to assess motivation for change is called Motivational Interviewing (MI). It helps people clarify their conviction and confidence to do things differently and uses questions to guide them through six stages of change. Ambivalence and uncertainty are the enemies of change.

When you meet a friend who . . . drinks too much; smokes a pack per day; is obese; doesn't exercise; or has high blood pressure and yet is unwilling to take your advice, change her lifestyle, or comply with recommendations from her doctor, *how do you feel?*

When your adolescent ADHD son . . . refuses to turn down the music and do homework, smells of cigarette smoke, hangs out with friends who drink, and stops participating in healthy activities, *how do you feel?*

If you are like most people, you feel sad, scared, helpless, frustrated, and unsure of how to help. You may respond with judgment, unwanted advice, or scary stories of the risks these people face, hoping to help them see the light. For those of you who have tried this approach (I certainly have), how's it been working for you? I want to help you become more effective at facilitating real behavioral change in yourself, your family, and your friends. Understanding these six stages of change will help you assess your own or someone else's readiness for change and increase your conviction and confidence to make it happen.

SIX STAGES OF CHANGE

Decisions to make lifestyle changes are the result of a natural process that takes place in stages over time. Each stage is the foundation for the next one. Let's talk about how to recognize, reinforce, and accelerate the natural process throughout these stages.

STAGES OF CHANGE

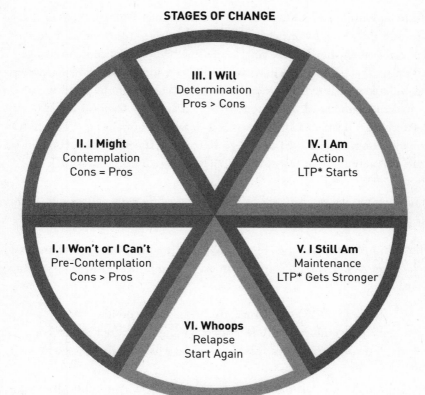

*Long-term potentiation

Change starts by determining a person's readiness for it. First, ask yourself (or a loved one) an open-ended question about the behavior to be changed: Would you consider . . .

- Losing weight?
- Quitting smoking?
- Getting more exercise?
- Changing your eating habits?
- Cutting back or abstaining from alcohol?
- Going to bed earlier?
- Limiting your e-mail?

If you answer "no," you're in Stage I, which is called the pre-contemplation stage. You are not thinking about a change, you are not ready for it, and you do not believe you can accomplish it.

Stage I: I Won't or I Can't. This is often called denial, when the cons of change outweigh the pros. "I won't change" means you have little to no motivation to change; "I can't change" means you lack the capability or confidence to change. In this stage either the negatives of changing the behavior (such as smoking, overeating, or looking at Internet pornography) seem to outweigh the positives, or you are in denial, lack knowledge or conviction to change, are skeptical, or feel powerless to change. If you or a loved one is in this stage, you can increase your conviction by asking, "If I decided to change, how would it benefit me?" Focusing on benefits is an important first strategy to help move someone to Stage II.

If you answer "maybe," you are in Stage II, called the contemplation stage. You are thinking about changing but have not yet decided.

Stage II: I Might. The cons of change equal the pros, but ambivalence and lack of confidence are still issues. To boost your confidence, ask yourself three questions:

1. If I really decide to change, do I think I can do it?
2. What would prevent me from changing; what are the barriers?
3. How do I think I can start changing; what are the strategies?

In this stage, it helps to focus on the benefits of changing and collect information that might help you develop solutions. I was once visiting my niece, who had just started seventh grade in a new school. She was struggling in music, and she told me the teacher was not helpful. Her instrument was the xylophone, and she had no idea how to play it. She lacked confidence. Together, we went to YouTube and searched the term "How to play the xylophone." In 20 minutes she was able to play a simple song, and her confidence soared.

If you answer "yes," you are in Stage III, called the determination stage. You are making the decision to change.

Stage III: I Will. The benefits of change now outweigh the drawbacks, and you can now develop a plan to make it happen.

If you answer, "I am doing it," you are in Stage IV, called the action stage.

Stage IV: I Am. In this stage you build confidence and look for any barriers that might derail you. Long-term potentiation (LTP) is beginning to occur in this phase, meaning that you are beginning to rewire your brain.

If you answer, "I am still doing it," you are in Stage V, called the maintenance stage.

Stage V: I Still Am. LTP is being strengthened and the new behavior feels more reflexive or automatic, but you are still on the lookout for barriers and traps.

If you answer, "I fell off the wagon," you are in Stage VI, called the relapse stage.

Stage VI: Whoops! Most people backslide at some point. It is a natural part of change. When you fall off the wagon, it is critical to ask why, learn from your mistake(s), and start again. Some people have to start over at Stage I. Most people jump back in at Stage III or IV.

In general, the job of people in Stages I and II is enhancing their motivation and conviction, while those in Stages III through V focus on sustaining motivation and engagement, eliminating obstacles, and overcoming barriers. If someone is in the "I Won't or I Can't" phase, the first step is to work on conviction and confidence until they make the decision "I Will." Then they can focus on the skills that will help them to engage in the new behavior.

For each behavior you want to change, ask yourself, "Which stage am I in?" and "How will it benefit me to change my behavior?"

By embracing change, we learn a principle inspired by Aristotle's teachings: "We are what we repeatedly do. Excellence, then, is not an act, but a habit."[13]

Strategy #4: Know what you need to do.

What are the new behaviors you need to master to be successful? For any problem, such as losing weight, overcoming an addiction, calming your temper, or avoiding distractions, it is critical to know which important behaviors will help you reach your goal, then practice them over and over. Here are a few general examples, followed by suggestions for specific issues:

- Make sure your blood sugar is stable to keep the PFC healthy
- Get enough sleep to keep the PFC healthy
- Take proper nutritional supplements

WEIGHT LOSS
- Start a food journal to monitor what you eat
- Stop drinking your calories; drink primarily water
- Upgrade the quality of your food
- Eliminate foods you may be intolerant of or allergic to, such as milk or wheat products
- Avoid places that trigger food cravings

- Add in exercise
- Learn to control your thoughts, so you don't have to medicate them with food or drugs
- Get your blood work done so you do not miss an important contributor, such as low vitamin D, thyroid, or testosterone levels

OVERCOMING ADDICTION
- Avoid friends who use substances
- HALT—don't let yourself get too hungry, angry, lonely, or tired
- Learn to control your thoughts, so you don't have to medicate them with drugs
- Attend 12-step groups on a regular basis if they help you
- Work to keep your temper under control
- Eliminate the ANTs (see discussion of automatic negative thoughts in chapter 5)
- Learn diaphragmatic breathing
- Consider SPECT to see if you had a brain injury in the past that needs to be treated
- Establish group support

ELIMINATING DISTRACTIONS
- Have defined periods where you turn off your gadgets
- Stop texting while walking
- Put away your tablet, smartphone, and other tech items at least an hour before bed

Just as in the story about my niece, you can google how to change virtually any behavior. Once you have the desire and motivation, learn the critical steps to take.

Strategy #5: Identify your most vulnerable moments and learn from your mistakes.

It's important to know when you are most vulnerable. Be curious about your behavior, not furious at your slipups or mistakes. Investigating setbacks can be extremely instructive if you take the time to really analyze them.

Eloise, 42, a highly successful realtor, came into my office feeling sad and ashamed. I initially saw her for panic attacks and drug use. Within a few months she had made great progress and completely stopped using drugs. But after a major fight with her boyfriend, she slipped and went on a weekend binge.

"I'll never be free of this behavior," Eloise told me. Then she stopped herself and said, "I know that's not true." We had worked on her thoughts. "I am just so mad at myself."

I went to the whiteboard in my office and drew the graph on how people change.

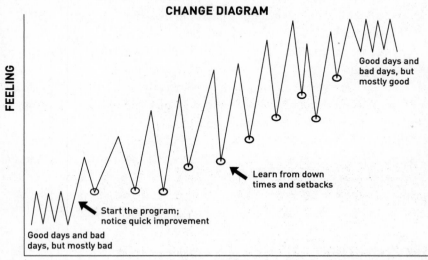

CHANGE DIAGRAM

"When people come to see me as patients, they have good days and bad days, but usually their days are not very good," I said. "Then we work together to change things, and they get better. But they never just get better and stay there. There is an up-and-down course. Over time they feel much better and usually stay that way. But it is the down times, the slipups, the setbacks that teach us most of what we need to know—if we embrace them and take time to learn from them. We have to turn bad days into useful information."

When Rahm Emanuel was the White House chief of staff, he once said that you never want a serious crisis to go to waste.[14] Slipups and setbacks are the same. Study them, learn from them, be curious. In my experience, the most successful people embrace their mistakes so they can learn from them.

Eloise and I investigated her relapse from a brain science perspective. The week before her relapse, a home fell through escrow and she lost sleep over it. In addition, her eating became more erratic, she did not take time to work out, and she skipped her supplements. Poor sleep, inconsistent eating habits, and a lack of exercise all contributed to lower activity in and blood flow to her brain. Combining those factors with a stressful week and relational conflict triggered more negative thoughts, and she relapsed. Rather than judge herself as a bad person, I encouraged her to be a good student and learn from the episode. She needed to be more diligent with sleep, exercise, and good food, along with learning how to master her mind (see Strategy #4).

I asked Eloise, "Do you have a GPS system in your car that talks to you?"

"Yes," she replied.

"When you make a wrong turn, what does the voice say to you?"

"'Make the next legal turn,' or something like that," she said.

"Does it start yelling or swearing at you?" I asked.

With a smile she said, "They wouldn't sell many of those GPS systems. Of course not."

"But isn't this what you are doing to yourself when you make a mistake? Instead of beating yourself up, whenever you make a mistake, learn from it, turn around, and go in a better direction."

Be both the investigator and the subject! Change is a process that occurs in steps. If you pay attention, the bad times can be more instructive than the good times. Journaling is key to helping keep track of both. Know when you are most vulnerable (not sleeping, forgetting to eat breakfast, waiting too long between meals, attending too many parties or social gatherings, etc.).

Strategy #6: Develop "if-then" plans to overcome your vulnerable moments.

:20-30 Once you know when you are vulnerable, you can create contin-
MINUTES gency plans to overcome unwanted behaviors. Psychology professor Peter Gollwitzer from New York University has published extensive research on behavior change. He recommends that people create "if-then" scenarios that spell out how they'll break unwanted habits.[15] For example, if *x* (situation) happens, then I will do *y* (preplanned action).

Dr. Gollwitzer wrote in *Fortune* magazine,

> The most effective plans are those that specify when, where and how you want to act on your goals by using an "if-then" format. Take drinking too much in the company of your friends as an example. In the "if" part of the plan, you identify the critical situation that usually triggers your bad habit. Perhaps the trigger is being offered a drink by your friends. In the "then" part, you specify an action that can halt accepting the offer such as responding to it by saying that you prefer a glass of water today. And then you link the "if" and the "then" parts together by making an "if-then" plan: "If on Friday evening

my friends offer me a drink, then I will answer: I prefer to have a glass of water today!"[16]

As insanely simple as it sounds, the research is impressive. If-then strategies have helped people reach their goals in dieting and athletics,[17] boosted physical activity in women by more than an hour a week compared to a control group,[18] increased the consumption of fruits and vegetables,[19] and helped to regulate emotions, including fear and disgust.[20] Using this simple technique has been shown to increase activity in the PFC,[21] which can help override the brain's automatic or reflexive behaviors from the ACG and BG. It has even been shown to help normalize the brain in children with ADHD.[22] Making your "if-then" plans known to others also improves your ability to stay on track.[23]

In a similar way, I often tell my patients that when it comes to brain health, the two most important words in the English language are *then what*. If I do this, then what happens? Thinking ahead helps to prevent a lot of unwanted trouble.

CREATE SIMPLE "IF-THEN" RULES FOR VULNERABLE TIMES, SUCH AS

1. *If* I am tempted to eat unhealthy foods, *then* I'll at least eat the healthy ones first.

2. *If* I find myself becoming irritated at someone, *then* I will take three deep belly breaths before I say anything else.

3. *If* I am anxious about a meeting, *then* I will write down my anxious thoughts, which helps to dispel them.

4. *If* I can cheat on my diet, *then* it can only be after reading my One-Page Miracle (see pages 190–193) and calling supportive friends (introduces delay and social support).

5. *If* I become aware of the impulse to eat something that is not healthy, *then* I will focus on something else—like taking a walk, reciting a poem, or drinking a glass of water—until the impulse goes away.

Strategy #7: Reframe your pain.

To succeed at changing, you have to disarm your impulses and make the right choices pleasurable.

The only way you can sustain change is to
change what brings you pleasure!

Learn how to find what you love about not being inebriated, or identify great low-calorie, highly nutritious food. Discover how good it feels when you're not tied up with anxiety. One of my friends told me she hated exercise, but she loved walking with her children. Mind-set is key.

Connect to who you are becoming, and think like a healthy person. How would a healthy person order this meal or act in this vulnerable situation? Willpower is a skill you can develop. If you can distract yourself for just a minute, temptations often go away.

Be careful about giving in to your own bad behavior! You may be causing your own behavior disorder. I was once with a patient who was struggling with her weight. She said she often felt as though she had to give in to her cravings. She had two teenage daughters, one of whom I was seeing because she had tantrums whenever she did not get her way. I asked this mother how her daughter would do if Mom always gave in to her temper tantrums—would she get better or worse? "Worse, of course," she replied. When you give in to your own tantrums or cravings, you are creating your own internal behavior disorder, which can ruin your health and kill you before your time. Be a loving, effective parent to yourself.

Strategy #8: Turn accomplices into friends.

Whom you spend time with matters! Cultivating bad habits—and good ones—is a team sport, and you need friends rather than accomplices. Accomplices encourage or are complicit with your negative behaviors, while friends, mentors, or coaches are people who support your positive behaviors. Ask for their help. Adding friends improves your chances for success up to 40 percent, and this is especially true for weight loss and fitness.

If you want to change your behavior, either you need to stop seeing your accomplices or turn them into friends, or you need to change your friends. Many accomplices can become friends if you have crucial conversations with them. Explain what they can start doing, stop doing, and continue doing to help you.

IN YOUR LIFE, ARE THESE PEOPLE ACCOMPLICES OR FRIENDS?

- Spouse
- Children
- Parents
- Grandparents
- Siblings
- In-laws

- Aunts, uncles, cousins
- Friends
- Neighbors
- Bosses
- Coworkers
- Teachers
- Classmates
- Students
- School administrators
- Church members or staff
- AA participants
- Community club members
- Gym friends

Identify your five most powerful friends who will support your good habits, as well as five accomplices who make it less likely you will succeed in changing your behavior. Spend more time with the people who will help you.

Strategy #9: Use tiny behaviors to create massive change.

Small daily improvements are the key to staggering long-term results.

As I mentioned in the introduction, Amen Clinics partnered with Professor BJ Fogg, director of the Persuasive Tech Lab at Stanford University, and his sister, Linda Fogg-Phillips, to help our patients with behavior change. One of their key suggestions is to take baby steps. We have been sprinkling these "Tiny Habits" throughout the book, since developing those small new behaviors is one of the best ways to make change a reality in your life and slowly builds new circuits or superhighways in your brain.

Based on his research, Dr. Fogg has found that change is easy when designed properly. He said,

> You don't have to be perfect. No one is. You just need to keep working on it.
>
> Change happens better and faster if you are playful, flexible, and iterative.
>
> Few people change all at once; change occurs most effectively when it is small and incremental over time. Relying solely on willpower is usually a prescription for failure.
>
> Know your motivation—when motivation is high you can do hard things. If you are just diagnosed with diabetes, for example, cutting out sugar becomes much easier than it would be if you simply want to lose a few pounds. When motivation is low, you have to make things as easy, simple, and "tiny" as possible. If

you just want to lose a few pounds, you could start by packing your lunch two days a week, instead of eating out.

When things don't work, be curious, not furious. Ask why and re-assess. It may take several tries.[24]

Our brains are wired to keep doing what we've always done—but we can change the ruts into superhighways of success. Making small changes is the secret to feeling better fast, and it can lead to taking on big changes that will ensure those feelings last.

NINE STRATEGIES TO EMBRACE CHANGE AND TURN YOUR RUTS INTO SUPERHIGHWAYS OF SUCCESS

1. Naturally boost serotonin.

2. Define what you want and why.

3. Assess your readiness for change.

4. Know what you need to do.

5. Identify your most vulnerable moments.

6. Develop "if-then" plans to overcome your vulnerable moments.

7. Reframe your pain.

8. Turn accomplices into friends.

9. Use tiny behaviors to create massive change.

TINY HABITS THAT CAN HELP YOU FEEL BETTER FAST—AND LEAD TO BIG CHANGES

:02- 15
MINUTES
Each of these habits takes just a few minutes. They are anchored to something you do (or think or feel) so that they are more likely to become automatic. Once you do the behaviors you want, find a way to make yourself feel good about them—draw a happy face, pump your fist, or do whatever feels natural. Emotion helps the brain to remember.

1. After I answer the phone, I will stand up and walk while I talk.

2. After I start to argue, I will ask myself, *Is my behavior getting me what I want?*

3. When I get out of bed in the morning, I will open the curtains/shades to let the sunshine in.

4. When I feel anxious, I will eat a complex carbohydrate, such as a sweet potato, to boost serotonin.

5. When I relapse or make a mistake with my health, I will ask myself, *What can I learn from my mistake?*

6. When I am tempted to eat unhealthy foods, I will eat the healthy ones on my plate first.

7. When I am dealing with someone who is stuck on a negative thought or arguing, I will ask them to go for a walk with me and will not bring up any charged topic for at least 10 minutes.

8. When I want to go out to eat, I will ask the healthiest person I know to go with me.

9. When I feel thoughts going over and over in my head, I will write them down, which helps to get rid of them.

PART 2

R IS FOR RATIONAL MIND

Once the physical functioning of your brain is healthy, it is critical to know how to program and strengthen your rational mind, which is an aspect of your psychological health. Where you bring your attention determines how you feel, and you can train your mind to work for you rather than against you. This section will show you how to quickly direct your thoughts in a way that elevates your mood rather than hurting it.

CHAPTER 5

MASTER YOUR RATIONAL MIND

HOW TO FEEL HAPPY AND PRESENT, WHILE CONQUERING WORRY AND NEGATIVITY

A thought is harmless unless we believe it. It's not our thoughts, but the attachment *to our thoughts, that causes suffering. Attaching to a thought means believing that it's true, without inquiring. A belief is a thought that we've been attaching to, often for years.*

BYRON KATIE, *LOVING WHAT IS: FOUR QUESTIONS THAT CAN CHANGE YOUR LIFE*

Dark thoughts in the mind are not "you," but are false messages from the brain. And because you are not your brain, you don't have to listen to them.

JEFFREY M. SCHWARTZ, MD, AUTHOR OF *YOU ARE NOT YOUR BRAIN*

Developing the habit of accurate, honest, and disciplined thinking is essential to feeling better fast and making it last. This is not positive thinking, which can actually inhibit feeling better over the long run. As I have noted before, people who live by the philosophy "Don't worry; be happy" die the earliest from accidents and preventable illnesses. Believing the future will be favorable without following a plan and putting in consistent effort can prevent people from taking the actions that will likely make that belief a reality.[1] This chapter will help you develop the mental discipline necessary for success, including eliminating the ANTs (automatic negative thoughts), quieting your mind, having an appropriate level of anxiety, and focusing on gratitude.

The human attention span is eight seconds, according to a 2015 study from Microsoft.[2] A goldfish's attention span has been estimated at nine seconds. Human development seems to be going the wrong way. With modern technology stealing our attention span and directing our minds to the will of corporate America, disciplining the habits of our moment-by-moment thoughts is an essential skill for achieving happiness and purpose. Our gadget addiction is feeding an old tendency of the human brain to be scattered, unfocused, and controlled by negativity and fear. Plus, it is making us feel worse.[3] People who have the most screen time (TV, texting, video games) have a higher incidence of feeling unhappy.

Monkey mind is a term that describes a mind that is unsettled, restless, indecisive, and uncontrollable. Monkey mind was described by Siddhartha Gautama (Buddha) in the sixth century BC, but it applies today more than ever. He said, "Just as a monkey swinging through the trees grabs one branch and lets it go only to seize another, so, too, that which is called thought, mind, or consciousness arises and disappears continually both day and night."

Thoughts that *you allow* to circle again and again in your mind build ruts or roads in the brain, making the thoughts more likely to dominate and control your life. Fortunately, as we've seen in the last few chapters, the brain can change. You can rebuild these neural network highways in a more productive way with focused effort.

MARCUS: TOO MANY NEGATIVE THOUGHTS

About 10 years ago, the parents of 14-year-old Marcus brought him to see me because he was struggling with schoolwork and with his temper. At his previous school, Marcus "barely had to try" to get good grades; but after moving to a new school for the athletics, he found the more academically rigorous program challenging, and his grades declined. He had trouble focusing, was easily distracted, procrastinated, and took longer to complete assignments than ever before. A prior psychiatrist diagnosed him with attention deficit hyperactivity disorder (ADHD), but the stimulant medications Ritalin and Adderall made him angry and more depressed, and for the first time he started to complain of suicidal thoughts. His SPECT scan revealed that his brain worked too hard, especially in the front, which was not consistent with a classic ADHD pattern. In research my team has published, we've seen that this pattern actually predicts a negative response to stimulant medications.

When I met Marcus, it was clear he struggled with many negative thoughts. He repeatedly referred to himself as stupid, and during our first session he told me,

"I hate school."

"I can never be as good as other kids."

"I'm a terrible person."

"I should try harder."

"I'm an idiot."

"I am a failure."

"My teachers hate me."

"It's my parents' fault for not letting me quit."

His thinking was in a rut. The highways in his brain were headed straight toward negativity, failure, and depression. When I showed Marcus his brain scan and compared it to a Ferrari whose engine was revved too high, he smiled, saying he liked that comparison. To help Marcus get control over his mind, I spent the next two months teaching him the six principles of disciplined thinking that we all should have learned in school.

Disciplined Thinking Principle #1:
Every time you have a thought, your brain releases chemicals.

That's how your brain works. You have a thought, your brain releases chemicals, electrical transmissions travel throughout your brain, and you become aware of what you're thinking. Thoughts are real, and they have a powerful impact on how you feel and behave. Just as a muscle that's exercised becomes stronger, repeatedly thinking the same thoughts makes them stronger too.

Every time you have an angry, unkind, hopeless, helpless, worthless, sad, or irritating thought, such as *I'm stupid*, your brain releases chemicals that make you feel bad. In this way, your body reacts to every negative thought you have. Marcus was exercising his brain to feel depression, sadness, and failure. I asked him to think about the last time he was mad. How did his body feel? When most people are angry, their muscles become tense, their hearts beat faster, their hands start to sweat, and they may even begin to feel a little dizzy. Marcus told me he got dizzy and sweaty and felt confused and stupid.

Similarly, every time you have a happy, hopeful, kind, optimistic, positive thought, your brain releases chemicals that make you feel good. I asked Marcus to think about the last time he had a happy thought. How did he feel inside his body? When most people are happy, their muscles relax, their hearts beat more slowly, their hands become dry, and they breathe more evenly. Marcus told me about an outing with his father, where they went fishing and had a great time. When he thought about it, he said he felt peaceful and happy. He didn't feel stupid.

Disciplined Thinking Principle #2:
Thoughts are powerful, and your body reacts to every single one you have.

Thoughts can make your mind and body feel good, or they can make you feel bad. Every cell in your body is affected by every thought you have. We know this from polygraph, or lie detector, tests. During a polygraph, a person is connected to instruments that measure

- hand temperature
- heart rate
- blood pressure
- breathing rate
- muscle tension
- sweat gland activity

The tester then asks questions, such as "Did you do that misdeed?" Almost immediately, the tested person's body reacts to every thought he has, whether he says anything or not. If the person did it and worries he'll be found out, his body is likely to have a stress response and react in the following ways:

- hand temperature drops
- heart rate speeds up
- blood pressure increases
- breathing rate increases, but breaths are more shallow
- muscle tension increases
- sweat gland activity increases

The opposite is also true. If he did not do the deed, his body will experience a relaxation response and react in the following ways:

- hand temperature increases
- heart rate slows
- blood pressure decreases
- breathing rate decreases and breaths become deeper
- muscle tension decreases
- sweat gland activity decreases

Again, your body reacts almost immediately to what you think—and not just when you're asked about telling the truth. Your body reacts to every thought you have, whether it is about work, friends, family, or anything else.

This is why when people become upset, they often develop physical symptoms, such as headaches, stomachaches, or diarrhea, or they become more susceptible to illness. Imagine what was happening in Marcus's young body as his mind was flooded with negative thoughts.

At Amen Clinics we have biofeedback equipment that measures the same physiological responses as polygraphs: hand temperature, heart rate, breathing rate, muscle tension, and sweat gland activity (see chapter 1, page 10). I hooked up Marcus to our equipment. When I asked him about baseball (a sport he loved), his baby sister, and his friends, his body showed an immediate relaxation response. Yet when I asked him about school, feeling stupid, or his history teacher (with whom he was having a particularly hard time), his hands immediately got colder, his heart rate and muscle tension increased, his breathing rate became disorganized, and his hands started to sweat more. Marcus and his mother were amazed to see the evidence of how his body responded to every thought he had.

I taught Marcus to think of his body as an "ecosystem" that contains everything in the environment, such as air, water, land, cars, people, animals, vegetation, houses, landfills, and more. A negative thought was like pollution to his whole system. Just as pollution in Los Angeles or Beijing affects everyone who goes outdoors, so, too, do negative thoughts pollute your mind and your body.

Disciplined Thinking Principle #3:
Your thoughts are hardwired to be negative.

In generations past, negative thoughts protected us from early death or becoming supper for powerful animals. From our earliest times on earth, being aware of and avoiding danger was crucial to survival. Unfortunately, even when the world became safer, negativity bias remained in our brains. Researchers have demonstrated that negative experiences have a greater impact on the brain than positive ones.[4] People pay more attention to negative than to positive news, which is why news outlets typically lead broadcasts with floods, murders, political disasters, and all forms of mayhem. According to research from the content marketing website Outbrain.com, in two periods of 2012 the average click-through rate on headlines with negative adjectives was an astounding 63 percent higher than for headlines with positive ones.[5] A negative perspective is more contagious than a positive one, which may be why political campaigns typically go negative at the end. Even our language is not exempt: 62 percent of the words in the English dictionary connote negative emotions, while 32 percent express positive ones.[6]

Psychologist and author Rick Hanson has written that the brain is wired for negativity bias. Bad news is quickly stored in the brain to keep us safe, but positive experiences have to be held in consciousness for more than 12 seconds before they stay with us. "The brain is like Velcro for negative experiences but Teflon for positive ones," Hanson wrote.[7] Psychologist Mihaly Csikszentmihalyi, author of *Flow: The Psychology of Optimal Experience*, suggested that without other thoughts to occupy us, our brains will always return to worry. The only way to escape this is to focus on what will bring "flow"— activities that increase our sense of purpose and achievement.

Negative emotions "trump" positive emotions, which is why it is critical to discipline our natural tendency toward the negative and amplify more helpful thoughts and emotions. I taught Marcus that his negative thought pattern was common but not helpful.

Disciplined Thinking Principle #4:
Thoughts are automatic and often lie.

Thoughts are based on complex chemical reactions in the brain; memories from the past; the quality of our sleep, hormones, and blood sugar; and many other factors. They are automatic, reflexive, random, and overwhelmingly negative. Plus, they are often erroneous. Unless disciplined and bridled, they will lie to you and wreak havoc in your life. Marcus thought he was stupid. He told himself so multiple times a day because he had trouble staying focused and didn't perform well on tests. Yet when we tested him, his IQ was 135—in the top one percent of all people. I told him it was critical to question every stupid thought that went through his head.

It's important to examine your thoughts to see if they are true and if they are helping you or hurting you. Unfortunately, if you never challenge your thoughts, you will simply believe them and then act out of that erroneous belief. If, for example, I thought, *My wife never listens to me*, I'd feel lonely, mad, and sad. I would give myself permission to be rude to her or ignore her. My reaction to the lie I was telling myself could cause a negative spiral in my marriage, which could then literally ruin the rest of my life.

By repeatedly allowing his undisciplined thoughts to invade his mind, telling himself he was stupid, a failure, and a terrible person who hated school and was hated by his teachers, Marcus was more likely to behave in ways that would make those terrible things happen. I told him that his brain makes happen what it sees, which is why it is critical to get control over your thoughts.

***Disciplined Thinking Principle #5: You can learn to eliminate the
ANTs, or automatic negative thoughts, that steal your happiness.***

I coined the term *ANTs* in the early 1990s after a hard day at the office, where
I had seen four suicidal patients, two teens who had run away from home, and
two couples who hated each other. That evening, when I arrived home and
walked into the kitchen, I was greeted by an ant infestation. There were thousands of the pesky invaders marching in lines on the floor and crawling in the
sink, on the countertops, and in the cabinets. Construction in our neighborhood had disturbed the earth, and the ants were looking for a new residence.
As I wetted paper towels and began wiping up the horde of ants, the acronym
ANT came to me—Automatic Negative Thought. Acronyms had been part
of my life since medical school, helping me remember the 50,000 new terms
I was learning. As I thought about my patients that day, I realized that, just
like my kitchen, they were also infested with ANTs that were robbing them
of their joy and stealing their happiness. A bizarre image came to me of ANTs
crawling on top of their heads and out of their eyes, noses, and ears. The ANTs
were setting up residence inside my patients' minds. The next day, I brought a
can of ant spray to work and placed it on my coffee table. As I started to talk
about the concept with patients, they understood it right away.

ANTs are thoughts that pop into your mind uninvited.
They make you feel mad, sad, worried, or upset.
And most of the time they're not even true!

Learning how to direct, question, and correct your automatic negative
thoughts is not a new concept. Two of my favorite New Testament verses from
the apostle Paul are Philippians 4:8 ("Whatever is true, whatever is noble, whatever is right, whatever is pure, whatever is lovely, whatever is admirable—if anything is excellent or praiseworthy—think about such things") and Romans 12:2
("Be transformed by the renewing of your mind"). Even 2,000 years ago, Paul
taught about the benefits of filling our minds with what is good and positive.
And more recently, in the 1960s, psychiatrist Aaron Beck formalized a school of
psychotherapy called cognitive behavioral therapy (CBT), which is a structured
way to teach patients to challenge and eliminate negative thoughts.

As the discussions about ANTs in my office continued, I replaced the can
of ant spray with a black ant puppet and an adorable, furry anteater puppet.
I then developed a simple exercise to help my patients eliminate the ANTs:
*Whenever you feel sad, mad, nervous, or out of control, write down your auto-
matic negative thoughts.* The act of writing down the ANTs helps to get the

invaders out of your head. People loved the concept and found it easy to follow. Early on, I taught ANT therapy to a nine-year-old boy who suffered with debilitating anxiety and depression. After several weeks he told me he was feeling much better. He said, "It's an ANT ghost town in my head." In 2017, I published a children's book, *Captain Snout and the Super Power Questions: Don't Let the ANTs Steal Your Happiness*, that explains the therapy to kids.

Think of automatic negative thoughts as you would the ants that might bother a couple at a romantic picnic. One negative thought, like one ant at a picnic, is not a big problem. Two or three automatic negative thoughts, like two or three ants at a picnic, become a bit more irritating. Twenty or thirty automatic negative thoughts, like twenty or thirty ants at a picnic, may cause the couple to pick up and leave. The more you allow the ANTs to stick around in your head, the more they will "mate" with other ANTs and produce offspring that drive school failure, anxiety, depression, anger, work strife, relationship turmoil, and even obesity.

You can learn to eliminate the automatic negative thoughts and replace them with more helpful thoughts that give you a more accurate, fair assessment of any situation. It's not positive thinking that ignores reality; instead, I advocate accurate, honest thinking. This skill alone can completely change your life if you embrace and practice it.

With a bit of practice, you can choose to think helpful thoughts and feel good, or you can choose to think toxic thoughts and feel lousy. It's up to you! One way to begin is to notice your thoughts when they are negative, write them down, and talk back to them. If you can correct negative thoughts, you take away their power. When you have a negative thought without challenging it, your mind believes it and your body reacts to it.

Whenever you notice these ANTs, you need to crush them, or they'll ruin your relationships, your self-esteem, and your personal power.

Disciplined Thinking Principle #6:
You can fight back against the seven different ANT species.

Over the years therapists have identified seven different types of negative thought patterns that keep your mind off balance. I think of these as "species" of ANTs. They go by various names, but these are the ones I like to use:

1. All-or-Nothing ANTs
2. Just the Bad ANTs
3. Guilt-Beating ANTs
4. Labeling ANTs

5. Fortune-Teller ANTs
6. Mind Reader ANTs
7. Blaming ANTs

1. ***All-or-Nothing ANTs.*** These sneaky ANTs make you feel sorry for yourself. They don't use words like *sometimes* or *maybe*. All-or-Nothing ANTs think in absolutes—words like *all, always, never, none, nothing, no one, everyone,* and *every time.*

I once met a woman on one of my tours for public television who told me she hated the gym so much that she would never exercise. I asked her, "Do you like to dance?" She replied, "Oh, I love to dance." "How about taking a walk on the beach?" I asked. "I like that too," she said. When I told her that dancing and walking on the beach are forms of exercise, she gave me a puzzled look. She had always equated "exercise" with the gym. When she realized that any type of physical activity qualified as exercise, she said, "Maybe I don't hate to exercise; maybe I just hate the gym."

This is an example of all-or-nothing thinking, when you believe that everything is either all good or all bad. It is the same as black-and-white thinking. When Marcus told me, "I can never be as good as other kids," that was an example of an All-or-Nothing ANT. When I asked if he was 100 percent sure he could never be as good as the other kids, he gave me several examples of areas in which he excelled. Questioning the ANTs helps to send them packing.

Here are a few more examples of All-or-Nothing ANTs:

> *We had an argument. I think it's over.*
> *My child isn't doing well at school. I've failed as a parent.*
> *One of my favorite employees just quit; I am an awful supervisor.*
> *I have always been fat; it will never change.*
> *Every time I try to exercise, I get injured.*
> *She's always in a bad mood.*
> *No one ever listens to me.*
> *I don't like any of the foods that are good for me.*

2. ***Just the Bad ANTs.*** This ANT can't see anything good! Its beady eyes zoom in on mistakes and problems, and it fills your head with failure, frustration, sadness, and fear. As discussed above, the brain is wired for negativity, and this ANT can take virtually any positive experience and taint it with negativity. It is the judge, jury, and executioner of new experiences, new relationships, and new habits.

I always hate school is an example of one of Marcus's Just the Bad ANTs. When I asked him if he always really hated school, he said no. He liked sports, time with his friends, and math.

Other examples of Just the Bad ANTs include

I wanted to lose 30 pounds in 10 weeks, but I've only lost 8 pounds. I'm a complete failure.

I went to the gym and did a hard workout, but the guy on the bike next to me was talking the whole time, so I'm never going back there.

I gave a presentation at work to 30 people. Even though people told me they liked it, one person fell asleep during my talk, so it must have really been terrible.

As we've seen, focusing on the negative releases brain chemicals that make you feel bad, and that reduces brain activity in the area involved with self-control, judgment, and planning. This increases the odds of your making bad choices, such as ordering a third drink, eating a bowlful of chips, or staying up so late updating your social networking site that you wake up exhausted and need to guzzle caffeine to get going. Focusing on Just the Bad ANTs sets you up for failure, while focusing on the positive will improve your mood and help you feel better about yourself. Putting a positive spin on your thoughts leads to positive changes in your brain that make you happier and smarter. Here's how one could think differently about those situations listed above:

I have already lost 8 pounds and have changed my lifestyle, so I will continue to lose weight until I reach my goal of losing 30 pounds.

After working out, I had a lot more energy for the rest of the day.

Most people told me they liked my presentation. I wonder if the person who fell asleep during it stayed up too late last night.

3. *Guilt-Beating ANTs.* Growing up Roman Catholic and going to parochial schools through ninth grade, I had to pass Guilt 101 and Advanced Guilt. Only kidding—but *should* and *shouldn't* were common words when I was growing up. Of course, there are many important *should* and *shouldn't* thoughts, but in my 35 years as a psychiatrist, I've found that guilt is generally not a helpful motivator of behavior. It often backfires and can be counterproductive to your goals. When Marcus told me he "should try harder in school," it wasn't helping him actually do better. In fact, to Marcus, it seemed

the harder he tried, the worse he performed. Thinking in words like *should, must, ought to*, and *have to* is typical of Guilt-Beating ANTs.

Here are some examples:

I should visit my parents.
I have to give up sugar.
I must start counting my calories.
I ought to go to the gym more.
I should be more giving.

What happens when you allow these ANTs to circle in your mind? Do they make you more inclined to visit your parents, cut the sugar, count calories, hit the gym, or be more giving? I doubt it. It is human nature to push back when we feel as if we "must" do something, even if it is to our benefit. It is better to replace the Guilt-Beating ANTs with phrases like *I want to do this, It fits with my goals to do that*, or *It would be helpful to do this*. In the examples above, it would be beneficial to change the phrases to

I want to visit my parents because they are special to me.

My goal is to stop eating sugar because it will reduce my cravings; prevent energy crashes, diabetes, and inflammation in my body; and get me off this emotional roller coaster.

I want to count my calories because it will help me learn to take control of my eating.

It is in my best interest to go to the gym because it will help me feel more energized.

I am a giving person, and it is my goal to give more to causes I believe are worthwhile.

4. **Labeling ANTs.** Whenever you label yourself or someone else with a negative term, you inhibit your ability to take an honest look at the situation. When Marcus thought, *I am an idiot*, he lumped himself in with all of the people he ever thought were idiots, which damaged his self-esteem and his ability to make progress in his life. Labeling ANTs strengthen negative pathways in the brain, making the ruts deeper and their walls thicker. These habitual ruts lead to troubled behaviors. If, for example, you label yourself as "lazy," then why bother trying to do better in school or at work? The Labeling ANT will cause you to give up before you try, and it will keep you stuck in your old ways. Examples of Labeling ANTs include

He's a jerk.
I'm lazy.
I'm a loser.
She's cold.
I'm a lousy businessperson.

Even positive labels can be harmful. I tell parents, for example, never to praise children for being smart; praise them instead for working hard. When you tell children they are smart, they become more performance oriented and assume that intelligence cannot be improved. If they start to struggle with a new task, they may feel "not smart" and give up. But if you praise children for working hard, when they come up against a difficult task, they will persist because "they work hard."

5. *Fortune-Teller ANTs.* Don't listen to these lying ANTs! Fortune-Teller ANTs think they can see what is going to happen in the future, but all they really do is think up bad stuff that makes you upset. They creep into your mind and predict the future with fear. Of course, it is helpful to prepare for potential problems, but if you spend all your time focused on a fearful future, you will be filled with anxiety. Marcus's anxiety was driven by his Fortune-Teller ANTs, such as *I will fail school . . . I'll never go to college . . . I will be a failure.* Other examples of this deceiver include

If I run, I'll sprain my ankle.
If I give that presentation, I will have a panic attack.
None of my investments will pay off.
If I go to bed earlier, I'm just going to lie there awake for hours.
After my divorce, I'll never find another love relationship.

Predicting the worst in a situation causes an immediate rise in heart and breathing rates and can make you feel anxious. It can trigger cravings for sugar or refined carbs and make you feel as if you need to eat to calm your anxiety. What makes Fortune-Teller ANTs even worse is that your mind is so powerful, it can make happen what you imagine. When you think you will sprain your ankle, for example, that thought may deactivate the cerebellum, making you more clumsy and likely to get hurt. Similarly, if you are convinced you won't get a good night's sleep or find a new relationship, you will be less likely to engage in the behaviors that might make it so. I helped Marcus eliminate this ANT by teaching him how to talk back to it: *I will find a way to succeed . . . I'll go to college if I want to . . . I will succeed with hard work.*

6. **Mind Reader ANTs.** This ANT is convinced it can see inside someone else's mind and know how others think and feel without even being told. It says things like "Everyone thinks I am stupid," or "They are laughing at me." When you're sure you know what others are thinking even though they have not told you and you have not asked them, you are feeding your Mind Reader ANTs. When Marcus told me, "My teachers hate me," he was allowing this ANT to torture him. I have 25 years of education, and I can't tell what anyone else is thinking unless they tell me. A glance in your direction doesn't mean somebody is talking about you or mad at you. I tell people that a negative look from someone else may mean nothing more than that he or she is constipated! You just don't know.

I teach all my patients the "18-40-60 Rule," which says that when you are 18 you worry about what everyone thinks of you; when you are 40 you don't care what anyone thinks about you; and when you are 60 you realize no one has been thinking about you at all. People spend their days worrying and thinking about themselves, not about you. Stop trying to read their minds. Examples include

> *My boss doesn't like me.*
> *My martial arts teacher doesn't respect me because I'm fat.*
> *My friends think I won't be able to keep up with them on our hike.*
> *My father thinks I'll never amount to much.*

Don't let this ANT erase your good feelings. When there are things you don't understand, ask for clarification. Mind Reader ANTs are infectious and cause trouble between people.

7. **Blaming ANTs.** When things go wrong, the Blaming ANT always sings the same old sad song: *He did it! She did it! It's not my fault! It's your fault!* This ANT doesn't want you to admit your mistakes or to learn how to fix things and make them right; it wants you to be a victim. Of all the ANTs, Blaming ANTs are the most toxic. I call them red ANTs, because they not only steal your happiness, they also drain you of your personal power. When you blame something or someone else for the problems in your life, you become a victim of circumstances who can't do anything to change the situation. When Marcus said, "It's my parents' fault for not letting me quit," he was

allowing the Blaming ANT to take hold in his brain. Be honest with yourself and ask yourself if you have a tendency to say things like

If only you hadn't done that, I would have been successful.
It's your fault I failed because you didn't do enough to help me.
It's not my fault I eat too much; my mom taught me to clean my plate.
I'm having trouble meeting this deadline because the client keeps changing his mind. I'm miserable, and it's all his fault!
My boyfriend didn't call on time, and now it's too late to go to that movie I wanted to see. He's ruined my night!

Beginning a sentence with "It is your fault that I . . ." can ruin your life. Blaming ANTs make you a victim, and when you are a victim, you are powerless to change your behavior. In order to break free from the Blaming ANT addiction, you have to change your thinking by making it your responsibility to change. It is your life. I love what author Vernon Howard once wrote: "Permitting your life to be taken over by another person is like *letting the waiter eat your dinner.*"

At the same time, self-blame is equally toxic. Always strive to be a good coach to yourself, rather than someone who is toxic or abusive.

Seven Different Types of ANTs (or How We Distort Reality to Make It Worse Than It Really Is)

1. All-or-Nothing ANTs: Thinking that things are either all good or all bad
2. Just the Bad ANTs: Seeing only the bad in a situation
3. Guilt-Beating ANTs: Thinking in words like *should*, *must*, *ought*, or *have to*
4. Labeling ANTs: Attaching a negative label to yourself or someone else
5. Fortune-Teller ANTs: Predicting the worst possible outcome for a situation with little or no evidence for it
6. Mind Reader ANTs: Believing you know what other people are thinking even though they haven't told you
7. Blaming ANTs: Blaming someone else for your problems

SEVEN STRATEGIES TO MASTER YOUR MIND

It is possible to learn how to listen to your thoughts and redirect them so that you feel happier and more positive. Here are seven strategies that will help you put what I have just discussed into practice.

Strategy #1: Eliminate ANTs as they attack.

:05- 15 Get a journal or use the note app on your phone, and whenever
MINUTES you feel sad, mad, nervous, or out of control,

1. Write down your automatic negative thoughts (ANTs).
2. Identify the ANT species. (It may be more than one.)
3. Ask yourself if you are 100 percent sure the thought is true.

Shining a beam of truth on the ANTs causes them to disintegrate. Here are six examples from my patients:

1. From a woman who was raped, who came to see me for anxiety and depression:

   ANT: *I am fractured.*

   ANT Species: She listed it as an All-or-Nothing and Labeling ANT.

   Is It True? "It is not true," she wrote. "I am a good person who was attacked. I can overcome it to become whole." Talking back to the thought takes away its power.

2. From a father whose adult son was a drug addict:

   ANT: *I am not a good father.*

   ANT Species: He listed it as an All-or-Nothing and Guilt-Beating ANT.

   Is It True? "It is not true," he wrote. "I was present and loving. Addiction runs in our family, but ultimately it was my son's choice to engage in behaviors where he lost control. I will be there to support him as I can, but I cannot control his life."

3. From a woman whose son was murdered:

   ANT: *I am evil for wanting his murderer to be punished.*

   ANT Species: She listed it as a Labeling ANT.

Is It True? "It is not true," she wrote. "I am a good person with a loving heart. I miss my son so much and have hope I will see him again in heaven."

4. From a woman having marital problems, who felt herself becoming more clinging and desperate:

    ANT: *My husband will leave me and I will be all alone.*

    ANT Species: She listed it as a Fortune-Teller ANT.

    Is It True? She wrote, "I don't know if it is true, but if I keep acting anxious and desperate, he will leave me. I need to be strong no matter what happens."

5. From a man who was fired from work because of his temper:

    ANT: *I am a bad person and will never find another job. My family will be destitute.*

    ANT Species: He listed it as a Labeling and Fortune-Teller ANT.

    Is It True? "I need to understand and fix my temper," he told me. "I am a good person and will work to find another job to care for my family and myself."

6. From a young adult who was struggling in college:

    ANT: *I'll never be as good as my friends.*

    ANT Species: He listed it as an All-or-Nothing ANT.

    Is It True? He told me, "I am better than my friends at some things and not at others. I need to stop being so hard on myself."

Confronting ANTs with truth is a powerful tool. Several months after Marcus learned to eliminate the ANTs, his anxiety and depression were remarkably reduced and his school performance improved. He went on to graduate from college with honors and eventually from law school. Don't believe every stupid thought you have.

Strategy #2: Stop monkey mind by paying attention to it.

: 🔟 We all deal with disjointed thoughts at times, but one of the best ways
MINUTES to stop the monkeys from ruining your mind with all their distractions is to start paying attention to them. When you ignore your inner life, like attention-starved children the monkeys start to misbehave, torture you,

belittle you, and wreak all sorts of havoc. However, when you start noticing your thoughts, evaluating them, or even being amused by them, they loosen their control over your emotional life.

Taking time to reflect and direct your inner life can help you train the monkeys to work for you, rather than threaten your sanity. Meditation is a wonderful way to get control of your mind (see chapter 1, pages 20–21). Research has shown that meditation can slow your heart rate, lower blood pressure, increase circulation, aid digestion, strengthen your immune system, improve cognition, focus, and memory, and decrease brain aging, addictions, anxiety, depression, and irritability.[8] Devoting a few minutes each day to this practice, whether by meditating on a Scripture passage or doing the Loving-Kindness Meditation, will help you quiet your mind.

Strategy #3: Start every day with the phrase "Today is going to be a great day."

10 SECONDS As soon as you awaken or your feet hit the floor in the morning, say these words out loud. Since your mind is prone to negativity, it will find stress in the upcoming day unless you train and discipline it. When you direct your thoughts to *Today is going to be a great day*, your brain will help you uncover the reasons why it will be so. When I'm on a tour for public television, for example, and I wake up in a different city every morning, my brain could anticipate everything that could go wrong, including the hassles of travel, causing me to feel lousy. Instead, when I say, "Today is going to be a great day," I think of all the wonderful people I'll meet or lives that may be changed by our work, and I enjoy the journey.

You have a choice in where you direct your attention, even in times of loss. This simple strategy can make a powerfully positive difference in your life.

Strategy #4: Record your moods and look for ways to increase gratitude.

15-30 MINUTES Business professionals frequently say, "You cannot change what you do not measure." That's why it's smart to keep a daily journal to record and measure the feeling(s) you want to decrease, such as anxiety, fear, sadness, anger, or grief, or that you want to increase, such as joy, happiness, or another emotion. Write down a feeling and evaluate it on a scale from 1 to 10, where 1 is "awful" and 10 is "great." Once you have established this baseline, you can see which of the interventions in *Feel Better Fast and Make It Last* work best for you. Whenever you have a difficult day or several days, you can look at your journal and try to spot trends, such as certain days of the week, times of the day, time of your menstrual cycle, whether you have eaten or not, and more.

One of the early lessons I learned as a psychiatrist was that I could make nearly anyone cry or feel upset by the questions I asked. If I asked people to think about their worst memories—the times they failed, the incidents where they were most embarrassed, or the day they lost someone they loved—within seconds they would feel bad. But the opposite was also true. If I asked them to think about their happiest moments—the times they succeeded or their experiences of falling in love—they generally started to smile. Here are six quick journaling exercises to help you change your focus.

1. **Write out three things for which you are grateful.** Gratitude helps direct your attention toward positive feelings and away from negative ones. Dr. Hans Selye, considered one of the pioneers of stress research, wrote, "Nothing erases unpleasant thoughts more effectively than conscious concentration on pleasant ones."[9] If I could bottle gratitude, I would. The benefits far outweigh almost all of the medications I prescribe, without any side effects. A wealth of research suggests that a daily practice of gratitude, which can be as simple as writing down several things we're grateful for every day, can improve our emotions, health, relationships, personalities, and careers. From a wonderful blog post by Amit Amin[10] at *Happier Human* and Courtney Ackerman at the Positive Psychology Program,[11] research suggests that gratitude can enhance

- Happiness
- Well-being
- Mood
- Self-esteem
- Resilience
- Sense of spirituality
- Impulse to give
- Optimism
- Reduction in materialism
- Reduction in self-centeredness
- Recovery from substance misuse
- Resistance to stress
- Resistance to envy
- Friendships
- Love relationships
- Career
- Networking ability
- Productivity
- Goal achievement
- Reduction in turnover
- Decision-making among physicians
- Physical health, including
  - Physical appearance
  - Better sleep
  - Fewer physical symptoms
  - More time exercising
  - Less physical pain
  - Lower blood pressure in people who were hypertensive
  - Recovery from coronary events
  - Vitality and energy
  - Longevity[12]

Focusing on gratitude has been found to increase the activity of the parasympathetic nervous system and decrease inflammatory markers;[13] improve depression, stress, and happiness;[14] reduce stress among caregivers;[15] and, among the elderly, significantly decrease state anxiety and depression as well as increase specific memories, life satisfaction, and subjective happiness.[16]

When you make a habit of bringing your attention to the things you're grateful for, you enhance how your brain works. In times of stress, take a minute to write down three things—big or small—you're grateful for. You might find you have trouble stopping at three.

2. **Share a gratitude letter.** Martin Seligman, PhD, considered the father of positive psychology, developed this powerful gratitude exercise along with his team at the University of Pennsylvania: Write a 300-word essay about someone you are grateful for, such as a teacher, mentor, friend, boss, or coworker. When you have finished, if possible, make an appointment with that person and read the essay aloud to him or her. Research has shown that doing this significantly increased life satisfaction scores and happiness and decreased symptoms of depression.[17]

3. **Express your appreciation.** To enhance gratitude, add appreciation, which is gratitude that is outwardly expressed and builds bridges between people. Expressing support and appreciation to others has been shown to decrease the stress response in the brain much more powerfully than receiving support.[18] *It is better for your brain to give than to receive.* To supercharge joyful thinking, get in the habit of writing down the name of one person whom you appreciate and why; then share your feelings with that person with a quick e-mail, text, or call. Do this once a week, and try not to repeat anyone for two months. This exercise will help you build many bridges of goodwill.

4. **Count your blessings.** You can boost your good feelings if you count your blessings instead of sheep at night. In a study of 221 teenagers, the group that focused on counting their blessings reported increases in gratitude, optimism, and life satisfaction and decreases in negative feelings.[19] At bedtime, write down as many good things in your life as you can think of in three minutes.

5. **Note down what went well.** Another exercise that has been shown to quickly increase your level of well-being is called "What Went Well." Research has shown that people who did this exercise were happier

and less depressed at one-month and six-month follow-ups than at the study's outset.[20] Right before bed, write down three things that went well that day; then ask yourself, "Why did this happen?" This simple exercise has been found to help people in stressful jobs develop more positive emotions.[21]

6. **Focus on your accomplishments.** I once treated a very successful businesswoman who made millions of dollars. She was struggling with anxiety and depression, and she felt that she was a failure and her life was worthless. She repeatedly focused on one incident where a reporter, who as far as I could tell accomplished little in his life except trashing successful people, had harshly criticized her in a magazine article. She played the article over and over in her mind. She had an obsessive pattern in her brain, where she tended to get stuck on negative thoughts and behaviors.

Her first homework assignment was to write out her accomplishments in as much detail as she liked. At her next session she brought eight pages full of accomplishments, including employing 500 people, doing charity work, and maintaining strong relationships. The exercise made her feel great and quickly changed her focus.

Write down the highest and most positive moments of your life. If you can find one moment, odds are you can find two. If you find two, you will likely find four, and so on. By bringing your attention to your successes, you are much more likely to feel better fast.

BENEFITS OF GRATITUDE

HAPPINESS

PERSONALITY
Less materialistic
Less self-centered
More optimistic
Increased self-esteem
More spiritual

SOCIAL HEALTH
More social connections
Healthier marriage
Kinder
More friendships
Deeper relationships

PHYSICAL HEALTH
Improved sleep
Less sickness
Increased longevity
Increased energy
More exercise

EMOTIONAL HEALTH
More good feelings
More relaxed
More resilient
Less envious
Happier memories

CAREER
Better management
Improved networking
More goals achieved
Improved decision-making
Increased productivity

Strategy #5: Create optimism with a dose of reality to build resilience fast.

Dr. Seligman developed a concept known as learned helplessness that has had a powerful influence over my career.[22] He found that when dogs, rats, mice, and even cockroaches experienced painful shocks over which they had no control, eventually they would just accept the pain without attempting to escape. Humans, he discovered, do the same thing. In a series of experiments, his research team randomly divided subjects into three groups: those who were exposed to a loud noise they could stop by pushing a button; those who heard the irritating noise but couldn't turn it off; and a control group who heard nothing at all. The following day the subjects faced a new research task that again involved painful sounds. To turn it off, all they had to do was move their hands about 12 inches. The people in the first and third groups figured this out quickly and were able to turn off the noise. But most of the people in the second group did nothing at all. Expecting failure, they didn't even try to escape the irritating noise. They had learned to be helpless.

Yet—and this is where it gets exciting—about one-third of the people in group two, who had been unable to escape the pain, never became helpless. Why? The answer turned out to be optimism. Dr. Seligman's team discovered that people who do not give up interpret the pain and setbacks as

- *temporary* as opposed to permanent;
- *limited* instead of pervasive; and
- *changeable* instead of out of their control.

Optimists would say things like "It will go away quickly; it's just this one situation, and I can do something about it." Dr. Seligman's team came to believe that teaching optimism could help inoculate people against anxiety, depression, posttraumatic stress disorder, and relationship problems. Here are some of his main ideas:

1. *Listen to yourself and others to see how things are explained.* Are the people powerful or victims? Do they have control or no control? Are hardships permanent or temporary? *Pessimists* describe *bad* things as permanent and pervasive and *good* things as temporary, while *optimists* describe things in just the reverse: the *bad* as temporary and the *good* as permanent and pervasive.

2. *Change your language and feelings around the situations you face.* You can stop being a victim, take control wherever possible, and understand that hardships are usually temporary.

3. *Allow mistakes to be learning experiences, rather than a final judgment on your self-worth.* Everyone makes mistakes; it's how you respond to them that determines how quickly you recover. Accepting a mistake and looking for the lesson you can take away from it will help you get over it and move on.

Pessimism and Optimism Are Habits of Thinking

PESSIMISTS (FEEL HELPLESS)	OPTIMISTS (FEEL HOPEFUL)
See problems as permanent	See problems as temporary
See problems as pervasive	See problems as limited
See no personal control	See personal control or influence
See failure as a statement about self	See failure as a lesson
Have low self-efficacy	Feel self-confident
Focus on problems	Are forward thinking
Tend to be hopeless	Tend to be hopeful
Tend to give up	Tend to stick with difficult things
Are less proactive with health	Are more proactive with health
Hold grudges	Forgive more easily
Focus on worries and negativity	Are less likely to dwell on the negative
Feel more stressed	Feel less stressed
Are more likely to have insomnia	Are more likely to sleep better
See glass as half-empty	See glass as half-full
Are more withholding	Are more altruistic

Strive to take control of your life, be forward thinking, and see possibilities. A huge study involving more than 97,000 people found that those who were optimistic had significantly lower heart disease than those who were pessimistic.[23] Women who scored highly on "cynical hostility" were also more likely to develop coronary heart disease. Optimism is also associated with a higher quality of life,[24] a lower incidence of stroke,[25] improved immune system function,[26] better pain tolerance,[27] and longer survival in lung cancer patients.[28]

Yet as we've seen, blind optimism can lead to early death. The Longevity Project from Stanford University found that people who were mindlessly optimistic died the earliest from accidents and preventable illnesses.[29] Being sleep-deprived led to increased optimism and poorer life choices.[30] College students who were too optimistic had more binge-drinking behavior,[31] and compulsive gamblers were often rated as too optimistic.[32] The bottom line: It is always best to balance optimism with planning for and preventing future trouble. Being optimistic about eating a third bowl of ice cream with caramel sauce will lead to early death, no matter how much you wish it wouldn't.

Strategy #6: Change the B stuff.

We are not controlled by events or people, but by our perceptions of them.

I once heard the following story: At the turn of the century a shoe company sent a representative to Africa. He wired back, "I'm coming home. No one wears shoes here." Another company sent their representative, who sold thousands of shoes. He wired back to his company, "Business is fantastic. No one has ever heard of shoes here." The two representatives perceived the same situation from markedly different perspectives, and they obtained dramatically different results.

Perception is the way we, as individuals, interpret ourselves and the world around us. Our five senses take in the world, but perception occurs as our brains process the incoming information through our "feeling filters." When our filters feel good, we translate information in a positive way. When our filters are angry or hostile, we perceive the world as negative toward us. Our perceptions of the outside world are based on our inner worlds. When we're feeling tired, for example, we're much more likely to be irritated by a child's behavior that usually doesn't bother us.

Our view of a situation has a greater impact on our lives than the situation itself. Noted psychiatrist Richard Gardner has said that the world is like a Rorschach test, where a person is asked to describe what he or she sees in 10 inkblots that mean absolutely nothing. What we see in the inkblot is based on our inner view of the world; our perceptions bear witness to our state of mind. As we think, so do we perceive. Therefore, in reality, we need not seek to change the outside world but rather to change our inner worlds. I teach all of my patients the *A-B-C* model:

A *is the actual event,*
B *is how we interpret or perceive the event, and*
C *is how we react to the event.*

Other people or events (*A*) can't make us do anything. It is our interpretation or perception (*B*) that causes our behavior (*C*). Consider, for instance, the time I yawned during a therapy session with a patient. He asked if I found him boring. I replied that it was important that he asked. I had been up most of the previous night with an emergency and was tired, but I found what he was saying very interesting. My yawning was *A*, his interpretation that I was bored was *B*, and his asking me about it was *C*. I was glad he asked about my yawn because some patients' *C* would have been to leave the therapy session with a negative feeling. When we can allow ourselves to look at the alternatives and challenge our initial negative perceptions, we've traveled a long way toward emotional health.

Questioning the *B* stuff is so important. It can make the difference between a meaningful life and death. Think about the two New Testament stories of Judas and Peter, two of Jesus' disciples, betraying Jesus on the night He was arrested (see Matthew 26:69–27:10). Judas accepted money to identify Jesus to the Temple guards, who arrested Him. Later that night Peter denied he even knew Jesus—three times. *A* was betrayal. *B* was their interpretation of the betrayal: Judas felt he had committed an unforgivable sin; Peter was ashamed and wept. *C* was each of their reactions: Judas returned the 30 pieces of silver and then hanged himself, while Peter asked for and was given forgiveness and later became a central figure in starting the Christian church. If we don't question our perceptions, they can take us to places we don't want to go.

Strategy #7: Watch the Disney movie Pollyanna.

One of my favorite movies of all time is the Disney movie *Pollyanna*, based on the 1913 book of the same name by Eleanor Porter. After her missionary parents died, Pollyanna came to live with her aunt Polly and was able to help turn a divided small town with many negative people into a positive community. She introduced them to "the glad game," which involved looking for things to be glad about in any situation. Her father had taught her this game once when she was very disappointed. She had always wanted a doll, but her parents never had enough money to buy one for her. When her father asked his missionary sponsors to send a secondhand doll, by mistake they sent

Pollyanna a pair of crutches. *How can I be glad about crutches?* she wondered. Then she decided she could be glad because she didn't need to use them. This simple game changed the attitudes and lives of many people in the movie. Pollyanna even told the minister what her father had taught her: The Bible had 800 "glad passages," and if God mentioned being glad that many times, it must be because He wants us to think that way.

Focusing on the negative in situations will make you feel bad. Playing the glad game, or looking for the positive, will help you feel better. This movie is worth the 134-minute investment.

It's no exaggeration to say that developing accurate, honest, and disciplined thinking can change your life. If you get rid of the ANTs, practice gratitude, manage your perceptions, and follow these other strategies, you'll see a decrease in worry, anxiety, anger, and negativity and be on your way to feeling better fast.

SEVEN STRATEGIES TO MASTER YOUR MIND

Developing strategies for accurate, honest, and disciplined thinking is critical to success. To accomplish this,

1. Eliminate ANTs as they attack.

2. Stop monkey mind by paying attention to it.

3. Start every day with the phrase "Today is going to be a great day."

4. Record your moods and look for ways to increase gratitude.

5. Create optimism with a dose of reality to build resilience fast.

6. Change the *B* stuff.

7. Watch the Disney movie *Pollyanna*.

TINY HABITS THAT CAN HELP YOU FEEL BETTER FAST—AND LEAD TO BIG CHANGES

10 -: 15
SECONDS   MINUTES   Each of these habits takes no more than a few minutes. They are anchored to something you do (or think or feel) so that they are more likely to become automatic. Once you do the behaviors you want, find a way to make yourself feel good about them—draw a happy face, pump your fist, or do whatever feels natural. Emotion helps the brain to remember.

1. When my feet hit the floor first thing in the morning, I will say to myself, "Today is going to be a great day."

2. After an ANT pops up, I will write down my negative thought and ask, "Is it true?"

3. After I get home and put away my keys, I will push play on a meditation audio.

4. Before I go to bed, I will count my blessings, listing at least three.

5. After I have a negative thought, I will think of what went well that day.

6. When I face a difficult situation, I will ask myself, "What is there to be glad about in this situation?"

7. After breakfast, I will think of one person I appreciate, and reach out and tell him or her in a quick text or note.

PART 3

A IS FOR ATTACHMENTS

As we discussed in the introduction, social connection is one of the four key aspects of health, along with the biological, psychological, and spiritual components. Our social attachments bring us our greatest joys and our most painful sorrows. When relationships are stressed or break apart, people become unhappy and are vulnerable to acting in counterproductive ways. To use a computer analogy, attachments are like network connections that link us to others in meaningful ways. Brain health is often the missing piece in understanding healthy or difficult relationships, trauma, and grief. These two chapters will give you powerful tools to improve any relationship and help eliminate the hurts that haunt you. In chapter 6 I'll look at habits that can elevate all of your relationships, and in chapter 7 I'll share helpful ways to deal with the grief and trauma that can come from loss, broken relationships, or other difficult circumstances.

CHAPTER 6

HEALING CONNECTIONS

HOW TO IMPROVE ANY RELATIONSHIP

The magic ratio is 5:1. We have found that as long as there are five positive interactions for every negative interaction, a couple can have a stable and happy relationship over time.

JOHN GOTTMAN, PhD

Truth is, everybody is going to hurt you: you just gotta find the ones worth suffering for.

ATTRIBUTED TO BOB MARLEY

Good relationships keep us happier and healthier, according to a 75-year longevity study from Harvard University. Positive social connections help us live longer, while loneliness kills us early. Sadly, one in five Americans is lonely, which means this is a public health problem too. Another lesson from the study: Being in positive, warm, satisfying relationships keeps our brains and bodies healthy into older age, while being in relationships filled with conflict is associated with sickness and early death.[1]

Emotional crises, panic attacks, depression, and obsessive behaviors are often triggered by the loss or threatened loss of a relationship. Marital problems, affairs, domestic violence, breakups—all of these relationship problems prompt people to come and see us at Amen Clinics. It is common for us to hear statements like "My marriage is falling apart," "All my relationships are failing," or "I want to be a better husband and stop hurting my family." Improving your social connections is one of the best ways to start to feel better fast and make it last.

Unlike polar bears, humans require social interaction to stay healthy. We have a fundamental need to belong that's just as essential as our need for food and water. People who are socially connected are happier and healthier, and they live longer.[2] People who are married are less likely to develop dementia than those who have never been married (lifelong singles have a 42 percent higher risk) or those who are widowed (their risk is 20 percent higher), according to recent research. (The association did not apply to divorced individuals.[3]) Loneliness or disconnection from others is also associated with an increased rate of depression, cognitive decline, and dementia.[4] Being in loving relationships is every bit as important as sleep, a healthy diet, and exercise.

Naomi Eisenberger, PhD, a professor in social psychology at the University of California, Los Angeles, has demonstrated in a fascinating series of studies that loss, or being socially excluded or rejected, activates the physical pain centers in the brain, and those who are more sensitive to physical pain are also more sensitive to social rejection. In addition, Eisenberger has shown that taking pain medication, such as acetaminophen (Tylenol), can help to ameliorate the pain of social rejection.[5] When it comes to the brain, a broken heart is not so different from a broken leg.

Rejection can also trigger aggression. Animals that are in physical pain often react toward others with aggression. Researchers who analyzed 15 school shooters in 2003 found that all but 2 suffered from social rejection.[6] Suicide, murder, and murder-suicides are often the consequence of broken social bonds.

Relating to others in healthy, effective ways is ultimately a brain-based skill, yet even most marital therapists get zero training on or about the brain. When your brain is healthy, you can perceive others more accurately, have good control over your emotions, and act in healthy ways that bring people closer to you. Your brain allows you to read social cues, listen, respond appropriately, deal with conflict, set effective boundaries, act inclusively, and be attentive in moments of interaction. A brain with short circuits, whether yours or someone else's, often interrupts effective relationships. Stop and think about it: Brains nurture, influence, stimulate, irritate, calm, and incite each other. Being raised by a parent with a difficult brain, having a spouse or boss with brain problems, or even dealing with a friend, teacher, or coworker who needs brain help can all cause immeasurable stress. Understanding the neuroscience of relationships will give you an uncommon advantage. As you care for your brain, all of your relationships are likely to improve.

EIGHT BRAIN-BASED HABITS
TO ELEVATE YOUR RELATIONSHIPS

Professor Howard Markman, director of the Center for Marital and Family Studies at the University of Denver, can predict with 90 percent accuracy if a couple will get divorced or stay married. He can make the prediction after watching a 15-minute conversation between the spouses where they are instructed to discuss an issue upon which they disagree. If the couple's argument involves the habits of blaming, belittling, escalation, invalidation, or withdrawal, their future is not likely to be happy. However, if the couple communicates respect and shared purpose and stops escalation in a civil way, the future looks much more positive. Markman also found that he could reduce divorce by one-third among couples to whom he taught several critical skills.[7] Good relationship habits can be learned and enhanced by a healthy brain that can remember and implement them.

This chapter will provide you with eight brain-based habits clinically proven to increase your relationship skills. In part, these techniques come from research in the field of interpersonal psychotherapy (IPT). Enhancing interpersonal skill has proven effective in reducing anxiety, depression, and stress, and in improving both business success and marital satisfaction. There are more than 125 studies showing IPT's effectiveness.[8] Even brain imaging studies have shown how improving relationships can help normalize the brain in people who are depressed.[9] The acronym RELATING will help you remember the essential relationship habits.

R is for Responsibility
E is for Empathy
L is for Listening and good communication skills
A is for appropriate Assertiveness
T is for actual, physical Time
I is for Inquiry and correcting negative thoughts
N is for Noticing what you like more than what you don't
G is for Grace and forgiveness

R IS FOR RESPONSIBILITY

Responsibility is not about blame. It is about your ability to respond to whatever situation you are in, as in these examples:

"It is my job to make this relationship better."

"I have the power to improve how we communicate and act toward each other."

"I have influence in my relationships that I exert in a positive way."

"I am responsible for my behaviors in our interactions."

People who take responsibility for their own behavior do better in relationships. Those who constantly blame others set themselves up for a lifetime of problems. Yet blame is fast and easy and even seems hardwired in the brain. In a Duke University study, researchers scanned the brains of volunteers while they were asked to judge the intent of others in multiple situations. One of the scenarios was "The CEO knew the plan would harm the environment, but he did not care at all about the effect the plan would have on it. He started the plan solely to increase profits. Did the CEO intentionally harm the environment?" Eighty-two percent of the volunteers said the CEO's action was deliberate. When researchers replaced the word *harm* with *help,* only 23 percent said it was intentional. The scientists discovered that when volunteers "blamed" the CEO, their brains reacted faster and more powerfully, activating the amygdala, which is involved with the feelings of fear and threat. Those who saw positive intention in the CEO's behavior reacted more slowly, with less activity in the amygdala and more activity in the prefrontal cortex (PFC), the brain region discussed in chapter 3 that's associated with forethought and executive function.[10]

Blame is quick, common, and possibly self-protective against aggression, but it is also the first and most devastating hallmark of self-defeating behavior in relationships. When you blame someone else and fail to take responsibility for your own behavior, you become a victim of other people and are powerless to change anything. If you struggle with blame, you'll typically hear yourself say things like

"It wasn't my fault that you took things the wrong way."

"That wouldn't have happened if you had listened to me."

"It's your fault that we are having trouble."

The bottom-line statement goes something like this: "If only you had done something differently, then I wouldn't be in the predicament I am in. It's your fault, and I am not responsible."

Deflecting responsibility for relationship troubles or making excuses when things don't go as you would like is the first step in a dangerous downhill slide. The slide typically follows this sequence:

Deflect responsibility
"It's your fault."

See life as beyond personal control
"My life would be better if you hadn't done . . ."

Feel like a victim
"If only you would be different, then . . ."

Give up trying
"It is never going to work. Why even try?"

Deflecting responsibility temporarily makes you feel better, but it also reinforces the idea that your life is out of your control, that others can determine how things will go for you. This causes inner turmoil, leading to anxiety and feelings of helplessness.

Sarah came to see me for marital stress. She had been in psychotherapy with another psychiatrist for more than three years but seemed to be getting nowhere. She complained that her husband was an alcoholic who mistreated her. She was often tearful and depressed and had problems concentrating. In our initial interview it was clear that she took no responsibility for how her life was turning out. She blamed her first husband for getting her pregnant at age 19 and felt "forced" to marry him, but she complained that he was unmotivated, so she divorced him. Then, in succession, she impulsively married two different men who were alcoholics and physically abusive. Tearfully, she expressed feelings of being continually victimized by men, including her current husband.

At the end of the session I asked her what she had done to contribute to her problems. Her mouth dropped open. Her previous psychiatrist had been a good paid listener, but he never challenged her notion of helplessness. At the beginning of the next session she told me that she almost didn't come back to see me. She said, "You think it's all my fault, don't you?" I replied, "I don't think it's all your fault, but I think you have contributed to your troubles more than you give yourself credit for; and if it's true that you've contributed to your problems, then you can do things to change them. As long as you stay an innocent victim of others, there is nothing you can do to help yourself."

Over several sessions Sarah got the message of personal responsibility and made a dramatic turnaround. She had grown up in a severely abusive alcoholic home, where she really was a victim of her circumstances, causing her amygdala to become overactive and making her feel constantly threatened. Unfortunately, she maintained that role in her adult relationships, including at work. Her unconscious continuation of her abusive childhood was ruining her ability to have control in her life.

Invariably, in classes where I teach this concept, some people will tell me that their problem is not deflecting responsibility but rather taking too much on themselves. These two concepts, deflecting responsibility and putting too much on oneself, are not mutually exclusive. A good "personal responsibility" statement goes something like this: "Bad things have happened in my life, some of which I had something to do with and some of which I did not. Either way, I need to learn how to respond effectively to whatever situation I am in." *Responsibility means you have the ability to respond in a positive, helpful way.*

Taking responsibility in relationships means continually asking yourself what you can do to make the relationship better. When my patients thoughtfully evaluate and change their own behavior, their relationships often dramatically improve. In my experience, the idea that we have no control or influence over the behavior of others is just not true. I often ask patients what they do to make their relationships better, and they usually can come up with a number of positive behaviors. Then I ask them what they do to make the relationships worse. Initially, they hesitate, not wanting to admit to their own negative actions, but after a bit of time they start to own up to the myriad behaviors they might need to work on. Here is an example.

Eight-year-old Carlos was sitting in my office because he had behavioral problems, especially at home. He started by telling me how much he hated his younger sister. "She irritates me all the time," he said. "I have no choice but to yell at her and hit her."

When he said he had no choice, my eyebrows raised.

Seeing my reaction, he justified his behavior further. "I have no choice; she irritates me all the time."

"What do you do to irritate her?" I asked softly.

"Nothing," he said. He paused and repeated, "Absolutely nothing."

I sat quietly.

"Well—" He paused, and then showed a wry smile. "Well, I take some of her things sometimes."

"Anything else?"

Carlos looked like he was thinking hard and then said, "I yell at her, tell her she cannot play with me, and ignore her when she talks to me."

"Okay," I said. "You do irritate her. I sort of suspected it. But what do you do that makes her happy?"

He then listed several things he did that helped them get along better, including playing with her, helping her with her kindergarten homework, saying thank you, and smiling at her. He had a lot more power than he believed. Helping Carlos tap into his power to make his relationship with his sister better, as well as know his ability to make things worse, helped change his victim mentality and ultimately his behavior.

What can you do today to make your relationships better? You win more in relationships when you ask yourself this question and stay away from blaming others.

E IS FOR EMPATHY

If, as a result of reading this book, you get only one thing—an increased tendency to think always in terms of the other person's point of view, and see things from that person's angle as well as your own—if you get only that one thing from this book, it may easily prove to be one of the stepping-stones of your career.

DALE CARNEGIE, *HOW TO WIN FRIENDS AND INFLUENCE PEOPLE*

Once when my family and I were on vacation in Hawaii, I was reading a book to our daughter Chloe, then four years old, when her mother walked into the room and accidentally bumped into the corner of the television armoire. Watching this happen, Chloe immediately said, "Ouch," as if she felt the pain herself. Touched by her caring, Tana gave Chloe a hug and told her she was okay. That simple interaction stayed with me for the whole trip. It was the essence of empathy, the human ability to feel what others feel. Chloe's mirror neurons were at work.

In the late 1990s, Italian neuroscientists Giacomo Rizzolatti, Leonardo Fogassi, and Vittorio Gallese were recording activity of the lower frontal lobes of the macaque monkey when they experienced a moment of research serendipity. As the scientists mapped the electrical activity of the monkey's actions, Dr. Fogassi selected a banana from a nearby fruit bowl. As he reached for the banana, the monkey's brain reacted as if he, too, were reaching for the fruit, even though he had not moved. He was playing out in his head what the researcher was doing. The researchers labeled the responsible cells "mirror neurons" and later discovered them in humans.[11] These neurons "allow us to grasp the minds of others," the researchers noted,[12] which is why we open our own mouths when we feed a baby or yawn when others start to yawn first. We "play" their minds in our brains.

THE MIRROR NEURON SYSTEM

MONKEY DOES ACTION   **MONKEY SEES ACTION**

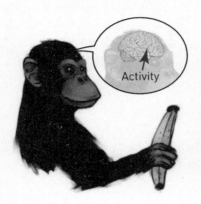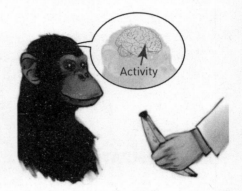

Researchers have found that children with autism, who often display social skill deficits, have problems in their mirror neuron systems. This system is important to empathy. When it is healthy, we can experience the feelings of others. When the system works too hard, we can become too sensitive, which would make us terrible doctors or nurses, as we could be crying all the time in response to others' pain. When it does not work hard enough, we could hurt others and it wouldn't bother us. As is true with so many parts of the brain, a healthy system helps us most.

Empathy helps us navigate the social environment and answer questions such as these: Is this person going to feed me? Love me? Attack me? Faint? Run away? Cry? The more accurately we can predict the actions and needs of others, the better off we are. The ability to "tune in" and empathize with others is a prerequisite for understanding, attachment, bonding, and love—all of which are important for our survival.

In several studies about why executives fail, "insensitivity to others" or a lack of empathy was cited more than any other flaw as a reason for derailment. Phrases like the following were used about those who did not succeed:

He never negotiated; there was no room for any views contrary to his.
She could follow a bull through a china shop and still break the china.
He made others feel stupid.
She was always talking down to her employees.
Whenever something went right, he took all the credit. Whenever things fell through, heads would roll.
It was her way or no way. If you disagreed with her, you were out.

Lack of empathy can cause failure in almost any endeavor. A lack of interpersonal skill not only causes others to avoid you; it can make them angry and feel active ill will toward you. Coworkers may look the other way if you are making serious mistakes; spouses may start finding fault in any area they can to retaliate for their hurt; and acquaintances may begin making excuses to decrease the time they spend with you. Lacking empathy also has a serious isolating effect that not only causes loneliness but also decreases honest feedback from others and cuts you off from coworkers' or friends' creativity and knowledge. One example from my practice was of a supervisor who returned to his office after being chewed out by the owner of a company. Upset, he snapped at his assistant for not having a report ready. She had just returned from taking her child to the emergency room because he had cut his head open falling against the corner of a table at day care. She started to cry and ran into the bathroom. The supervisor and assistant didn't speak to each other for a week, and she finally quit a job she needed. If instead of thinking only of their own trying days, each had taken a minute to think about what was going on with the other (empathy), this fight could have been avoided and her job saved.

How is your empathy? Can you feel what others feel? Do you sabotage your relationships by being insensitive? Do you take the behavior of others too personally? Or instead, when someone dumps on you, do you wonder what might be going on that caused him or her to act that way? Of course, you can carry that last question to an extreme and attribute any negative criticism directed at you to someone else's problem. Balance is the key. *When negative behavior comes your way, ask yourself two questions: 1) Did I do anything to cause it? 2) What is going on with the other person?* Those two questions will help you to be more sensitive to other people and improve your relationships, which will help you feel better overall—now and in the long run.

Developing empathy involves a number of important skills, including mirroring, treating others in a way you would like to be treated, and being able to get outside of yourself. The following three exercises are designed to help you increase your empathic skills.

Exercise #1: Mirroring

Your ability to understand and communicate with others will be enhanced by learning what therapists call the "mirroring technique." You can use this technique in any interpersonal situation to increase rapport. When you mirror someone, you assume or imitate his or her body language—posture, eye contact, and facial expression—and you use the same words and phrases in conversation that the other person uses. If, for example, someone is leaning forward in his chair, looking at you intensely, you do the same without making a big point of it. If you note that she uses the same phrase several times, such as "I believe we have a winner here," pick it up and make it part of your vocabulary for that conversation. This is not mimicry, which implies ridicule; rather, this technique allows the other person to identify with you, albeit unconsciously.

Holding Hands Can Be a Pain Reliever

In an example of the mirroring technique at work, researchers at the University of Colorado Boulder and the University of Haifa recently found that holding the hand of a loved one who is in pain can help take away the discomfort. Their experiments have shown that when your spouse is in pain and you hold his or her hand, your breathing rates, heart rates, and even brain-wave patterns sync up too. Plus, the more empathy you feel for your partner in pain, the more in tune your brain waves become and the greater the pain-relieving effect.[13]

:0: Try it: The next time your partner is in pain, hold her or his
MINUTES hand while you focus in a heartfelt way on feeling empathetic about the pain.

On a side note: Be careful whom you allow to hold your hand. If that person's brain waves are the result of anger or anxiety, you may pick up those patterns and feelings too. People are contagious.

Exercise #2: The Golden Rule

Another exercise that will help you look beyond yourself and into the feelings of others is found in the New Testament book of Luke: "Do to others as you would have them do to you" (6:31). In at least one interaction per day, consciously choose to treat someone else as you would like to be treated in that situation. If your spouse has a headache when you feel romantic, for example, instead of feeling rejected, make an effort to understand. You might say something like "It must be awful to have a headache before going to bed. Can I get anything for you?" This empathetic line will get you more passion than the accusation "You always have a headache!"

Exercise #3: Get Outside of Yourself

The next couple of times you get into a disagreement, try taking the other person's side of the argument. At least verbally, begin to agree with their point of view. Argue for it, understand it, see where they're coming from. Although this can be a difficult exercise, it will pay off royally if you use it to learn to understand others better. In order to do this effectively, you must first listen to the opposing viewpoint without interrupting. When you do this exercise, difficult people often become less difficult. By agreeing with them, you'll take the wind out of their sails and deflate their anger.

L IS FOR LISTENING AND GOOD COMMUNICATION

Poor communication is at the core of many relationship problems. Jumping to conclusions, trying to read minds, and needing to be right are only a few traits that doom communication. When people do not connect with each other in a meaningful way, their own minds take over the relationship and many imaginary problems arise. This can occur at home, with friends, and at work.

Donna was frequently angry at her husband. During the day, she would spend time imagining their evening together, in which they would spend time talking and being attentive to each other's needs. When her husband came home tired and preoccupied by a hard day at work, she felt disappointed and reacted angrily toward him. Her husband felt bewildered. He was unaware of his wife's thoughts during the day and didn't know he was disappointing her. After a few couple's therapy sessions, Donna learned how to express her needs up front and found a very receptive husband.

Too often in relationships we have expectations and hopes that we never explicitly communicate to our partners or colleagues. We assume they should know what we need and become disappointed when they don't accurately read our minds. Clear communication is essential if relationships are to be mutually satisfying.

10 Ways Communication Is Sabotaged in Relationships

1. *Poor attitude.* You expect the conversation to go nowhere, and subsequently you don't even try to direct it in a positive way. Negative assumptions about others feed into this poor attitude. Because you don't trust them from the beginning, you remain stiff and guarded when you are together.

2. *Unclear expectations and needs.* Do you expect people to guess what you want or need? It is great when others can anticipate our needs, but most people are too busy to be able to do it effectively. That does not make them good or bad; it simply means it's important to speak up about what you need.

3. *No reinforcing body language.* Body language is critical because it sends both conscious and unconscious messages. When you fail to make eye contact or acknowledge others with facial expressions or body gestures, they begin to feel lost, alone, and unenthusiastic about continuing the conversation. Eye contact and physical acknowledgment are essential to good communication.

4. *Competing with distractions.* Distractions frequently doom communication. It's not a good idea, for example, for my daughter to talk to me about something important during the fourth quarter of a Lakers basketball playoff game. Decrease distractions to have clear communication.

5. *Never asking for feedback on what you're saying.* You might assume that you are sending clear messages to the other person when, in fact, what he or she understands is completely different from what you meant. Feedback is essential to clear communication.

6. *"Kitchen sinking."* When people feel backed into a corner, they may bring up unrelated issues from the past in order to protect themselves or intensify the disagreement. Stay on track until an issue is fully discussed.

7. **Mind reading.** You arbitrarily predict what another person is thinking and then react to that imagined information. Mind reading is often just a projection of what you think. Even after couples have been married for 30 years, it's impossible for them to always be right about what is going on in the other person's head. Asking for clarification is essential to good communication.

8. **Having to be right.** When a person has to be right in a conversation, there is no communication, only a debate. Needing to be right destroys effective communication.

9. **Sparring.** Using put-downs or sarcasm or discounting someone else's ideas erodes meaningful dialogue and sets up distance in relationships.

10. **Lack of monitoring and follow-up.** Often it takes repeated efforts to get what you need, but it's very important not to give up on communication. When you stop asking for what you need, you often silently resent the other person, which subverts the whole relationship. Persistence will help you get what you want.

As a consultant to organizations and businesses, I have found that the underlying problem in employer-employee disputes is often a lack of clear communication. In many cases, when the communication improves, other problems are also quickly resolved.

One brief example: Billie Jo was an administrative assistant who was frequently angry at her boss. He would give her general guidelines for projects and then become irritated with her when something wasn't done to his satisfaction. Because of his gruff manner, she was too afraid to ask him specific questions about the work. She began to really hate her job. She developed frequent headaches and neck tension and was constantly looking for another position. A friend pushed Billie Jo to tell her boss about her frustrations, saying, "If you're going to quit anyway, you have little to lose." To Billie Jo's surprise, her boss was receptive to her direct approach and encouraged her to ask more questions about the projects he assigned.

Here are six keys to effective communication in relationships:

1. Have a good attitude and assume the other person wants the relation-ship to work as much as you do. Doing so can set the mood for a positive outcome. I call this having "positive basic assumptions" about the relationship.

2. State what you need clearly and in a positive way. In most situations being direct is the best approach, but the way you ask is important. You can demand and get hostility, you can ask in a meek manner and not be taken seriously, or you can be firm yet kind and get what you need. How you approach someone has a lot to do with your success rate.

3. Decrease distractions and make sure you have the other person's attention before you begin a conversation. Find a time when the person is not busy or in a hurry to go somewhere.

4. Ask for feedback to ensure the other person correctly understands you. Clear communication is a two-way street, and it's important to know if you got your message across. A simple "Tell me what you understood I said" is often all that is needed.

5. Be a good listener. Before you respond to others, repeat back what you think they've said to ensure that you've correctly heard them. Statements such as "I hear you saying . . ." or "You mean to say . . ." are the gold standard of good communication. Doing this allows you to check out what you heard before you respond.

6. Monitor and follow up on your communication. It's very important not to give up.

Learn and Practice Active Listening

"I hear you saying . . . ," or active listening, is a technique therapists are taught to increase healthy communication. This technique involves repeating back what you understand the other person to be saying, which gives you the opportunity to check whether the message you received is the one the speaker intended to convey. Communication often breaks down because of distortions between intention and understanding, especially in emotionally charged encounters.

:0 1-02 Simply saying, "I hear you saying . . . is that what you meant?" can MINUTES help you avoid misunderstandings. This technique is particularly helpful when you suspect a breakdown in communication.

Other phrases you could use with this technique include

1. "I heard you say . . . am I right?"
2. "Did you mean to say . . . ?"
3. "I'm not sure I understand what you said. Did you say . . . ?"
4. "Did I understand you correctly? Are you saying that . . . ?"
5. "Let me see if I understand what you're saying to me. You said that . . . ?"

Advantages to "active listening" include

1. You receive more accurate messages.
2. Misunderstandings are cleared up immediately.
3. You are forced to give your full attention to the other person.
4. Both parties are now responsible for accurate communication.
5. The speaker is likely to be more careful with what he says.
6. It increases your ability to really hear the other person and thus learn from her.
7. It stops you from thinking about what you're going to say next so that you can understand what the other person is saying.
8. It increases communication.
9. It tends to cool down conflicts.

When I teach active listening to parenting classes, I often use the following example: If my son came home when he was a teenager and said he wanted to have blue hair, how would I respond *without* the active listening skill versus *with* the active listening skill?

STEP 1: REACT VS. REPEAT BACK WHAT YOU HEAR
Without active listening: Just react. My father, for example, would have said, "No way as long as you live in my house are you going to have blue hair!" This only ends the conversation or starts a fight.

With active listening: Repeat back what you hear. I might say, "You want blue hair?" and then stay quiet long enough for my teen to explain.

STEP 2: STICK TO YOUR GUNS VS. LISTEN FOR THE FEELINGS BEHIND THE WORDS
My son might say, "All the kids are wearing their hair that way" (as if he had somehow taken a scientific poll).

Without active listening: My dad would likely say, "I don't care what anyone else does; you're not going to have blue hair. If they are going to jump off a bridge, are you going to go with them?" Again, this sets up a fight with the teen or causes him to withdraw.

With active listening: I would listen for the feeling behind the words and say, "Sounds like you want to be like the other kids." This encourages understanding and further communication.

STEP 3: DENY YOUR CHILD'S FEELINGS VS. REFLECT BACK WHAT YOU HEAR YOUR CHILD SAYING AND FEELING

My son might say, "Sometimes I feel like I don't fit in. Maybe changing my appearance will help."

Without active listening: "Don't be silly. Of course you fit in. Your appearance has nothing to do with it!"

With active listening: "You think your appearance prevents you from fitting in?"

As you can see, these are two completely different conversations. One is demeaning and limits communication, while the other promotes communication and understanding. At the end of a half hour, if my son still wants to have blue hair, I will tell him, "No way as long as you live in my house." But at least now I know why he wants it, and he is much more likely to accept the answer.

Active listening in a relationship increases its level of understanding and communication. And when people feel understood by you, they feel closer to you. Begin practicing this technique on at least two people every day for a week. See if it doesn't increase your communication abilities—and thus your ability to learn from others.

The Benefits of Active and Constructive Communication

When your daughter reads you her speech, which she is scheduled to deliver at school the next day, and asks for your opinion, how do you respond? How about when your spouse wants to tell you about his day at work? As we have seen, the way you communicate with others can help or hurt your relationships. Studies have shown that a technique called *active and constructive communication* can quickly strengthen your relationships and improve your mood.[14]

Marty Seligman and his colleagues at the University of Pennsylvania have written about four typical styles of communication:

- Active and Destructive: pointing out negative aspects of a situation
- Passive and Destructive: ignoring the person completely

- Passive and Constructive: supporting someone but in an understated way
- Active and Constructive: giving both authentic and enthusiastic support[15]

If you want to improve your relationships, research shows that active constructive communication works, while the other styles do not. Let's say your daughter just got her first acting audition. Here are examples of how you could respond:

- Active and Destructive: "That is such a hard profession. Why would you ever want to do that?"
- Passive and Destructive: Little to no response.
- Passive and Constructive: "That's nice."
- Active and Constructive: "Wow! That's amazing. Congratulations! Tell me all about it."

15 SECONDS Use active constructive communication when responding to someone.

Communicating actively, positively, and constructively helps us build positive relationships and enhance self-esteem.[16]

FOUR TYPICAL COMMUNICATION STYLES

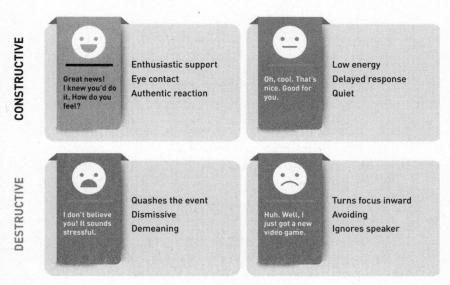

	ACTIVE	**PASSIVE**
CONSTRUCTIVE	Great news! I knew you'd do it. How do you feel? — Enthusiastic support / Eye contact / Authentic reaction	Oh, cool. That's nice. Good for you. — Low energy / Delayed response / Quiet
DESTRUCTIVE	I don't believe you! It sounds stressful. — Quashes the event / Dismissive / Demeaning	Huh. Well, I just got a new video game. — Turns focus inward / Avoiding / Ignores speaker

A IS FOR ASSERTIVENESS

Assertiveness involves standing up for one's rights without infringing upon those of others, whereas aggression involves the use of verbal and nonverbal noxious stimuli to maintain rights.
DRS. MARSHA RICHINS AND BRONISLAW VERHAGE

In healthy relationships it's important to say what you mean. In that way, assertiveness and communication go hand in hand. Being assertive means you express your thoughts and feelings in a firm yet reasonable way, not allowing others to run over you emotionally, and not saying yes when that's not what you mean. Assertiveness never equates with being mean or aggressive.

Here are five simple rules to help you assert yourself in a healthy manner:

1. *Do not give in to the anger of others just because it makes you uncomfortable.* Anxious people do this a lot. They are so anxious that they agree in order to avoid the tension. Unfortunately, doing this teaches others to bully you to get their way. *We teach others how to treat us by what we allow in our lives.* Being assertive in the face of another's anger doesn't mean you have to be angry back, but it does mean you don't agree with someone simply because you're uncomfortable. When you are feeling anxious about another person's anger, it is a good time to do the deep breathing techniques I taught you earlier (see chapter 1, page 17). Take three deep, slow breaths and really think about what your opinion is; then state it clearly without much emotion.

2. *Say what you mean and stick up for what you believe is right.* People will respect you more. People like others who are real and who say exactly what's on their minds.

3. *Maintain self-control.* Being angry, mean, or aggressive is not being assertive. You can be assertive in a calm and clear way.

4. *Be firm and kind, if possible.* Above all, be firm in your stance. Again, we teach other people how to treat us, so when we give in to their temper tantrums, we actually teach them the way to control us. When we assert ourselves in a firm yet kind way, others have more respect for us and will treat us accordingly. Now, if you've allowed others to emotionally run over you for a long time, they're going to be resistant to change. If you stick to your guns, you will help them learn a new way of relating to you, and the relationship will improve. Ultimately, you also will respect yourself more.

5. *Be assertive only when it is necessary.* If you assert yourself all the time for unimportant issues, you'll be perceived as controlling, which invites oppositional behavior.

T IS FOR TIME

Relationships require actual, physical time. In this era of commuting, traffic, two-working-parent households, e-mail, the Internet, television, and video games, we have seriously diminished the time we have with the people in our lives. Spending actual, physical time with the people who are important to us will make a huge difference in our relationships. When I teach the parenting course we give at Amen Clinics (one of the most effective things I've ever done to help children), I say that relationships really require just two things—time and a willingness to listen. Focused time, even if there's not a lot of it, is critically important to relationships.

:05 MINUTES *Special time.* I teach an exercise in my parenting course called "special time," which involves spending 20 minutes a day doing something with your child that he or she wants to do. Twenty minutes is not much time, but this exercise makes a huge difference in the quality of your relationships. I have one rule for this exercise: no commands, no questions, and no directions. It's not a time to try to resolve issues; it is just a time to be together and do something your child wants to do, whether it's playing a game or taking a walk. The difference it made in parent-child relationships was much more dramatic than anything else I did for them, including prescribing medicine. Look for ways to spend time with the people who are important to you. Think of this time as an investment in the health of the relationship.

In a similar way, be present when you are spending time with others at work or at home. We encounter so many distractions that we are rarely present anywhere we are. In the powerful book *Influencer: The Power to Change Anything*, the authors tell a story about a large health care organization that went from having terrible customer satisfaction to becoming one of the region's first-class organizations. In studying the employees who ranked "great" versus those who were "poor," the researchers found only five simple differences. The effective employees

1. Smiled
2. Made eye contact

3. Identified themselves by name
4. Let people know what they were doing and why
5. Ended every interaction by asking, "Is there anything else you need?"[17]

These things were easy to do, and they indicated that the service providers were present and focused on the interaction at hand. Being present in the moment with your spouse, friend, or colleague can help make the other person feel appreciated and secure.

I IS FOR INQUIRING

Earlier in the book we discussed eliminating the ANTs (automatic negative thoughts) that invade your mind. When you're suffering in a relationship, it's important to inquire into the thoughts that are making you suffer. Ask yourself what thoughts are repeatedly going through your mind, and then consider how accurate they might be. If you are fighting with your husband, for example, and you hear yourself thinking *He never listens to me*, write that down. Then ask yourself if it is true: Does he really "never" listen to you? Often when we tell ourselves little lies about other people, it puts unnecessary wedges between us and them. Relationships require accurate thinking in order to thrive. Whenever you feel sad, mad, or nervous in relationships, check out your thoughts. If there are ANTs or lies, stomp them out.

N IS FOR NOTICING WHAT YOU LIKE

Noticing what you like a lot more than what you don't like is one of the secrets to having great relationships. Paying attention to what you like encourages more of that behavior. I learned this concept for the first time when my son was seven years old and we were living in Hawaii. I was in my child psychiatry fellowship-training program.

One day I wanted to have special time with my son, so I took him to a place called Sea Life Park, which is like SeaWorld. We had a great day together. We went to the orca show and the dolphin show, and we saw sea lion antics onstage. Toward the end of the day my son sort of grabbed my shirt and said, "Daddy, take me to see Fat Freddie." I said, "Who's Fat Freddie?" "It's the penguin, Dad," he said. Fat Freddie was an emperor penguin who performed in the large stadium at Sea Life Park. I looked on the show schedule and saw there was one more Fat Freddie show that day. When we got to our seats, the stadium was filled.

Freddie was amazing. To start the show, he climbed a ladder to a high diving board. He went to the end of the board, bounced up and down, and then jumped into the water. When he got out of the water, on command he bowled with his nose, counted with his flippers, and jumped through a hoop of fire. I was thinking to myself, *How cool is this?* My son was clapping, very happy that we were at the show. Toward the end, the trainer asked Freddie to go get something. Freddie immediately brought it to the trainer. When I saw this, I thought, *I ask this kid to get me something, and he wants to have a discussion for 20 minutes, and then he doesn't do it.* I used to find myself frequently frustrated and angry at my son, but I knew he was smarter than the penguin.

After the show I went up to the trainer and asked her how she got Fat Freddie to do all the things he did. The trainer understood what I was asking her, because she looked at my son and then she looked at me and said, "Unlike parents with their kids, I notice Freddie whenever he does anything like what I want him to do. I give him a hug and a fish." The light went on in my head: Whenever my son did what I wanted him to do, I paid no attention to him because I'm a busy guy. But when he didn't do what I wanted him to do, I gave him a ton of attention because I didn't want to raise bad kids. I was inadvertently teaching him to be a little monster in order to get my attention. I started collecting penguins to remind myself to notice what I like about others more than what I do not like. I now have more than 2,000 penguins.

What do you think Fat Freddie would have done if he was having a bad day and didn't do what the trainer asked him to do? Imagine if, all of a sudden, the trainer started screaming at him, "You stupid penguin. I can't believe I ever met a penguin as stupid as you. We ought to ship you off to the Antarctic and get a replacement." Depending on his temperament, if he understood her, Fat Freddie would have either bitten her or gone off to a corner and cried.

What do you do when the important people in your life do not do what you want them to do? Do you criticize them and make them feel miserable? Or do you just pause and decide to notice what you like more than what you don't like? This is a critical point that's important for changing behavior: Focus on the behaviors you like more than the behaviors you don't.

It turns out there is also a great deal of science behind this concept:

- A marriage with *five times* more positive comments than negative ones is *significantly less likely to result in divorce.*
- A business team with *five times* more positive comments than negative ones is *significantly more likely to make money.*
- College students who receive *three times* more positive comments than negative ones are *significantly more likely to have flourishing mental health.*[18]

The amount of positivity in a system divided by the amount of negativity is called the *Gottman ratio* after marital therapist John Gottman, who discovered that the number of positive comments to negative ones significantly predicts marital satisfaction and the chances of staying together versus getting divorced. It is also called the *Losada ratio* after Marcial Losada, who applied Gottman's ratio to the workplace. Keep in mind that balance is important. When comments are too positive, they lose their impact, especially if the ratio is above nine.

G IS FOR GRACE AND FORGIVENESS

Amazing grace! How sweet the sound
That saved a wretch like me!
I once was lost, but now am found;
Was blind, but now I see.
JOHN NEWTON, "AMAZING GRACE"

Forgive us our sins, as we have forgiven those who sin against us.
MATTHEW 6:12, NLT, FROM THE LORD'S PRAYER

The first definition of *grace* in the *Merriam-Webster Dictionary* is "unmerited divine assistance given to humans for their regeneration or sanctification."[19] It is a gift from God that we do not deserve. Grace and forgiveness go hand in hand. One of the most famous prayers in history commands us to forgive others if we ourselves want to be forgiven. Forgiveness is powerful medicine. Holding on to grudges and hurts, even if they are small, increases stress hormones that negatively impact our moods, immunity, and overall health. Giving grace and forgiveness can be hard, but when done properly it can also be powerfully healing. Research has linked forgiveness to mental health outcomes such as reduced anxiety, depression, and major psychiatric disorders, and with having fewer physical health symptoms and lower mortality rates.[20] I often tell my patients that the person who forgives also usually ends the argument.

Grace and forgiveness do not mean letting someone off the hook or con-doning bad behavior. They are not the same as justice and do not require being reconciled with the person who has given offense or done harm. More often than not, a former victim of abuse should not reconcile with the abuser, especially if the abuser has not sought serious help. Grace and forgiveness are acts of strength, not weakness.

Psychologist Everett Worthington of Virginia Commonwealth University has studied forgiveness for years and developed a model called REACH for-giveness, which stands for

Recall the hurt—This time recall it differently, without feeling victimized or holding a grudge. This moves you toward relating to the offense from the point of view of the offender.

Empathize—Replace negative emotions with positive, other-oriented emotions. This involves empathizing—putting yourself in the shoes of the person who hurt you and imagining what he or she might have been feeling.

Altruistic gift—Give the gift of your forgiveness to the person who hurt you. Think about a time in your past when you wronged someone and that person forgave you; remember how much freer you felt afterward. That freedom is your gift to your offender.

Commit to the forgiveness that you experience—When you have forgiven, write a note to yourself about it. You can also cement your feelings by engaging in a ritual, such as completing a forgiveness certificate or writing a word symbolizing the offense in ink on your hand and then washing it off.

Hold on to the forgiveness—If or when you encounter the offender, you may feel anger and fear, and you may worry that you haven't really forgiven him or her. But that is just your body's response as a warning to be careful. Reread your notes to remind yourself that you have laid aside the offense.[21]

In 1996, Dr. Worthington's research was put to the worst possible test: His mother was murdered in a home invasion. Although police believed they had found the murderer, he was never prosecuted. Despite the awful tragedy, Dr. Worthington said, "I had applied the forgiveness model many times, but never to such a big event. As it turned out, I was able to forgive the young man quite quickly." This is an amazing testimony to the power of forgiveness.

Is there someone in your life who needs your grace, whom you could forgive? It may help you feel better. Just keep in mind that forgiveness is usually not a quick process. The REACH forgiveness model, for example, focuses on changing from the inside, which can take time. (To see a presentation on this topic from Dr. Worthington, search YouTube for "Helping People Reach Forgiveness—Everett Worthington.")

My wife, Tana, tells a story about her involvement in a brain health program we were asked to develop for the Salvation Army's largest chemical addiction recovery program. She helped re-create the food portion of our plan for the participants. After her first visit to the campus, she was suddenly filled with horrible, judgmental thoughts about the addicts in the program. It's clear that clean eating helps people with addictions make better decisions, so she wanted to participate. But how could she help people who brought up feelings of fear and loathing inside her? Most of the participants (beneficiaries) are court ordered to be in the program, and many go there after having served time in jail for some pretty serious criminal offenses.

Growing up, Tana directly experienced the consequences that drugs can have on people's lives. Her uncle was murdered in a drug deal gone wrong. She hated drugs and had no tolerance for anyone who used them. When she told me she didn't think she could follow through with helping at the Salvation Army, that God had picked the wrong person this time, I smiled and said, "God picked the perfect person." I was right. Working with that population gave Tana new empathy for the clients' backgrounds, which were not that much different from her own. And she realized that for every person she helped who was a parent, there would be one less scared child in the world.

The eight keys we've discussed in this chapter will improve almost any relationship. Being responsible and empathic, listening, being assertive, spending time, inquiring into negative thoughts, noticing what you like more than what you don't, and giving grace and forgiveness are tools you can use today to bring those in your life closer to you.

THE BRAIN AND RELATIONSHIPS

In addition to developing great habits to help people connect, our brain imaging work has taught us that the physical functioning of the brain is an often-overlooked component of why relationships succeed or fail. Over the past three decades I have scanned hundreds of couples who have had serious marital problems. In my training as a marital therapist, and in the training of almost all marital therapists on the planet, there was not one lecture on how the physical functioning of your brain impacts the relationship. Yet, since your brain is involved in everything you do and everything you are, if it doesn't function right, you are likely to have significant problems relating to people you care about. At Amen Clinics, we look at relationships and relationship conflict in a whole new way, involving compatible and incompatible brain patterns. I have come to realize that many relationships do not work because of brain misfires that have nothing to do with character, free will, or desire. Many relationships are sabotaged by factors beyond conscious or even unconscious control. Sometimes a little targeted brain intervention can make all the difference between love and hate, staying together and divorce, effective problem-solving and prolonged litigation. See my book *Change Your Brain, Change Your Life* for a detailed look at this topic.

EIGHT STRATEGIES TO ENHANCE YOUR ABILITY TO CONNECT BY RELATING

1. Ask yourself if you are taking RESPONSIBILITY in your relationships: "How can I respond in a positive, helpful way?"

2. Practice EMPATHY: Treat others as you would like to be treated.

3. In conversations, LISTEN and practice good communication skills.

4. Be ASSERTIVE: Say what you mean and stick up for what you believe is right in a calm, clear, kind way.

5. Spend TIME: Remember that actual, physical time with others is critical to healthy relationships.

6. INQUIRE into the negative thoughts that make you suffer in a relationship, and decide if they're true.

7. NOTICE what you like in the behavior of those around you more than you notice (and complain about) what you don't like.

8. Give the altruistic gift of GRACE and forgiveness whenever you can.

TINY HABITS THAT CAN HELP YOU FEEL BETTER FAST—AND LEAD TO BIG CHANGES

:03-20
MINUTES

Each of these habits takes just a few minutes. They are anchored to something you do (or think or feel) so that they are more likely to become automatic. Once you do the behaviors you want, find a way to make yourself feel good about them—draw a happy face, pump your fist, or do whatever feels natural. Emotion helps the brain to remember.

1. After I've had a fight with a loved one, I will take responsibility for my part and apologize (responsibility).

2. When someone acts negatively toward me, I will ask myself, *Did I do anything to cause it? What is going on with this person?* (empathy).

3. When I am in a conversation with someone, before responding with my input, I will reflect back what I heard him or her saying (active listening).

4. When I am challenged or bullied, I will state the case for what I believe, calmly and clearly (assertiveness).

5. When I set aside time to be with my child, I will spend 20 minutes doing whatever he or she wants to do, with no agenda (time).

6. When I have a negative thought about my spouse, such as *He never listens to me*, I will write it down and ask myself, *Is that true?* If it is not, I will quash the thought (inquiry).

7. When a friend does something annoying, I will turn my attention to the things I like about her rather than dwelling on the annoyance (noticing).

8. When someone is mean or hurtful to me, I will try to create grace in my heart to forgive them (grace and forgiveness).

CHAPTER 7

OVERCOMING TRAUMA AND GRIEF

ELIMINATE THE HURTS THAT HAUNT YOU

Sometimes the bad things that happen in our lives put us directly on the path to the most wonderful things that will ever happen to us.
NICOLE REED, *RUINING YOU*

The brain you bring into a trauma will often determine the life that comes out of it.
DANIEL AMEN

On July 16, 2003, Steven, a 33-year-old bicycle repair mechanic working in Santa Monica, California, insisted on having an early lunch. He was not sure why, but he felt drawn to the Santa Monica Farmers' Market, so he headed there on foot. As he arrived, George Russell Weller, 86, lost control of his 1992 Buick LeSabre and barreled through the three-block-long farmers' market. Bodies went flying and people screamed as Weller's car headed straight for Steven. He knew he would be hit. Steven later said, "I thought he was going to run over my legs. . . . I thought I would lose my legs." At the last possible moment, he managed to jump out of the way. In the chaos, 10 people were killed, and more than 50 were injured. Steven, who had been a military tank commander in the first Gulf War, used the medical skills he had learned to help save others. Still, a woman died in his arms.

Traumatized, Steven went back to work that same day. But for months afterward he couldn't sleep and couldn't stop his hands from shaking. By chance—or fate, if you believe in such things—Linda Alvarez, a Los Angeles CBS News anchor, took her bicycle to Steven's shop shortly after the disaster and discussed it with him in a brief conversation. As they talked, Linda noticed that Steven was shaking. "It started that day," Steven said, showing her his trembling hands, "and it won't stop." The image of Steven's hands stayed with Linda. A month later, while working on another story, Linda learned about work I was doing with a treatment technique called Eye Movement Desensitization and Reprocessing, or EMDR, planting the seed for a story about the treatment and Steven's trauma.

EMDR: A POWERFUL TOOL TO FEEL BETTER FAST

EMDR is an effective psychological treatment developed by my friend Francine Shapiro, a psychologist. In 1987, during a walk around a lake, she noticed that a disturbing thought disappeared when her eyes spontaneously started to move back and forth from the lower left to the upper right visual fields. She tried the eye movements again with another anxiety-provoking thought and found that the anxious feeling went away. In the days that followed, Francine tried the technique with friends, acquaintances, and interested students and found that it was helpful in relieving anxiety. She went on to work with patients and developed a technique that is now used worldwide.

This form of therapy is based on research suggesting that traumatic events can prevent the brain from processing information as it normally does, which results in these events getting "stuck" in the brain's information processing center. Then, when someone who experienced a trauma recalls it, the memory triggers an intense re-experiencing of the original event, complete with all of its upsetting sights, sounds, smells, thoughts, and feelings. New incidents can have the same effect. During EMDR, to "unlock" the brain's processing center, a client brings up emotionally troubling memories while his or her eyes follow a trained therapist's hand moving horizontally back and forth. Employing a specific protocol, the clinician helps the client identify the images, negative beliefs, emotions, and body sensations associated with a targeted memory or event. Positive statements and beliefs replace negative ones, and the client rates the believability of a new thought while thinking of the disturbing event.

The goal of EMDR treatment is to help clients rapidly process information about a negative experience and move toward an adaptive resolution. When EMDR is effective, people who undergo it come to understand, both consciously in their minds and unconsciously in the physical functioning of their brains, that the event is in the past and no longer a threat. This means a reduction in distress, a shift from a negative belief to a more positive one, and the possibility of more optimal behavior in relationships and at work. It is often used with people who suffer from posttraumatic stress disorder (PTSD), a lasting emotional response to severe trauma that changes the nervous system.

HEALING MULTIPLE LAYERS OF TRAUMA

When CBS producer Angeline Chew called to ask if I would be interested in doing a segment about EMDR and using Steven's story as an example, I was happy to help. I had just finished a study with therapist Karen Lansing on police officers who were involved in shootings and developed PTSD afterward.[1] EMDR was very effective in quickly alleviating the officers' symptoms, as well as normalizing their brain function on SPECT scans. My colleagues and I have published several brain SPECT imaging studies on posttraumatic stress disorder that show significant increases in activity in the limbic or emotional areas in a pattern that looks like a diamond. The affected brain areas are the anterior cingulate gyrus, which indicates a fixation on negative thoughts or behaviors; the basal ganglia and amygdala, involved with anxiety; and the thalamus, which shows a heightened sensory awareness. In addition, we see increased activity in the right lateral temporal lobe, an area of the brain involved in reading the intentions of other people.

NORMAL "ACTIVE" BRAIN SPECT SCAN	CLASSIC POSTTRAUMATIC STRESS DISORDER SCAN
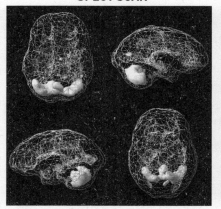	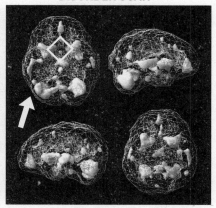
Most active areas are in the cerebellum at the back of the brain.	"Diamond plus" pattern shows increased activity in the anterior cingulate gyrus (top of diamond), basal ganglia/amygdala (middle), and thalamus (bottom), as well as in the right lateral temporal lobe (indicated by the arrow).

After talking to Steven and discovering that he was willing to participate, we felt he would be a good candidate for EMDR and that his story of healing could be an inspiration to others. As is often the case in people who develop PTSD, Steven had experienced other traumas besides the one at the Santa Monica Farmers' Market. He grew up in a severely abusive alcoholic home. One of his earliest memories was of his father burning down the family home, and he also remembered that his father had once dangled him over the side of a 400-foot-high bridge. When he was 11, his favorite firefighter uncle died in a fire set by an arsonist, and Steven faced death as a tank commander during the Gulf War. He had many layers of trauma.

As part of his evaluation, we scanned Steven three times: before treatment, during his first EMDR session, and after eight hours of treatments. Initially, Steven's brain showed the classic PTSD pattern, with his limbic or emotional brain being extremely hyperactive. Using EMDR with him, we cleared out the traumas one by one. His brain actually showed benefit during the first treatment and was markedly improved after eight hours of treatment (see the scans below). Steven's shaking subsided, and he felt calmer and less stressed. One of the most healing insights Steven shared with me was that during the process, he started to forgive his father and wondered what *his* brain might have looked like. Steven had held deep and understandable resentment toward his father, but the brain science gave him a new perspective on himself and his dad. When we helped Steven calm and balance his brain, he was happier and able to sleep better.

STEVEN'S BASELINE "ACTIVE" SPECT SCAN	DURING FIRST EMDR SESSION

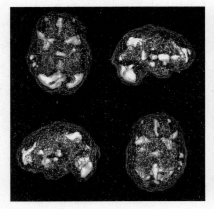
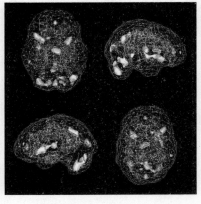

Strong "diamond plus" pattern	Calming starting to occur

AFTER EIGHT HOURS OF TREATMENT

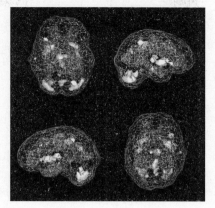

Most active areas are in the cerebellum at the back of the brain.

GETTING THE RIGHT DIAGNOSIS IS CRITICAL TO FEELING BETTER FAST

Going through emotional trauma or grief can leave a lasting imprint on the brain. In order to properly heal it, it is critical to get the right diagnosis. In 2015, we published two studies on more than 21,000 patients, including veterans, that demonstrated we could distinguish between PTSD (emotional trauma) and traumatic brain injuries (physical trauma) with high levels of accuracy based on SPECT scans.[2] In January 2016, *Discover* magazine awarded this research 19th place among the top 100 stories in 2015 in all of science—between Tesla's entry into the energy market (number 18) and the discovery of a new vegan dinosaur species (number 20). It was critically important because the symptoms of PTSD and traumatic brain injury (TBI) often overlap (anxiety, depression, irritability, headaches, and insomnia), but the treatments are very different. In fact, treating PTSD as if it is a TBI, or vice versa, can actually make people worse, which is why I believe neuroimaging studies are so important when people struggle and find that the simple treatments to feel better fast are ineffective.

Grief is often mislabeled as depression, ADHD, PTSD, panic disorder, and other psychiatric conditions. If you experience symptoms of these conditions after a loss, consider doing grief work before taking medication. If grief is misdiagnosed, psychotropic medications can get in the way of or even prolong recovery.

SEVEN STRATEGIES TO ELIMINATE THE HURTS THAT HAUNT YOU

Brain imaging research has shown that PTSD is associated with hyperactivity in the amygdala and other emotional parts of the brain, but it also leads to decreased activity in parts of the prefrontal cortex (PFC). This means that people who suffer from trauma have heightened fear responses (high amygdala activity) and lower self-control (lower PFC activity). The combination of heightened fear and lowered self-control is a prescription for trouble. Common forms of self-medication, such as alcohol, opiates, marijuana, or a diet laden with sugar and foods that turn to sugar, can help to calm the amygdala and anxiety in the short run, but they also reduce the activity of the PFC even more, giving someone less control over these behaviors. That leads to further trouble, including addictions and obesity.

Research has also found that the brains of those experiencing grief tend to show greater activity in the limbic system and parts of the PFC. The pain of grief is often so brutal that people will do anything to escape it. In so doing—just as for PTSD—they often choose strategies that hurt rather than help them. Alcohol, marijuana, or unhealthy food may lessen the pain for a short while, but unfortunately it returns even worse. Similarly, taking opiates or benzodiazepines, such as Valium or Xanax, can calm the pain briefly but actually will make it worse in the long run.[3]

Integrating my clinical experience with patients, extensive brain imaging work, and the science of healing from trauma and grief (see "Recovering from Grief: Additional Suggestions" on page 166), I've come up with seven strategies that will help you feel better fast. Whether you have PTSD because of past trauma, are mourning the loss of a family member or friend, or are dealing with significant stress in your life, the relief will be lasting.

Strategy #1: Consider EMDR (Eye Movement Desensitization and Reprocessing).

As discussed earlier, EMDR is especially helpful in dealing with intrusive memories and anxiety that interfere with joy. It also helps control the triggers that make you feel upset. Initially used for people with PTSD,[4] EMDR has also been shown to be effective for grief,[5] anxiety,[6] panic disorders,[7] depression,[8] chronic pain,[9] phantom limb pain,[10] addictions,[11] and performance enhancement.[12] It was found to be helpful when used in groups of teenagers after the earthquake in Italy in 2016.[13] EMDR is one of the most rapid and effective treatments I have ever personally witnessed. I have my patients keep a journal of the times that are hard for them, then work with an EMDR therapist to help eliminate their anxious reactions. It is important that this technique be done by an EMDR certified therapist. You can find one at the EMDR International Association website (www.EMDRIA.org).

EMDR: A Personal Reflection

I have a personal history with EMDR, which I've talked about in my book *Healing the Hardware of the Soul* and other places. In late 1996, I was invited to give the State-of-the-Art Lecture in Medicine to the Society of Developmental Pediatrics on brain SPECT imaging. The lecture generated a heated discussion. A pediatrician from the Bay Area stood up and criticized my work, saying that people quoted me and my brain imaging research as a justification to prescribe medication to children with ADHD. "We give glasses to children who can't see," I replied. "If you can see physical brain problems on SPECT in people who have ADHD, doesn't it make sense to treat them?" Shortly after the meeting, someone (I suspected this pediatrician) anonymously reported me to the California medical board.

In California, if you do anything in medical practice outside the "standard of care," you can have your license revoked. The law is designed to protect the public, but it can also stifle innovation. What I was doing with brain SPECT imaging was certainly different from my colleagues' work. For a year, I answered questions, gave the medical board copies of research articles, hired an attorney, and appeared at interviews. Many times I felt like running away, and I was more anxious than I had ever been in my life. I had trouble sleeping, developed nightmares for the first time, and constantly had an upset stomach. When I talked about the stress with my friend and colleague Dr. Jennifer Lendl, an EMDR trainer, she suggested the treatment for me. "We're studying EMDR in others; it looks as though you need it too," she said. My SPECT study before EMDR showed the "diamond plus" pattern, which was different from my baseline scan a couple of years earlier.

I found the EMDR process fascinating. As Dr. Lendl moved

her fingers horizontally left and right, I felt as if I were on a train watching all of the events related to the investigation. I thought about the fear of failure, losing my medical license, being unable to further develop the brain science I loved, and being embarrassed in front of my family and friends. As Dr. Lendl continued to move her fingers, I felt the anxiety diminishing, and I spontaneously began to replace the negative images with healthier ones. "I have a wonderful attorney to help me; what I am doing helps many people; even if I lose, I will have helped many people; my family and friends will always love me whether I'm a doctor or work in a grocery store; it will be okay; God will always be there for me." Four EMDR sessions eliminated the anxiety. I slept better and my stomach stopped being upset. My follow-up scan showed overall calming of my emotional brain. After a year, the medical board found no violation and dismissed the complaint, allowing me to continue the work I loved.[14]

Strategy #2: Try trauma-focused cognitive behavioral therapy (TF-CBT).

TF-CBT was developed in the 1990s by psychiatrist Judith Cohen and psychologists Esther Deblinger and Anthony Mannarino. As they note, trauma can lead to guilt, anger, feelings of powerlessness, self-abuse, acting-out behavior, and mental health issues, such as depression and anxiety. It is common for PTSD to manifest itself with bothersome recurring thoughts about the traumatic experience. Similar to the ANT-elimination strategy discussed in chapter 5 (pages 107–108), the idea of TF-CBT is that learning to correct these thoughts is critical to getting and staying well. TF-CBT has been shown to be particularly effective with children and teens[15] and in group therapy settings,[16] and the results last over time.[17] You can find a TF-CBT therapist at www.tfcbt.org.

Strategy #3: Write the story of what happened in the context of your life.

Narrative exposure therapy (NET) is a brief psychotherapy for trauma developed by Drs. Maggie Schauer, Frank Neuner, and Thomas Elbert that has been shown in studies to be effective.[18] It has been used most often with individuals, groups, and communities that have experienced multiple traumas as a result of political or cultural forces (such as refugee groups or people affected by a natural disaster). NET has been shown to reduce PTSD symptoms after 4 to 10 sessions with a therapist.

The stories people tell themselves about trauma and their lives in general influence their health and well-being. Seeing yourself solely around traumatic experiences leads to lasting feelings of trauma and stress. NET therapy involves writing a chronological story of your life, including detailed accounts of the traumas you have experienced, and reliving the emotions without losing connection with the present moment. You include positive events in your story, which helps add balance and context to what you believe about your life. One of my patients, for example, grew up with an abusive alcoholic mother, but my patient also remembered the times her mother would put towels in the dryer to warm them before getting her and her siblings out of the bathtub. When treatment ends, the therapist will create a documented autobiography for the patient.

NET is different from other treatments in that it focuses on creating an account of what happened in a balanced way that helps to recapture a person's self-respect. For more information, see the Narrative Exposure Therapy channel on the Vivo International website (www.vivo.org). NET is similar to written exposure therapy (WET), which has also been found to be effective for PTSD.[19]

Strategy #4: Don't block your painful feelings.

Let painful feelings wash over you, cry or scream (not at others!), and then challenge the thoughts that underlie the feelings to see if they are true. Avoiding painful thoughts, feelings, and memories creates more harm than good in the long run. Many research studies have shown that avoidance increases the likelihood of a host of psychological issues, such as PTSD,[20] depression,[21] anxiety disorders,[22] binge eating,[23] chronic pain,[24] low academic performance,[25] and more. Whenever you are suffering with trauma or grief, write out your feelings or find a friend or therapist you can talk them out to. This can help bring perspective, which often gets lost during emotional crises. Blocking your feelings leads to engaging in negative behaviors to deal with the excess negative emotional energy.

One of my favorite poems about not blocking thoughts or emotions is by Rumi, a 13th-century Persian poet. In "The Guest House," he describes being human as akin to a guest house that receives new "arrivals"—new emotions—every day. While some of these visitors are positive and some are negative, we can welcome them all, knowing that experiencing them may help us grow. Rumi wrote,

Still, treat each guest honorably.
He may be clearing you out
for some new delight.[26]

Strategy #5: Break the bonds of the past.

One of the most powerful "feel better fast" techniques I've used with patients is what I call "breaking the bonds of the past." It stems from the belief that negative feelings and behaviors are often based on past memories that are either toxic or misinterpreted, and evaluating the truth of these memories can help us feel better. This technique requires only five simple steps. Whenever you have a painful or disruptive memory or feeling, write out the answers to the following questions:

1. When was the last time you struggled with the painful or disruptive memory or feeling, experienced it, or felt suffering because of it? Write down the details.
2. What were you feeling at the time? Describe the predominant feeling.
3. When was the first time you had that feeling? Imagine yourself on a train going backward through time. Go back to when you first experienced the feeling and write down the incident in detail.
4. Can you go back even further to a time when you had that original feeling? Write down the details of the original incident.
5. If you have a clear idea of the origins of the feelings, can you disconnect them from the past by reprocessing them through an adult or parent mind-set, or reframing them in light of new information? Consciously disconnect the emotional bridge to the past with the idea that what happened in the past belongs in the past, and what happens now is what matters.

Here are three examples of how this can work.

NATE: ADDRESSING PANIC ATTACKS

Nate, 15, came to see me for panic attacks. He had several episodes a day when he felt as if he were choking or drowning. His breathing became shallow, fast, and labored. His heart raced, he broke out in a sweat, and he felt as though he were dying. Nate hated these episodes. The fear of having them was so overwhelming that he stopped going to school. I went through the following steps with him during our second visit.

1. *Tell me about the last time you had a panic attack.* Nate said it was the day before. He was eating dinner when all of a sudden he felt as if he were starting to choke, and he had all the familiar awful symptoms— a sense of suffocation, racing heart, sweating, and feeling as if he were going to die.

2. *Tell me what you were feeling at the time. Describe the predominant feeling.* Nate said he felt as though he were going to die.

3. *Imagine yourself on a train going backward through time. Go back to a time when you first had that feeling.* I asked Nate to go back in time to remember the first time he felt he was going to die. He sat there for a minute and then started to choke. I thought he was having a panic attack in front of me. I asked him to breathe slowly and tell me what was going on. He slowed his breathing, wiped his brow, and told me about a time when he was six years old. He was sitting at a lunch table at school and accidentally swallowed a plastic wrapper from a candy bar. He started to choke on the wrapper. Initially no one saw him. He couldn't breathe, and no one noticed. He thought he was going to die. After what seemed an eternity, a teacher saw him and did the Heimlich maneuver on him, dislodging the wrapper. Nate said he had forgotten about the event until now.

4. *After he settled down and composed himself, I asked him to go back even further in his mind to see if there was an earlier time when he had the feeling he was going to die.* He closed his eyes and said he remembered a time when he was very young. He was coming out of somewhere dark into a place filled with bright lights, lights that felt hot. People were moving around. He felt fear. He couldn't breathe, and something awful covered his face. He felt as though he were going to die. To my amazement, Nate had just described a birth experience. When he opened his eyes, I asked him if he knew anything about his birth. He said no, no one had ever talked to him about it. I asked his mother to come into the room, and then I asked her about his birth experience. She told me that he was a meconium baby (this means the infant's feces get into the amniotic fluid, which is very dangerous for the newborn). He was born blue and had to be resuscitated by the doctor. His mother said she had never talked about it with Nate because she didn't want to worry him.

5. *Break the bonds of the past through an adult or parent mind-set, or reframe them in light of new information.* With Nate's mother in the

room, I took him back to both of those times. First, with the birth experience, I had the teenage Nate go back and explain to the baby what had happened. The baby was in trouble for a short time, but the doctors helped clean him up so he could breathe normally. I then took him through the candy wrapper incident and had the teenage Nate tell six-year-old Nate that he is grateful to the teacher who helped him and that he is alive, well, and healthy (and he needed to stop eating candy wrappers).

After that session, Nate's panic attacks disappeared. I saw him a few more times, but essentially disconnecting his present symptoms from the past sensitizing event took care of them.

CHUCK: GETTING FREE FROM IMPOTENCE

Chuck, 35, came to see me for impotence. He felt he was going to lose the woman he loved, who was getting frustrated over the issue.

1. *Tell me about the last time you were impotent.* Two nights ago.

2. *Tell me what you were feeling at the time. Describe the predominant feeling.* Chuck said, "I feel as if I am a failure."

3. *Imagine yourself on a train going backward through time. Go back to a time when you first had that feeling.* I asked Chuck to go back in time to when he first felt as if he were a failure. After about two minutes he started to sob. As he gained a measure of control, he told me of a time when he was seven years old and having trouble with his homework, especially reading. His father repeatedly hit him, called him stupid, and told Chuck he would never amount to anything. He would be a failure. Chuck said he had completely blocked the memory until that moment.

4. *I then asked Chuck to go back even further in his mind to see if there was an earlier time when he felt like a failure.* After several minutes, he said no.

5. *Break the bonds of the past through an adult or parent mind-set, or reframe them in light of new information.* I took Chuck back to the traumatizing incident and had the adult Chuck talk to his seven-year-old self. His father didn't understand dyslexia, which Chuck was diagnosed with in the fourth grade. Once he was diagnosed, his father became more understanding and supportive.

After that session, Chuck's issue with impotence was resolved, which improved his relationship.

JENNY: OVERCOMING ANNOYANCE AND ALCOHOLISM

Jenny, 42, struggled with alcohol use and lost her marriage in the process. During her recovery, she joined the Christian program Celebrate Recovery. She found that when she went, she usually showed up at meetings 30 minutes late to avoid the worship music. I asked her why.

1. *Tell me about the last time you were late to a meeting.* A week ago.

2. *Tell me what you were feeling at the time. Describe the predominant feeling.* Jenny said, "Annoyed."

3. *Imagine yourself on a train going backward through time. Go back to a time when you first had that feeling.* I asked Jenny to go back in time to when she first felt annoyed. After about 30 seconds, she said, "About age seven, when my mother wanted me to enter piano contests. I spent hours and hours practicing. Initially, I loved it, but the pressure was insane. All I did was go to school, practice music, and go to church. My dad was the minister, and my mom played the piano. And it went on and on for like 20 hours. There were times I would fall asleep in church and then get beaten with the belt when I got home." "No wonder you get annoyed with the music at church," I replied. Jenny laughed.

4. *I then asked Jenny to go back even further in her mind to see if there was an earlier time when she felt annoyed.* After several minutes, she said there was a time when she was three when her father hit her mother and broke her lip, splattering blood all over Jenny's new clothes. It made her feel really annoyed.

5. *Break the bonds of the past through an adult or parent mind-set, or reframe them in light of new information.* Jenny's adult self talked to her three- and seven-year-old selves. She told them her mom and dad were not healthy and had no business raising children under that level of stress. But she did not have to be like her parents and could start to enjoy the music at church. What happened in the past belongs in the past, and what happens now is what matters.

Jenny's recovery has gone much better, and Celebrate Recovery is an integral part of her program.

Note: If this process brings up painful memories that do not go away in a short period of time, seek professional help from a licensed psychotherapist.

Strategy #6: Strive for "posttraumatic growth."

One of the most exciting areas of trauma research is in posttraumatic growth (PTG). The term was coined in the mid-1990s by psychologists Richard Tedeschi and Lawrence Calhoun at the University of North Carolina at Charlotte.[27] According to Dr. Tedeschi, as many as 90 percent of trauma survivors report at least one aspect of posttraumatic growth, such as a renewed appreciation for life. Whenever a group of people are traumatized, about 10 percent will develop PTSD, while 80 percent will return to their normal baseline within a few months. Another 10 percent will actually be stronger than they were before the trauma happened—those who experience PTG.

POSTTRAUMATIC GROWTH CURVE

Most | People

PTSD
Depression
Anxiety
Suicide

Posttraumatic
Growth

RESILIENCE

Research suggests that PTG is based on five factors that can improve symptoms of distress.[28] I've adapted them slightly to form the acronym SPARK:

1. A deepening of **spiritual life**, including a significant change in one's belief system or a new or stronger sense of meaning and purpose. Martin Luther gave his life to God and a religious order after he survived a life-threatening thunderstorm.

2. Seeing new **possibilities** because of the trauma or grief. New opportunities have emerged from the situation, opening up possibilities

that were not present before. One of my friends, for instance, lost her daughter to a drunk driver and now has traveled the country helping other families who have had similar experiences.

3. Increased **appreciation of life** in general; becoming better at appreciating each moment. After a near-death experience, one of my patients lost her fear of death but also started putting in fewer hours at work to spend more time with her family.

4. A change in **relationships** or **relating to others** in more meaningful ways than before the trauma occurred. There is an increased sense of connection, and people appreciate family and friends more. One of my friends who has experienced many challenges parenting a child with autism started Talk About Curing Autism, a support group with more than 50,000 members. She has a huge group of new friends who bring meaning and purpose to her life.

5. **Kick-start greatness through increased personal strength.** This is seen in expressions such as "If I lived through that, I can live through anything!"

COMPONENTS OF POSTTRAUMATIC GROWTH

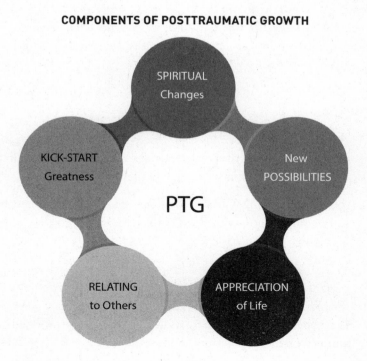

Eight sessions of EMDR helped to promote PTG in survivors of the large-scale ferry disaster that occurred in the Yellow Sea off South Korea in April 2014.[29] To encourage PTG in yourself, look back over your own traumas and, using these five criteria, ask yourself how your life may have changed in a positive way as a result of those events.

CHARLEY: THE HEALTHIEST PERSON I'VE EVER MET

Charley had anxiety and trouble breathing when he first came to see me. The 16-year-old had a condition known as Goldenhar syndrome, a deformity that usually affects just one side of the face. He was born without his left jawbone and had undergone 21 surgeries to fix the deformity, leaving his face scarred and looking like an old railroad yard. His panic started when the doctor put the anesthesia mask over his face for the 20th surgery. His mother brought Charley to see me. He had always been a resilient boy, and she was worried because he had at least two more surgeries to go. A few sessions of hypnosis easily cleared up his anxiety.

As I got to know Charley, I came to believe that despite his anxiety, he was the healthiest person I had ever met. He was president of his 10th-grade class, got straight As in school, and had a girlfriend he adored. He also had clear goals and a great attitude. After his anxiety had lifted, I continued to see him at no cost. For the most part, doctors study illness, not resilience, but I had to know why he was so healthy despite his circumstances. I came to believe that there were five reasons for Charley's emotional strength, which paralleled the research of PTG.

1. *Spiritual changes:* Charley had a deep sense of purpose and believed he was on the planet to make it better.

2. *Possibilities:* Because of his experience, Charley had developed great empathy for others who suffered, and he was considering training to be a physician to help others like himself.

3. *Appreciation of life:* Charley loved life. Each year he found he was more competent in school and relationships and more excited about his future.

4. *Relationships:* He developed close relationships, especially with his mother, even though she never allowed his disability to be an excuse for anything. She suffered for her son, but early in his life she realized that babying him would only handicap him. Charley still did chores, was expected to do well at school, and participated with other kids

even when they made fun of him. She helped him rehearse what to say when other kids were cruel, which they were. When he didn't get upset by the teasing, the other kids became his friends and protected him against any further teasing.

5. *Kick-start greatness through personal strength:* Charley was an optimist. In listening to him speak, I found that he almost always saw the positive side of things. He did not see his condition as a handicap. When we talked about it, he said everyone has something. "This is my problem. At least I don't have cancer."

THE IMPORTANCE OF BRAIN RESERVE

Another explanation for PTG is a concept I call brain reserve. Brain reserve is the extra cushion of brain function you have that helps you deal with whatever stresses come your way. The more reserve you have, the more resilient you are and the less impact trauma and grief will have on your life. To explain brain reserve to my patients, I often go to the whiteboard in my office and draw the image below.

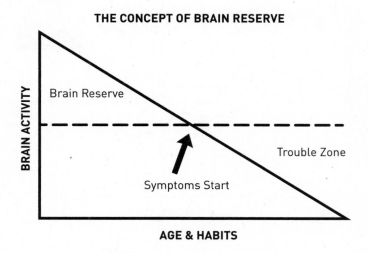

When you were conceived, your brain had a lot of potential for reserve, but if your mom smoked, ate unhealthy food, was chronically stressed, or had infections, your reserve was being depleted even before you were born. If, however, your mother was healthy, ate well, took her vitamins, and was not terribly stressed, she was helping to increase your reserve. Over the course of the rest of your life, you are either increasing or decreasing your brain reserve. If, for example, you fell down a flight of stairs at age three and hit your head, even if you had no symptoms, you decreased your reserve. If you started smoking marijuana as a teenager, you decreased your reserve further, and if you played tackle football or hit a lot of soccer balls with your head, you have even less reserve—even though you might not yet be symptomatic.

Think of it this way: Take two soldiers engaged in a war who are in the same tank and are both exposed to the same blast injury at the same angles. One of them walks away psychologically unharmed, while the other is permanently disabled by trauma. Why? It depends on the level of brain reserve that each of them had prior to the accident. One soldier had more reserve because he took good care of his brain, his parents fed him well, he had lots of educational opportunities, and he didn't play football. The other soldier started lower on the line with less reserve. Both soldiers are effective at their jobs, but they started at different places. Even though the blast diminished the reserve of both, the one with a higher reserve remained functional.

WHY SOME WALK AWAY FROM ACCIDENTS UNHARMED AND OTHERS DO NOT

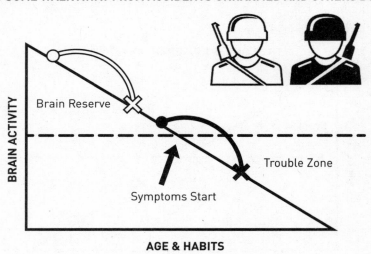

Most of the people we see at the Amen Clinics start below the dotted line and are symptomatic. Getting well is not just about becoming symptom-free; it's also about boosting your brain reserve and getting back above the line. That requires the three simple strategies discussed in chapter 2 (pages 30–44): developing brain envy (you have to really care about your brain); avoiding anything that hurts your brain; and engaging in regular brain-healthy habits. Every day you are either boosting or stealing from your brain's reserve; you are either aging your brain or rejuvenating it. When you truly understand this concept, you will have a lot more influence over how you deal with trauma and grief.

Strategy #7: Consider using the hormone oxytocin, which has been found to be helpful for both grief and emotional trauma.

Oxytocin is produced in both women and men. Although it's often associated with female reproduction, more recently it has become known as "the love hormone," as it brings forth feelings of trust, security, connection, calmness, and contentment. I first became aware of oxytocin's unique ability to help with trauma and grief after reading a book by Dr. Ken Stoller, who worked with us at Amen Clinics for several years. In *Oxytocin: The Hormone of Healing and Hope*, Ken wrote about his own firsthand experience with oxytocin and grief. His 16-year-old son, Galen, had been killed in a train accident, and Ken was overwhelmed with what he termed pathological grief—a mixture of debilitating fear, anxiety, and panic permeating his grief. He was consumed with obsessive thoughts about how Galen had died and what he might have experienced in his last moments.

Ken had been prescribing oxytocin to treat fear and anxiety in children on the autism spectrum, but it was several weeks before he realized that it might help him as well. His greatest fear and panic were during the predawn hours, when he would have terrible nightmares. He wrote,

One night, I set my alarm to wake up before this period and dosed myself with oxytocin, and the outcome felt nearly miraculous. The severity of obsessive negative thoughts during this acute grieving period was altered within minutes after the application of an oxytocin nasal spray. Whereas before I had to breathe through this emotionally difficult hour as if I were in a Lamaze class, that survival strategy became unnecessary with the use of oxytocin. This time, I was actually able to play music until the sun came up.

It took about ten minutes to experience the full effect, and with each passing minute a great sense of emotional equanimity took place. The panic and fear dropped away from me as if I were shedding clothing. If I wanted to think about my son's train accident, I could. But the moment I didn't want to think about it, the accident faded into the background of my mind. It wasn't there hammering away at me as if it had a life of its own. By successfully diverting these negative feelings from wherever they would have taken me, I was able to process my grief without the interference of negative obsessions. This was invaluable, to say the very least, and kept me from developing severe post-traumatic stress disorder (PTSD) . . . because that was certainly where I was headed.[30]

Oxytocin helped Ken get through the worst of his emotional pain, and he was able to stop using it after a few weeks. He has since prescribed oxytocin for other patients facing grief and has seen it benefit each one.

Other researchers have also recently shown the benefit of oxytocin for trauma.[31] Dr. J. L. Frijling and colleagues from Holland found that giving intranasal oxytocin calmed the fear circuit in the brain (amygdala) and decreased the symptoms of acute PTSD.[32] Oxytocin has also been shown to increase compassion in people who suffer with emotional trauma.[33] Any physician can write a prescription for it, and most compounding pharmacies can make the intranasal or sublingual (under the tongue) form. The typical adult dosage is 10–40 IUs two to three times a day. Dr. Stoller and others recommend it for short-term use only, as long-term use has the potential to change oxytocin receptors in the brain.

RECOVERING FROM GRIEF: ADDITIONAL SUGGESTIONS

The emotion of grief affects nearly all of us at some point in life. Eight million people become new grievers every year due to the death of someone they love. Nearly 50 percent of marriages end in divorce, leaving the broken couple, their children, and their families grieving.

Grief is the normal response to a significant loss. And it is often accompanied by regret and the pain of being unable to connect with someone (or something) who has been there for you for a period of time. Other common symptoms of grief include sadness, trouble concentrating, memory problems, insomnia, irritability, diarrhea, headaches, a loss of appetite, and feeling numb. Complicated grief, which is marked by intense and ongoing longing for the departed, is often associated with conflicting feelings—happiness that a loved one is no longer suffering, but yearning because you miss him or her terribly.

But grief is not just about losing a loved one to death, divorce, an empty nest, or another method. It can occur after losing one's health, freedom, financial stability, a home, a job or career (with retirement), or even following a loss of trust or safety. When parents have a disabled child, they often experience intense grief over the loss of what they had dreamed for their son or daughter. Losing pets is also extremely painful for many people. One of the only times I've seen my very tough father cry was when he lost Vinnie, his dog and best friend of nine years.

The symptoms of unresolved grief may include

- Inability to accept the loss
- Emotional numbness
- Unwillingness to think or talk about someone who has died, or a loss you experienced
- Happy memories that frequently turn painful
- Talking only about the positive aspects of the relationship and ignoring the negative ones
- Talking only about the negative aspects of the relationship and ignoring the positive ones
- Feeling life is meaningless
- Loss of identity or purpose
- Inability to perform tasks of daily living
- Delusions or hallucinations

Be Intentional with Overcoming Grief

Overcoming grief takes time because humans are wired for connection. We become attached to others because that helps us to survive and thrive. When someone we are attached to goes away, either by death or by choice, our emotional brains become overfired through looking for him or her, leaving us vulnerable to depression. Therefore, to overcome grief we must be intentional. Healing will be easier if your brain is better, so make sure to keep a watchful eye on behaviors that either help healing or prevent it. Here are some simple additional steps:

- *Start as soon as possible.* People may tell you to wait, but if you fell and broke your arm, when would you want to start healing? Immediately! There's no advantage to putting off the healing process.

- *Keep a brain-healthy routine.* It's especially important to eat brain-healthy food, take supplements, exercise, and sleep.

- *Discover what was left unsaid or unfinished, and write it down.* That way it will not endlessly spin in your mind. Talk to others about what you wish had been different so you can learn from it.

- *Be on the alert for an ANT invasion*—especially the Guilt-Beating and Blaming species (see chapter 5, pages 102–106).

- : **15** *Write out the story of what happened.* Each day for four days,
  MINUTES   spend 15 minutes getting the story out, making sure to list
  both the positives ("He is no longer suffering") and negatives
  ("I miss her so much it hurts") of the situation. Writing has helped
  children and refugees deal with grief,[34] and it has been shown to
  decrease feelings of loneliness and help improve mood.[35] In one study,
  bereaved people who had lost someone to an accidental death or
  homicide wrote for 15 minutes a day for four days, either about the
  loss or about something trivial. Afterward, those who had written
  about the loss reported less anxiety and depression and greater grief
  recovery than those who had written about trivialities.[36]

- *Reach out for social support.* Therapy and support groups can help you
  build skills to overcome grief.

- *Breathe with your belly.* When you get anxious or short of breath,
  belly breathing can help you calm down or catch your breath (see
  chapter 1, pages 14–16).

- *Consider supplements.* As discussed in the last chapter, loss and rejection
  are felt in the same part of the brain as physical pain. Supplements such
  as s-adenosyl-methionine (SAMe), curcumins, magnesium, and omega-3
  fatty acids help physical pain and may also help emotional pain.

- *Get any chest pain checked out.* Chest pain is particularly common
  in grief.[37] Stress hormones can make our hearts beat in an abnormal
  rhythm,[38] which can cause chest pain. When I went through a
  period of grief, my chest hurt so badly I thought I had heart disease.
  I didn't. But after my assistant Kim lost her fiancé to a heart attack,
  she started to have chest pain. When she had it evaluated, the doctors
  discovered her coronary arteries were more than 90 percent blocked.
  She did have heart disease, which responded very well to treatment. It
  turned out that the death of her fiancé may have saved her life. If you
  experience chest pain, get a physical. If your heart is fine, practicing
  deep breathing, hand warming, guided imagery, and hypnosis can
  calm your brain, as can taking 250–400 mg of magnesium glycinate
  two to three times a day.

- *Deal with triggers as they come up.* Getting triggered is particularly common in grief, especially when the person or pet you lost can occupy every fun place in your brain. Whenever you get triggered by an anniversary, birthday, holiday, place, song, or smell, don't try to block the feeling. Allow it to wash over you, cry if tears start to flow, and let yourself be grateful for the memory. Make sure to correct any negative thoughts that tag along with the painful feelings.

- *Be patient.* No one does grief perfectly. I lost someone important to me about 12 years ago. I knew many of the right things to do, but I still suffered for several months and could not get the person out of my head. Ultimately, reading Byron Katie's book *Loving What Is*, which elegantly teaches you not to believe every stupid thought you have, was incredibly helpful. Be patient and forgive yourself as you work through the hard times.

What Would the Other Person Want for You?

Recently, my wife, Tana, and I took our 14-year-old daughter Chloe to see the movie *The Shack*. It's a beautiful movie but hard to watch because it's about a little girl who is kidnapped and killed by a sex offender. A parent's greatest fear is losing a child, and this was particularly upsetting for Tana. During an episode of *The Brain Warrior's Way Podcast* that we record together, Tana said, "Losing Chloe has always been my biggest fear. Why? Because I not only love her, I'm a sheepdog and protective by nature. It's my responsibility to protect her. *The Shack* is about forgiveness, and as I watched, I kept wrestling with myself [about what I would do if this happened to Chloe]. *No, I wouldn't be able to do it.* Then the movie would make an impactful point, and I would waver . . . *I'd forgive this person.* Then, all of a sudden, I'm back to *No, I wouldn't be able to do it* . . . I'm watching this with my daughter, and she saw me crying and she looked at me; it was almost like she could read my mind. She said something so powerful to me."

What Chloe had said to Tana was this: "I know you're thinking that you would want to go find that person and do something awful to him. You can't do that; I'm telling you, you can never do that."

Tana was stunned and said, "You can't say that . . . you can't say that . . . take it back."

Chloe responded, "No, you can't, because I would be so disappointed. I would be so upset."

Tana said, "Take it back right now."

Chloe said, "No, because if I did have any way of knowing, I would be so disappointed, because it would ruin your life. The only thing that would ever make me happy is knowing you found some way to make sense of it and some way to be happy again."

When my patients are experiencing grief, I often ask them what their loved one would have wanted for them: "Would they want you to spend your life angry, miserable, and seeking revenge; or would they want you to find peace? Would they want you to find love and joy?" Chloe's message to her mother blew my mind.

19 Things Not to Say to a Grieving Person

- "How are you doing?" (This may come across as dismissive of what he or she is going through.)
- "You'll be okay after a while."
- "I understand how you feel."
- "You shouldn't feel that way."
- "Stop crying."
- "At least he's in a better place; his suffering is over."
- "At least she lived a long life; many people die young."
- "She brought this on herself."
- "Aren't you over him yet? He has been dead for a while now."
- "There is a reason for everything."
- "God's in charge."
- "She was such a good person that God wanted her to be with Him."
- "Just give it time. Time heals." (Time alone does not heal; taking the right steps heals.)
- "You're young; you can still have other children."
- "You'll do better next time in love."
- "It was just a dog or cat. You can get another one."
- "Stay busy. Don't think about it."
- "You have to be strong for your spouse, children, mother, etc." (This diminishes the person's need to take time to heal.)
- "Just move on."

Grief and trauma, at varying levels of intensity, are an inescapable part of the human experience. But we don't have to passively endure the suffering that comes with them. The strategies I've talked about in this chapter will help you get a handle on your pain and begin to feel better.

---

13 Things to Say to (or Do for) a Grieving Person

- "I am so sorry for your loss."
- "I wish I had the right words. Please know I care and am here for you."
- "You and your loved ones are in my prayers."
- "I can't imagine how you feel." Then be quiet and let them tell you about their feelings.
- "I can't imagine how you feel. When I lost my father, I felt . . ." Then listen without judgment or criticism. Use the active listening technique discussed in chapter 6 (see pages 134–136).
- "I'm here for you." Better yet, if there is something specific they need, ask if you can do it for them. Ask if you can make phone calls or send e-mails on their behalf.
- "I'd like to attend the funeral." Going to the service is often an important sign of support.
- "Want to talk about what happened?" Many people avoid this question, but it helps grieving people to explain their feelings, if they desire, and having a compassionate ear can help them process it more accurately.
- Just be present.
- Share a memory.
- Be empathetic. It is okay for you to show your feelings.
- Continue connecting, even after a few months. Many people are inundated with cards, calls, or visits in the first few weeks, but they need support long after the funeral is over.
- Listen for guilt. People who are grieving often feel guilty and wish they had done something differently. *The Grief Recovery Handbook* by John James and Russell Friedman, which has a wealth of information to help people with grief, includes

a wonderful example of helping someone with guilt. This is a dialogue between a grieving parent and a grief specialist with the authors' Grief Recovery Institute:

Griever: My son committed suicide. I feel so guilty.
Institute: Did you ever do anything with intent to harm your son?
Griever: No. (*This is an almost universal response.*)
Institute: The dictionary definition of guilt implies intent to harm. Since you had no intent to harm, can you put the "G" word back in the dictionary? You are probably devastated enough by the death of your son, you don't need to add to it by hurting yourself with an incorrect word that distorts your feelings.
Griever: Really? I never thought of it that way.
Institute: Are there some things that you wish had ended *different, better, or more?*
Griever: Oh, yes.[39]

SEVEN STRATEGIES TO ELIMINATE THE HURTS THAT HAUNT YOU

1. Consider Eye Movement Desensitization and Reprocessing (EMDR).

2. Try trauma-focused cognitive behavioral therapy (TF-CBT).

3. Write the story of what happened in the context of your life.

4. Don't block your painful feelings.

5. Break the bonds of the past.

6. Strive for "posttraumatic growth."

7. Consider using oxytocin, which has been found to be helpful for both grief and emotional trauma.

TINY HABITS THAT CAN HELP YOU FEEL BETTER FAST—AND LEAD TO BIG CHANGES

:03-45
MINUTES

Each of these habits takes just a few minutes. They are anchored to something you do (or think or feel) so that they are more likely to become automatic. Once you do the behaviors you want, find a way to make yourself feel good about them—draw a happy face, pump your fist, or do whatever feels natural. Emotion helps the brain to remember.

1. Whenever I feel upset, I will cross my arms and stroke down from my shoulders to my lower forearms. (This stimulates both sides of the brain and helps to have a calming effect on the mind.)

2. When I feel a wave of a traumatic memory or grief coming on, I will observe myself and write down any negative thoughts that come to my mind and challenge them.

3. When painful memories from the past get stuck in my brain, I will write them out from an adult perspective, which can stop the thoughts from circling in my head.

4. When I struggle with grief or a traumatic memory, I will read Rumi's poem "The Guest House."

5. When I feel anxious, I will practice five diaphragmatic breaths to calm myself.

6. When memories of a traumatic event surface, I will ask myself what I am thinking or feeling. Then in my mind, I will go back to the very first time in my life that I can remember thinking those thoughts or feeling those feelings to see if my past is infecting the present. If it is, I will say to myself, "That was then and this is now."

7. When a lost loved one's birthday (or other anniversary) arrives, I will spend time recalling happy memories and be grateful for the time we had together.

8. When I feel upset or lonely, I will call a friend and ask for his or her support.

PART 4

I IS FOR INSPIRATION

True inspiration gets at the spiritual side of health. It's about knowing why you are on the planet, and the meaning and purpose underlying why you do what you do. Knowing and acting on your "why" is critical to living each day with joy. This section will introduce you to the neuroscience of passion and show you how to know your purpose in just a few minutes.

CHAPTER 8

CREATE IMMEDIATE AND LASTING JOY

PROTECT YOUR BRAIN'S PLEASURE CENTERS TO LIVE WITH PASSION AND PURPOSE AND AVOID ADDICTIONS AND DEPRESSION

Nothing is as important as passion. No matter what
you want to do with your life, be passionate.

JON BON JOVI

On October 15, 1988, Kirk Gibson came to the plate as a pinch hitter in the ninth inning of Game One of the World Series between the Los Angeles Dodgers and the Oakland A's. Gibson, who was a star for the Dodgers that year, had injured both of his legs and didn't play in the earlier innings of the game. Now he was facing Dennis Eckersley, one of the best closers in the American League, who had saved 45 games. The Dodgers were behind four runs to three, and there were two outs and a runner on first base.

When Gibson came to the plate, famed Dodger announcer Vin Scully said, "All year long, they looked to him to light the fire . . . and all year long he answered the demands, until he was physically unable to start tonight with two bad legs—the bad left hamstring and the swollen right knee. And with two outs, you talk about a roll of the dice . . . this is it."

Gibson worked the count to three balls and two strikes, and then the whole world heard Scully's incredible voice cry, "High fly ball into right field. She i-i-i-is . . . GONE!" Scully then said nothing for more than a minute, while the cameras told the story of the Dodgers' win: pandemonium on the field at Chavez Ravine in Los Angeles, the crowd going wild, and players pouring out of the dugout, jumping into the air, and hugging one another.[1] Over and over, sports fans have watched the clip of Kirk Gibson double pumping his right arm as he rounds second base with a look of pure joy on his face—an iconic play that will forever be remembered in sports history. I have thought about that moment many times in the past 30 years.

In 1991, when we first started the brain imaging work we do at Amen Clinics, all of us were very excited. The scans gave us insights that allowed us to help many treatment-resistant patients get better, faster than ever before. In one case, we treated a boy who had violent episodes that had led to three psychiatric hospitalizations. His scan showed he was likely having seizure activity on the left side of his brain. Once put on antiseizure medication, he became calmer, sweeter, and more in control of his emotions. The treatment literally changed the trajectory of his life. That gave us a home-run feeling. We also treated a woman who had been diagnosed with Alzheimer's disease, whose children were about to put her in a senior care facility to ensure her safety. She had left something cooking on the stove and almost burned her house down. Her scan revealed that she did not have Alzheimer's disease. Instead, she was likely suffering from a severe depression that masqueraded as Alzheimer's. With treatment for depression, she got her memory and independence back. A double arm-pump moment of joy for us, the patient, and her family. There was another patient diagnosed with Alzheimer's disease, this time a man, who was deteriorating month by month, but his scan showed he had enlarged, fluid-filled spaces in his brain. When the pressure on his brain was relieved by shunting out the excess fluid, his memory and cognitive function returned and he had another decade of high-quality life. Pure joy—for him and for us.

There were many moments when we felt like Gibson as he rounded second base. Of course, it wasn't always like that. But the stories of change imprinted lasting joy in the brains of our team members, which caused us to pay close attention to what we were learning. Those incredible feelings helped us develop passion for and purpose in our work, despite brutal criticism in the beginning from some of our colleagues. The word *passion* comes from the Latin word *passionem*, which means "suffering" or "enduring." Pursuing your passion requires endurance and may involve suffering, thanks to the way our brains work.

The passion and love I had for our patients and work helped me deal with the criticism, as did a quotation from Dr. Viktor Frankl, a psychiatrist, a Nazi concentration camp survivor, and the author of *Man's Search for Meaning*: "Life is never made unbearable by circumstances, but only by lack of meaning and purpose."[2]

Living with passion and purpose is a critical "feel better fast" strategy. This chapter will look at what neuroscience says about purpose, meaning, passion, and love (including new love) and the impact these have on the health of your brain. It will also look at what helps and hurts your pleasure centers, so you can avoid addictions and depression, and what happens when love, passion, or purpose goes wrong. It will help you find out how to know your purpose and actualize it in your life.

PURPOSE CAN HELP YOU FEEL BETTER FAST

Does having meaning and purpose help you feel better fast and make it last? In her research, University of Wisconsin psychologist Carol Ryff found that those who had a higher sense of purpose in life—defined as "the psychological tendency to derive meaning from life's experiences and to possess a sense of intentionality and goal directedness that guides behavior"—had

- Better mental health
- Less depression
- Greater happiness
- More satisfaction
- More personal growth and self-acceptance
- Better-quality sleep
- Longevity

Over time, researcher Patricia Boyle and colleagues from Rush University in Chicago studied more than 900 people and found that higher scores on this "purpose" scale were associated with

- A reduced risk of Alzheimer's disease
- Less mild cognitive impairment
- A slower rate of cognitive decline in old age[3]

Other researchers have also associated purpose in life with a longer lifespan. One group measured "eudemonic wellbeing," a type of well-being that relates to your sense of control and purpose, and to feeling that what you do is worthwhile. The scientists followed 9,050 people over eight and a half years and found that those who had higher scores on eudemonic wellbeing were

30 percent less likely to die during the follow-up period compared to those with the lowest scores. They also walked faster and had greater grip strength, two signs of healthy vigor.[4] As strength of purpose increases, so do physical strength and endurance. Purpose in life has also been associated with lower risk of cardiovascular disease[5] and stroke, higher levels of immunity, and better-quality sleep, with less sleep apnea and fewer restless leg symptoms.[6] Scoring higher in "purpose in life" also makes it less likely that negative social media issues (such as not getting the number of likes you might want on a post) will affect your self-esteem.[7] A lack of purpose has been associated with negative health indicators, including higher levels of the stress hormone cortisol, increased markers of inflammation, lower HDL cholesterol levels, and greater amounts of abdominal fat.

WHERE PASSION LIVES IN THE BRAIN

Purpose helps us find meaning in life, which in turn fuels our passion for the things we find meaningful. Passion, purpose, and meaning all work in the drive, motivation, and pleasure centers deep in the brain. These areas include the ventral tegmental area (VTA), nucleus accumbens and caudate nucleus (both part of the basal ganglia), and substantia nigra (see figure on page 182). These regions are powered by the neurotransmitter dopamine. When Gibson hit his ninth-inning home run, dopamine flooded his pleasure centers, prompting him to double pump his fist. The basal ganglia integrate emotion and movement, which is why we jump when we're excited or freeze when we get scared. When dopamine floods the basal ganglia, players throw up their arms, yell with joy, or run onto the baseball diamond as a group. Likewise, when an actor gets a standing ovation, an attorney wins an important case, a child brings home an excellent report card, or a pastor delivers a passionate sermon, dopamine is released, activating the pleasure centers—and triggering good feelings.

Along with dopamine, the neurotransmitter serotonin also plays an important role in love, passion, and pleasure. Serotonin, released by the raphe nuclei deep in the brain, is involved with mood, sleep, shifting attention, appetite, bowel function, and social relationships. It also helps to regulate anxiety and happiness.

Dopamine and serotonin tend to counterbalance each other in the brain. As one goes up, the other generally goes down. Antidepressants that increase serotonin, such as Lexapro (escitalopram), Prozac (fluoxetine), and Zoloft

HOW DIFFERENT LEVELS OF DOPAMINE AND SEROTONIN AFFECT BEHAVIOR AND MOOD

NEUROTRANSMITTER LEVEL	DOPAMINE* EFFECTS	SEROTONIN† EFFECTS
Healthy	Feelings of pleasure; feeling motivated and focused	Feeling happy and optimistic, with healthy sleep and bowel function
Too Low	Higher incidence of depression and apathy; low levels are common in Parkinson's disease due to the death of dopamine-producing cells in the brain's substantia nigra	Depression, anxiety, obsession, insomnia, irritable bowel issues, and cravings for sweets, which increase serotonin in the brain but also can make you gain weight
Too High	Feeling anxious, agitated, aggressive; confusion; racing thoughts; trouble sleeping; poor decision-making	Feeling passive, apathetic; lower motivation; decreased sexual desire
Supplements	S-adenosyl-methionine (SAMe), L-tyrosine, bacopa, mucuna	5-hydroxytryptophan (5-HTP), saffron, L-tryptophan

* Methamphetamine abuse releases massive amounts of dopamine and can make someone paranoid and aggressive. Of the 100 murderers I have scanned, 40 of them committed the crime under the influence of methamphetamine.

† Ecstasy use releases high amounts of serotonin and can increase empathy, decrease anxiety, enhance sensory experiences, and make people feel blissful, but when the effects wear off, it can leave users feeling very depressed and foggy-headed or confused.

(sertraline), can improve mood and decrease anxiety but can also decrease sexual desire and motivation. Antidepressants that increase dopamine, such as Wellbutrin (bupropion), boost sex drive and can enhance focus and motivation, but they may trigger anxiety. Stimulant medications that boost dopamine, such as Adderall (amphetamine salts) or Ritalin (methylphenidate), can increase focus and motivation but can also decrease appetite and cause some people to feel obsessed.

DOPAMINE AND SEROTONIN PATHWAY

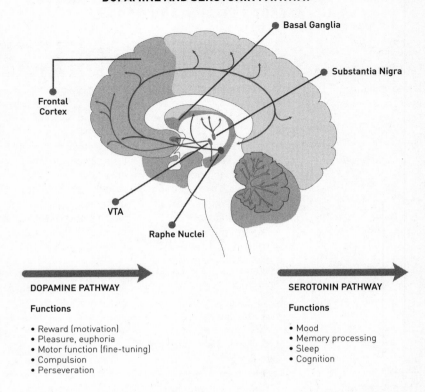

DOPAMINE PATHWAY

Functions

• Reward (motivation)
• Pleasure, euphoria
• Motor function (fine-tuning)
• Compulsion
• Perseveration

SEROTONIN PATHWAY

Functions

• Mood
• Memory processing
• Sleep
• Cognition

SEX, DRUGS, ROCK 'N' ROLL, SMARTPHONES, VIDEO GAMES, . . . AND THE BRAIN

Living in Southern California, I've had the opportunity to treat many famous performers, including rock stars, singers, songwriters, actors, athletes, and pastors. Many have experienced worldwide fame, which releases massive amounts of dopamine, stimulating their pleasure centers over and over as strangers recognize them everywhere they go, often begging for autographs or screaming their names. Repeated, intense activation of the pleasure centers wears them out, much like a cocaine high that lessens with frequent use of the drug. Over time, if these stars are not careful, it takes more and more dopamine-producing activities—more fame, falling in love, affairs with multiple partners, drugs, racing cars, and even stealing—just to feel normal or not to feel depressed. So many Hollywood actors, singers, sports figures, and celebrity pastors have followed this tragic pattern that I have a prayer for young stars-in-the-making: "God, please don't let them be famous before their brains develop"—which, as we have seen, is usually around the age of 25.

If the pleasure centers become damaged by overuse, toxins, or head trauma, or if dopamine is excessively high for prolonged periods, the ventral tegmental area, nucleus accumbens, and basal ganglia become less responsive. The dopamine high stops being as intense as it once was. This increases the risk of depression—or addiction to substances that people turn to in order to fix the bad feelings caused by the numbing of these brain regions. The addictive substances include nicotine, alcohol, methamphetamines, cocaine, pornography, and food (specifically, foods high in sugar and fat). When a powerful release of dopamine hits the pleasure centers, increases euphoria, and then wears off, people can feel flat or depressed and start craving a way out of the bad feelings. As a result, they reengage in the actions that intensely ramped up their dopamine levels in the first place. Over time, it takes more and more of the substance to get the same response. This is the cycle of addiction.

THE ADDICTION CYCLE

Engage in actions to increase dopamine

Feel high or pleasure

When dopamine wears off, experience withdrawal, leaving you feeling flat or depressed

Reengage in dopamine-producing behavior, even if it is bad for you

With intense stimulation, pleasure centers need more and more excitement in order to feel anything at all

THE CYCLE OF ADDICTION

Many forces in our changing society, besides fame, are putting excessive demands on our pleasure centers. Text messaging, e-mail, video games, social media, television, and using multiple electronic devices can overstimulate our pleasure centers in the same way that cocaine does, psychologist Archibald Hart warned in *Thrilled to Death: How the Endless Pursuit of Pleasure Is Leaving Us Numb*.[8] We all know people who are glued to their smartphones even while they are talking to others. For these people, every time their devices ping to signal a new incoming message, it causes a small release of dopamine. Television is all about "breaking news" and quick, high-intensity action (think *Game of Thrones*). Dopamine is constantly released in video gamers as they play, and the games were specifically designed to hook your attention, according to Nir Eyal's *Hooked*. As video game and technology usage goes up, so do depression and obesity.[9] Ian Bogost, famed video game designer (Cow Clicker and Cruel 2 B Kind) and chair of media studies and professor of interactive computing at the Georgia Institute of Technology, called these new habit-forming technologies "the cigarette of this century" and warned of their "equally addictive and potentially destructive side effects."[10]

And that's not all. Have you ever wondered why there are so many horror films? Why, in addition to the movie *Saw*, are there also *Saw II*, *Saw III*, *Saw IV*, *Saw V*, *Saw VI*, *Saw 3D* (VII), and *Jigsaw* (VIII)? I once asked a producer why he made *Piranha 3D*, a horror film about a horde of razor-teeth-equipped prehistoric piranhas, released by a tremor beneath a lake, that wreak havoc on bikini-clad coeds on spring break. He said, "People want them, they go see them, and they make money." Even just watching the trailer will give you a dopamine jolt.

In short, our devices,[11] online communities, games, TV-watching habits, and scary movies are wearing out our pleasure centers and changing our brains. Our fast-paced, pleasure-seeking lifestyle is robbing us of the ability to experience joy from the simple things in life. Things that once made us happy—such as a smile from a friend, a glorious sunset, or a great tennis match—have lost the power to move us. Our excessive pursuit of constant thrills, Archibald Hart suggested, may contribute to emotional problems, such as depression and anxiety, as well as addictions to drugs, alcohol, Internet gambling, pornography, and compulsive shopping.[12]

Even new love, for millennials at least, has turned into a video game. Amen Clinics collaborated with *The Dr. Oz Show* on a brain imaging–Tinder experiment with several thirtysomething men and women to determine the effect of the dating app on mood and focus. If they were lucky enough to get a "swipe right"—meaning someone using the dating app liked their pictures and short bio—it increased activity in the pleasure and mood centers of their brains. If, however, there were fewer "swipes right" and more "swipes left," indicating rejection, their brains were more vulnerable to pain and depression.

In 2005, anthropologist Helen Fisher from Rutgers University published a groundbreaking study using functional MRI (fMRI) brain scans of college students who viewed pictures of someone who was special to them along with those of acquaintances. The pictures of their loved ones activated the pleasure centers in their brains, rich in the "feel-good" neurotransmitter dopamine that's involved with attention and the motivation to pursue and acquire rewards.[13] That is why, when you do find a match on a dating site or at work or church, the high of new love can feel like an addiction with its euphoria, craving, withdrawal, and the need for more and more to feel good.[14] New love works in the same areas of the brain as cocaine and can cause people to feel giddy, anxious, uncertain, or obsessed; irrationally notice the positive and completely miss the negative; make poor decisions; have trouble sleeping; and feel as if they are on a roller coaster.

When new love is rejected, the brain's pain centers are activated, making it more likely that people will drink alcohol or use drugs to counteract the negative feelings. Alternatively, if the high of new love simply wears off, the other person's faults become easy to see, and couples can more rationally decide whether to stay together or separate. It is for this reason that you should be very cautious about marrying someone within the first few months of meeting. You can't be certain if you're marrying the actual person or a dopamine-induced illusion.

New research also shows that lasting love, even after 20 years or more, can still activate the brain's pleasure centers, but in different ways than new love. Lasting love provides a deeper sense of bonding and connection, peace, happiness, and warmth—more akin to the warmth of heroin than the jolt of cocaine. The feeling of being high on heroin was once anonymously described as "being cradled to sleep by God, wrapped up in a warm, luxurious blanket that shields you from all your worldly fears, angers, and pains." While the pain of a new-love breakup feels awful, leaving a long-term love relationship is typically much worse, more akin to heroin withdrawal. Many people describe it as having their skin ripped off while they are awake. It is often associated with symptoms similar to heroin withdrawal as well—diarrhea, nausea, depression, and a sense of hopelessness that can go on for months, together with anxiety, panic, and sleeplessness. Cleary, love's connection with our pleasure centers is powerful.

Research has also shown that having passion for your work[15] and even being a sports fanatic[16] can activate the reward or pleasure circuits deep within the brain, and like love, these experiences can be extremely positive—or negative. They can make us feel balanced or unbalanced. As we mentioned in chapter 3, at Amen Clinics we did the first and largest brain imaging study on active and retired NFL players. As you might imagine, we saw high levels of brain damage in players, but we also saw the possibility of recovery in 80 percent of them.[17] In addition, depression was very high in these players— four times the national average. Brain trauma (from hits and concussions) is certainly one of the causes of depression, but many of the players also clearly missed football. They missed the camaraderie, the game itself, the competition, the money, the adulation of the crowds, and the fame. When the game was gone from their lives, the dopamine drip of positive football pleasure chemicals was also gone, which contributed to their depression.

Whenever one door of love, passion, or purpose closes, it is critical to find others to replace it with in order to keep your pleasure centers functioning and releasing dopamine in a healthy way. If you don't, you are more prone to low feelings and depression. That's why depression is more common after retirement, especially when retirees don't find a new source of passion and purpose. In fact, although retirement can initially boost your health, it later increases your risk of clinical depression by 40 percent while raising your chances of being diagnosed with a physical condition or illness by 60 percent.[18]

HOW TO PROTECT YOUR PLEASURE CENTERS TO FEEL BETTER FAST AND CREATE LIFELONG JOY

With so many diversions in our lives that have the potential to negatively affect our pleasure centers and keep us from experiencing purpose and passion for the things we value most, we need to act. Here are some simple steps to take in order to protect your pleasure centers and keep them healthy:

- Limit or completely eliminate the use of constantly stimulating devices and activities, such as smartphones, gaming, shopping, pornography, scary movies, and high-risk activities (see page 187 for a longer list).
- Engage in regular physical exercise, especially something you love that does not endanger your brain, such as dancing, swimming, or tennis.
- Meditate—it protects the brain while enhancing a sense of well-being.
- Make time to laugh—humor enhances the pleasure centers without wearing them out.
- Connect meaningful activities with pleasure, such as volunteering for activities you love. One example: I love table tennis and enjoy keeping score for others during tournaments.

- **:02**
  MINUTES Start every day by thinking of three things for which you are grateful (a small dopamine drip) and one person you appreciate (another small dopamine drip), then reach out through text or e-mail to tell that person you appreciate him or her. (See chapter 5, pages 110–111.) You are building a bridge of gratitude. If the person responds, it is yet another, maybe bigger, dopamine drip.
- Seek pleasure in the little things in your life, such as a walk with a friend, holding hands with your spouse, a great meal, or a meaningful church service.
- Eat foods that contain dopamine-boosting properties, such as chicken, turkey, seafood, almonds, pumpkin and sesame seeds, turmeric, oregano,[19] vegetables (for folate and magnesium), olive oil, and green tea.
- Consider supplements to support dopamine, such as omega-3 fatty acids, SAMe, and green tea extract. Don't try them all at once; try them one at a time to see which ones work best for you. For more information, see chapter 10.

POSITIVE THINGS THAT ACTIVATE DOPAMINE	POTENTIALLY NEGATIVE THINGS THAT ACTIVATE DOPAMINE
Meaning and purpose	Jumping out of airplanes
Lasting love	Repeatedly falling in love
Volunteering	High-risk sports (e.g., helicopter skiing)
Relationships	Extramarital affairs
New learning	Excessive video games
Traveling	Pornography
Spiritual experiences	Cocaine
Gratitude/appreciation	Fame
Winning by striving to be your best	Winning by hurting others
Losing (when it motivates practice)	Losing (when it causes pain)
Digital discipline	Undisciplined digital behavior
Pumpkin seeds	Methamphetamines
Green tea	Alcohol
SAMe	Scary movies
L-tyrosine	Gossiping
Bacopa	
Omega-3 fatty acids	

FINDING PURPOSE AND MEANING: DR. VIKTOR FRANKL'S CONTRIBUTION

He who has a why to live can bear almost any how.
FRIEDRICH NIETZSCHE

Having purpose in life will give you a constant, never-ending drip of dopamine. This has been my personal experience over the past three decades. It starts by knowing what gives your life a deep sense of meaning. As we've mentioned, Dr. Viktor Frankl was a psychiatrist and World War II concentration camp survivor. He was also the father of logotherapy, a form of psychotherapy based on the idea that humans are strongly motivated to live with purpose. He believed that we can find meaning as a result of responding genuinely and compassionately to life's challenges. My friend Dr. Jeff Zeig, who personally knew Dr. Frankl, told me that he heard Dr. Frankl say, "If it is meaningful, I do it. If it is not meaningful, I don't have time for it."[20]

> *"If it is meaningful, I do it.*
> *If it is not meaningful, I don't have time for it."*
> *—Dr. Viktor Frankl*

> *In a world of constant, meaningless distractions, this is*
> *incredibly important advice. Ask yourself, What am I doing*
> *that is meaningful that I could do more of, and what am*
> *I doing that is meaningless that I could do less of?*

Before World War II, Frankl, who was living in Austria, applied for and received a visa to go to the United States. His sister also got a visa and emigrated to Australia just as Hitler's power was growing and the barbarism in Austria was increasing. With his visa in hand, Frankl was in a quandary about whether to stay or leave. One day he was ruminating about his choice—staying to protect his parents or leaving to escape the concentration camps and continue with his work. At his parents' home he saw a piece of marble marked with one of the Hebrew letters from the Ten Commandments. His father had found it at the site of the largest synagogue in Vienna, which had been burned.[21] Frankl asked his father, "What letter is this?" His father said, "Well, it could only be one of the Commandments, 'Honor thy father and mother.'" At that moment, Frankl decided to give up his visa. As he explained to Dr. Zeig, "You could look at [the marble] as just a piece of calcium carbonate—it was nothing." But when he could project meaning into that moment, it changed the direction and destiny of his life.[22]

When Frankl was taken to his first concentration camp, he brought a manuscript, which he hid inside the lining of his coat in an attempt to save it. Of course, as soon as he arrived at the camp, the guards stripped him and he lost everything. This experience led him to break from the then-popular theories of Dr. Abraham Maslow. If you remember your college introductory psychology course, you may recall that Maslow created a "hierarchy of needs." He theorized that unless your basic needs were met, you could not do things that were transcendent. Frankl believed that Maslow was wrong—that even in the most horrific, barbaric circumstances, there was still the possibility that you could create meaning. In the camps, Frankl saw people who were not safe, were without proper clothing, had little food, and were stripped of every dignity still make heroic contributions if they could find the purpose in their situations. He believed that people in all circumstances have a choice in how they respond, even to suffering. He also disagreed with the behaviorists at the time, who believed that humans responded to a stimulus with a predictable response. Stephen Covey has written about finding words that he believed crystallize Frankl's teaching on suffering: "Between stimulus and response, there is a space. In that space lies our freedom and our power to choose our response. In our response lies our growth and our happiness."[23]

Resilience, Frankl believed, stemmed from love. When he was dealing with frostbite and swollen legs, didn't have warm clothes, and had to work in ice-cold conditions, Frankl said that he survived by looking up at the sky and thinking of his wife, Tilly. He would focus on love and recognize that it was the most profound and meaningful virtue. It was the central point that could help him survive the horrors he was living through. When you are facing a difficult situation, having something purposeful to focus on, particularly love, crystallizes resilience. To recover from the horror of being in the camps, Frankl knew that meaning and purpose were a critical part of the healing process.

Frankl believed there were three ways to create meaning:

- Purposeful work, or being productive—asking questions such as "Why is the world a better place because I am here?" or "What do I contribute?"
- Love—loving the people who are central to our lives
- Courage in the face of difficulty—shouldering whatever difficult fate we have and helping others shoulder theirs[24]

In the midst of difficulty, Frankl said, "everything can be taken from a man but one thing: the last of the human freedoms—to choose one's attitude in any given set of circumstances, to choose one's own way."[25] He encouraged his patients to see meaning in life's moments and to direct their focus away from painful ones to more appealing circumstances. "Love is the ultimate and the highest goal to which man can aspire," Frankl said.[26] "Self-transcendence provides a pathway to ultimate meaning."[27]

He also helped people find meaning through

- Creative values—what we create, achieve, and accomplish
- Experiential values—experiencing what is good, true, and beautiful, or fully knowing another human
- Attitudinal values—looking for meaning in situations, even those that appear meaningless[28]

There is a story, for example, about Frankl treating an older doctor who could not stop grieving the loss of his wife. He asked the man, "What would have happened, Doctor, if you had died first, and your wife would have had to survive you?"

"Oh," the man replied, "for her this would have been terrible; how she would have suffered!"

Frankl said, "You see, Doctor, such a suffering has been spared her, and it was you who have spared her this suffering—to be sure, at the price that now you have to survive and mourn her."

The man said nothing but shook Frankl's hand and left his office. Frankl said, "When we are no longer able to change a situation . . . we are challenged to change ourselves. . . . In some way, suffering ceases to be suffering at the moment it finds a meaning, such as the meaning of a sacrifice."[29] While we can't avoid suffering, we can choose how to respond to it. When we discover meaning in it, we can move forward.

ONE-PAGE MIRACLE: HOW TO FOCUS ON LOVE, MEANING, AND PURPOSE

In my work with patients, I ask all of them to get clarity of purpose by completing an exercise I call the One-Page Miracle (OPM). Completing it allows you to define what you want and to focus like a laser on your life's meaning and purpose.

When you tell your brain what you want, your balanced brain will help you align your behavior to get it! Whatever your brain sees, it helps to make happen. If you focus on negativity, you will feel depressed. If you focus on fear, you are likely to feel anxious. If you focus on achieving your goals with passion and purpose, you are much more likely to achieve them. Too many people are thrown around by the whims of the day, rather than using their brains to guide their paths.

The OPM will help guide your thoughts, words, and actions. I call it the One-Page Miracle because I have seen this exercise quickly focus and change many people's lives.

To develop your own OPM, ask yourself what you truly want in the following areas, including how those areas give you love, meaning, and purpose.

What do I want in my relationships with my

partner _____

_____

children _____

_____

parents _____

_____

siblings _____

_____

extended family _____

_____

friends _____

_____

What do I want in my work? _____

_____

_____

What do I want in my finances? _____

_____

_____

What do I want for myself in these arenas?

Physical _____

_____

Emotional _____

_____

Spiritual _____

_____

Creative _____

_____

Experiential _____

_____

Attitudinal _____

_____

Also, ask yourself,

What makes me happy? _____

_____

What do I naturally pay attention to? _____

_____

What kind of books do I read? _____

_____

CREATE IMMEDIATE AND LASTING JOY   *   193

What do I love to talk or learn about? _____

_____

What work would I do for free? _____

_____

What boosts dopamine for me—gives me a jolt of joy and pleasure?

_____

_____

What are my strengths? _____

_____

Where can I add value or make a difference? _____

_____

How do I believe my life will be measured—by my friends, my family, and my God?

_____

_____

_____

KNOW YOUR PURPOSE IN FIVE MINUTES

:05
MINUTES One of my favorite TEDx talks is on how to find your life's purpose in five minutes, by Adam Leipzig, CEO of Entertainment Media Partners; it has more than 10 million views.[30] Leipzig started by telling a story about his 25th college reunion at Yale University. He said he made an astounding discovery: 80 percent of his privileged, well-off, powerful friends were unhappy with their lives, despite being on their second spouses and second houses. The difference between them and the 20 percent who were happy was "knowing their purpose," which makes sense given the research we've discussed. To know your purpose, Leipzig said, you have to know the answers to five simple questions:

1. Who are you? What is your name?
2. What do you love to do? Examples include writing, cooking, designing, creating, speaking, teaching, crunching numbers, etc. To get clarity of purpose, ask yourself, "What is the one thing I do where I feel supremely qualified to teach others?"
3. Whom do you do it for? Or, how does your work connect you to others?
4. What do those people want or need from you?
5. How do they change as a result of what you do?

When I answer these questions, it looks like this:

1. My name is Daniel.
2. I love optimizing people's brains and inspiring people to care about their brains. I love doing it within the context of our team at Amen Clinics.
3. We do it for our families as well as for those who come to our clinics, read our books, or watch our shows.
4. The people we touch want to suffer less, feel better, be sharper, and have greater control over their lives. They want better brains and better lives.
5. As a result of what we do, people change by having better brains and better lives. They suffer less, become happier and healthier, and pass it on to others.

Notice that only two of the five questions are about you; three are about others.

There is a Chinese saying that goes, "If you want happiness for an hour, take a nap. If you want happiness for a day, go fishing. If you want happiness for a year, inherit a fortune. If you want happiness for a lifetime, help somebody." For centuries, the greatest thinkers have suggested the same thing: Happiness is found in helping others.

Leipzig closed the talk by teaching us a powerful technique. He said, "When you're at a gathering and someone asks you, 'What do you do?' answer by telling them the answer to question number five." In my example, when people ask me what I do, I say, "As a result of what we do, people have better brains and better lives. They suffer less, become happier and healthier, and pass it on to others." By answering that simple question, I get to share my life purpose with everyone I meet, which certainly produces a bit of dopamine to press on my pleasure centers. How would you answer that question?

FIVE STRATEGIES TO CREATE LASTING JOY AND FEEL BETTER FAST

This is the true joy in life, the being used for a purpose recognized by yourself as a mighty one; the being thoroughly worn out before you are thrown on the scrapheap; the being a force of Nature instead of a feverish, selfish little clod of ailments and grievances complaining that the world will not devote itself to making you happy.

GEORGE BERNARD SHAW

1. Focus on what you want—on what gives you passion and purpose.

:02 MINUTES Read your OPM daily and ask yourself, *Is my behavior getting me what I want?* With my wife, Tana, for example, I deeply desire a lifelong relationship that is kind, caring, loving, supportive, and passionate. I don't always feel like it in the moment, but that is what I always want. Having a close relationship with her will help me feel happy and stable and is incredibly important to my sense of meaning and purpose. Know what you want, write it down, and look at it every day. It will encourage your brain to help make it happen.

2. Limit or completely eliminate low-value dopamine-producing activities or substances that wear out your pleasure centers.

These include

- Caffeine
- Nicotine
- Excessive television
- Excessive video games
- Pornography
- Undisciplined digital behavior
- Scary movies

3. Engage in high-value activities that increase dopamine and strengthen your brain.

Here are a number of examples:[32]

- Sunlight (vitamin D)
- Exercise
- Meditation
- Yoga
- Touch
- Massage therapy
- Pleasurable music
- DHA from fish oil
- Olive oil
- Green tea
- Protein-rich diet
- Turmeric
- Oregano
- Magnesium
- Resveratrol

4. Focus each moment on living with meaning and purpose.

Ask yourself, *Do the foods I am eating, the exercises I am doing, the conversations I am having, and the activities I am engaging in have meaning?* Toward the end of his life, Viktor Frankl would only do things that were deeply significant to him. He received thousands of requests but focused his efforts on just those that were the most meaningful to him. He was afraid of flying, so he actually took up flying small planes to overcome his fear. He once said, "There are some things about myself I don't have to tolerate."[32] His is such a powerful model for living. Look at your day—where are you spending your time? Does it help you reach your OPM goals? Get rid of the things in your life that do not fit your goals.

One of my friends, Larry, an attorney in New York, complained that his three-year-old daughter, Lara, wanted nothing to do with him when he came home. He said, "That must be a girl thing. At that age, they just want their mothers."

"Nonsense," I replied, "you're not spending enough time with her." I knew he was working too late and just using "It's a girl thing" as a rationalization.

He complained that there were too many things happening at work that he could not let go. I had Larry do the One-Page Miracle exercise, and afterward it was clear that his wife and daughter were very important to him. Then I asked him to be aware of all his activities at work for a week. Keeping detailed notes on his activities each day, he could tell he was wasting a lot of time: He walked to the coffee shop twice a day for drinks; three or four times a week he went to lunch with friends; and he constantly took phone calls from colleagues who had questions about their businesses. I asked him to define his work goals and figure out what were the most important things for him to be doing at work. What were the tasks and activities that built and sustained his business? He wrote three things:

1. Take great care of my current clients,
2. Develop new clients, and
3. Spend 10 percent of my time on pro bono work.

I suggested he let go of anything unrelated to these three goals. Then I told him about one of the most powerful exercises I have ever given parents—"special time," where you spend 20 minutes a day with a child, doing something he or she chooses to do. (I describe it in chapter 6, page 139.) Larry did it faithfully every day with Lara, and at work he focused on what was truly important to him. He brought his coffee to work, he limited lunch with friends to once a week, and he screened calls. Within a month, he was coming home earlier, and whenever he walked through the door, Lara ran to her daddy, wrapped her tiny arms around his legs, and hugged him closely. He was happier than ever. Be sure you spend time on the things that matter.

5. Live with the end in mind.

Psychiatrist Elisabeth Kübler-Ross, a pioneer in near-death studies and the author of the groundbreaking book *On Death and Dying*, said, "It is the denial of death that is partially responsible for people living empty, purpose-less lives; for when you live as if you'll live forever, it becomes too easy to postpone the things you know that you must do."[33] If you truly want to live a purposeful life, live with the end in mind. None of us knows when death is going to come, but if you knew you would be dead in a week, a month, a year, or five years, what would matter to you most? Where and with whom would you spend your time? In college I took a death and dying course in which we studied Dr. Kübler-Ross's work. Our final paper was writing our own funeral service, which has had an impact on me ever since. I picked Louis Armstrong's song "When the Saints Go Marching In" as one of the music pieces.

What will matter toward the end of your life? What will you want to be doing? Whom will you want to be with? What will have mattered in your life? If you live that way along the journey, you'll find your life more purposeful, more meaningful, and more filled with love.

TINY HABITS THAT CAN HELP YOU FEEL BETTER FAST—AND LEAD TO BIG CHANGES

:03-30 MINUTES   Each of these habits takes just a few minutes. They are anchored to something you do (or think or feel) so that they are more likely to become automatic. Once you do the behaviors you want, find a way to make yourself feel good about them— draw a happy face, pump your fist, or do whatever feels natural. Emotion helps the brain to remember.

1. When I need to get work done, I will put my smartphone on "Do not disturb" as a discipline to be more focused and to stop the constant pings or drips of dopamine it tries to addict me to.

2. When I am on the train or bus to work, I will read my One-Page Miracle and ask myself, "Will my behavior today get me what I want?"

3. When I start getting upset about something happening in my day, I'll ask myself, "Does this have eternal value?"

4. When it is sunny outdoors, I will take a walk to soak up the sunshine and boost my vitamin D level.

5. When I start the coffee or tea in the morning, I'll think of three things for which I'm grateful.

6. Once a week, I will watch a comedy to boost my dopamine level (*Whose Line Is It Anyway?* is a great show to start with).

7. Before I go to bed, I will write down one purposeful thing I did that day.

FIVE STRATEGIES TO CREATE LASTING JOY AND FEEL BETTER FAST

To live with love, passion, meaning, and purpose over a prolonged period of time,

1. Focus on what you want—on what gives you passion and purpose.

2. Limit or completely eliminate low-value dopamine-producing activities or substances that wear out your pleasure centers.

3. Engage in high-value activities that increase dopamine and strengthen your brain.

4. Focus each moment on living with meaning and purpose.

5. Live with the end in mind.

PART 5

N IS FOR NOURISHMENT

Your brain and mind need a constant source of energy to run your life. Think of nourishment as the battery that powers your body. Certain foods can make you feel great now but not later, while others can help you feel good now *and* later. In chapter 9 we'll look at the Feel Better Fast diet and talk about learning to love the foods that love you. In chapter 10 we'll turn our attention to nutraceuticals (supplements with health benefits) and discuss those that will help boost your focus, memory, and mood—immediately and for a lifetime.

CHAPTER 9

THE FEEL BETTER FAST DIET

FOODS THAT HELP YOU FEEL GREAT NOW AND LATER

The real "weapons of mass destruction" are highly processed, pesticide-sprayed, high-glycemic, low-fiber foodlike substances in plastic containers.

MEMORY RESCUE

With the help of my wife and coworker, I traded the fast food for more nutritious options. At first I was very fearful that I wouldn't be satisfied, or that my cravings would just drive me back to the same old foods and huge portions. But something amazing happened—my cravings disappeared virtually OVERNIGHT. I had no idea that nutritious foods could be so satisfying! It's like someone flipped a switch in my brain!

**RICK, WHO LOST 100 POUNDS IN A YEAR
AND HAS KEPT IT OFF FOR FIVE YEARS**

Victor, 53, had suffered with anxiety, depression, and insomnia for decades. He had seen endocrinologists, psychiatrists, cardiologists, and sleep doctors with no relief. He had tried multiple medications after a suicide attempt, but none of them had helped.

One of the strategies we commonly use at Amen Clinics is to change our patients' diets. We help them eat foods that nourish their brains and bodies—such as colorful vegetables and fruits as well as healthy proteins and fats—and eliminate, at least temporarily, all of the potential troublemaker foods that could be causing negative reactions in their bodies, such as gluten, dairy, corn, soy, food additives and preservatives, and artificial sweeteners. I first heard of this idea more than 25 years ago from my friend Dr. Doris Rapp, who saw remarkable improvements in children with ADHD, aggression, and even autism when they eliminated these foods. Subsequently, I have read a growing number of studies in journals, such as the *Lancet*, reporting significant benefits from dietary interventions.[1] Some of our patients resist—remember, the brain hates change—but we reassure them that when this strategy is conscientiously applied, it can be more effective than almost anything else they could do for their health.

In medical school, like most of my colleagues, I received minimal nutrition education, equivalent to two days out of the 140 weeks it takes to get a medical degree. This state of affairs is insane given that 75 percent of the health care dollars in the United States are spent on chronic, preventable illnesses[2] that stem from our diet and lifestyle choices. Research suggests that our poor choices account for *90 percent* of type 2 diabetes, *80 percent* of coronary artery disease, *70 percent* of strokes, and *70 percent* of colon cancer.[3] Poor diets are also associated with depression,[4] anxiety,[5] ADHD,[6] dementia,[7] and even suicide.[8] But there is good news: Brain-healthy diets have been shown to be effective treatments for depression,[9] ADHD,[10] and cognitive decline.[11]

When I first attended Alcoholics Anonymous (AA) meetings as part of my psychiatric training, I was dismayed to see that many recovering alcoholics continued to smoke cigarettes, drink loads of coffee filled with fake creamers and sugar, and eat donuts and other unhealthy foods. In their attempts to get better, they were perpetuating inflammation and making themselves worse. Even today, when I speak at churches, schools, hospitals, addiction treatment centers, and businesses—places that are supposed to be serving the health of others—I'm routinely horrified by the food that's served, which is toxic to brain health.

Victor, whose story I opened with, was a vegetarian, which put him at a higher risk of depression,[12] and his diet consisted mostly of beans, rice, corn, and cheese. He told our nutritionist he was willing to try a healthier diet and gave up gluten, dairy, corn, and all the other potential problem foods mentioned earlier. As I wrote in *Memory Rescue*, after a week on the new eating plan, his mood was better than it had been in years. Then he added back each of the foods, one at a time. He added back gluten, and nothing happened. The same was true of dairy, except he had more gas and a queasy stomach, and of soy. But when he added back corn, he said he knew "within a couple of bites" that it was the problem. He had an image of putting a gun in his mouth and pulling the trigger, something that had not happened since before he went on the diet. Even though Victor loved corn chips, corn tortillas, and popcorn, they obviously did not love him back. He decided that this bad relationship was not worth the pain, so he kicked corn out of his life. He was shocked that after suffering for so long he could feel normal with so little effort. You can too—by eliminating foods that are potentially harmful for you and only eating those that serve your health.

Food can be medicine or poison. Intuitively, most people know that certain foods affect their energy and moods. Having a big plate of pasta at lunch, for example, causes a blood sugar spike that makes you feel great for a short while. But it also stimulates your pancreas to produce lots of insulin, which will ultimately make your blood sugar fall so you feel tired and lethargic, as if your mind were swimming in mud.

This chapter will give you a dietary plan in five straightforward strategies to help you feel better fast.

THE FEEL BETTER FAST DIET: FIVE SIMPLE STRATEGIES

1. Give yourself an attitude makeover.
2. Learn the Feel Better Fast food rules.
3. Time your meals to get healthier.
4. Choose 20 foods you love that love you back.
5. Know which foods to lose and which to choose to help attention, energy, mood, memory, anxiety, pain, and sleep.

Strategy #1: Give yourself an attitude makeover.

Your attitude, or mind-set, may be the single most important factor in feeling better fast. When your mind-set is one of deprivation and your focus is on what you cannot have, you are more likely to remain mired in illness and brain fog. Yes, you may be giving up sugary fast foods and beverages you enjoy—which are often, by the way, pesticide-laden—but these are the very things that drive inflammation and illnesses such as diabetes, heart disease, cancer, depression, dementia, and early death. To feel better fast and make it last for a lifetime, it is critical to develop an abundance mind-set, where you focus on the high-quality, nutritious, and delicious foods you *can* have that build and sustain your health. If you are able to change your attitude about this, everything else will be easier.

Think for a moment about the advertising slogans that swirl on the airwaves and Internet and on food packaging, targeted at you and your children:

- "I'm lovin' it"
- "It's finger lickin' good!"
- "Have it your way"
- "Open happiness"
- "You deserve a break today"
- "Oh, I wish I were an Oscar Mayer wiener . . ."
- "They're gr-r-reat!"
- "They're magically delicious!"

- "The Breakfast of Champions"
- "Melts in your mouth, not in your hand"
- "Betcha can't eat just one"

Big business has purposefully designed these catchy jingles and phrases to target your mind and trigger the "bliss point" in your brain. Yes, you are being brainwashed. In the 1970s, Howard Moskowitz, a mathematician, discovered the perfect combination of sugar, salt, and fat that would optimize the human brain's pleasure experience—what he dubbed the "bliss point." Triggering it not only increases sensory experiences like taste and texture but activates the nucleus accumbens and other centers deep in the brain that are associated with motivation and pleasure. As discussed in chapter 8 (see page 183), the nucleus accumbens is the same part of the brain that is activated by certain drugs, such as cocaine, methamphetamines, nicotine, and morphine. In other words, the job of food designers is to create foods that hook your brain, just as addictive drugs do. "Betcha can't eat just one"! They were not kidding.

Here are a few of the weapons food scientists have discovered or manipulated to hook your brain:

- *Vanishing caloric density or "meltiness":* Foods that melt quickly make the brain think there are fewer calories; hence you eat more.

- *Sensory-specific satiety:* This refers to our tendency to become bored with eating the same food multiple times. Researchers discovered how to override the brain signal behind it by not including one distinct, overwhelming flavor. (Cooking with a variety of healthy herbs and spices does the same thing, only in a healthy way.)

- *Perfect crunchiness:* The perfect break point for this pleasure signal is four pounds of pressure.

- *Texture:* Removing fiber helps food slide down the throat more easily and increases the pleasure sensation. Fiberless food also means you can eat your food more quickly and get out of the fast food restaurant in less time, meaning these food emporiums can serve more bodies in a single day.

- *Aroma:* Flavor is enhanced by aroma. In fact, humans have only five major taste sensations—sweet, sour, bitter, salty, and umami, or savory, as in meat broth or tomato sauce. Other nuances are created through smell. That's why Cinnabon, for example, places ovens at the front of its stores and bakes fresh rolls every 30 minutes on a schedule. Between times, the chain eatery often bakes brown sugar and cinnamon just to create the enticing aroma that patrons seem helpless to resist.

- *Sugar:* In animal and human studies, sugar has been found to be an addictive substance that prompts bingeing, reward-seeking, craving, and tolerance (it takes more and more to get the same response).[13]

Society and corporations blame *you* for being overweight or sick because you lack self-control and portion control, or because your level of exercise is inadequate. But how can you have self-control when food scientists have been using sophisticated neuroscience and plotting against your brain for decades?

The first step in reorienting your eating habits is to stop being a victim of the food companies and start taking control of the food you put in your body. Start by changing your attitude. Why do I buy only healthy food for my family and team members at Amen Clinics? These are behaviors that help fuel success in every area of our lives. Plus, I love my family, the people I work with, and myself. Doing the right things for our health is never about deprivation; it is always about the abundance of what we really want—happiness, mental clarity, energy, effectiveness, and longevity. Why should you be serious about the quality of the nutrients you put in your body and the bodies of those you care about? Because doing so gives all of you the best chances at feeling great now and later, and because you love your friends, your family, and yourself. It's really that simple. Making consistently good decisions about food is an act of love. Damaging your most precious assets (brain and body) with poor-quality foodlike substances is an act of pure sabotage toward yourself and others.

Over the years, many people have told me this position is extreme and I should lighten up. Their reasoning includes responses like these:

- *"It's best to practice moderation."* I believe this is usually an excuse or rationalization to make poor decisions.

- *"Relax! We are all dying, so why not have a little fun along the way?"* Yes, we are all dying, but why accelerate it? Doesn't the quality of your life, now and into the future, matter? This response also reveals a lack of understanding that high-quality food can taste amazing.

- *"I can't afford to eat healthy."* In truth, you can't afford *not* to eat healthy. Consuming low-quality, cheap food ends up being far more expensive in the long run in terms of elevated health care costs and poor decision-making. According to the Harvard School of Public Health, eating healthy costs about an extra $1.50 a day.[14] You can make that up with one less coffee run.

- *"I don't have time."* Sure, grabbing a donut or ordering take-out burritos or deep-fried wings provides a speedy meal, but it's just as fast to grab an apple or orange or to order take-out salad bowls—and they will help you feel better fast and stay healthier. It takes some planning to eat food that is good for you, but meal kits from AmazonFresh, Walmart (Takeout Kit and Home Chef), and others can help without breaking your budget or requiring a lot of time.

- *"It's too hard."* Being disciplined about eating is not the easiest habit to incorporate in a world of toxic choices, but it's worth the effort. Think of it this way: Whatever you are doing now is a habit, and you can develop new habits that serve your health rather than steal from it.

- *"Why be so radical?"* I am convinced we need to be more serious now than ever. Low-quality diets are clearly associated with poor school performance in childhood and dementia in the elderly, and virtually every illness in between, including depression, diabetes, heart disease, cancer, autoimmune diseases, and obesity. My wife, Tana, and I wrote about this in *The Brain Warrior's Way*, detailing how you are literally in a war for the health of your brain. Everywhere you go, someone is trying to entice you to swallow unhealthy food that can lead to an early death.

Research is uncovering ever more reasons for urgency. In a recent study in mice at the University of Bonn, scientists found that a high-fat, high-calorie Western diet appears to make the immune system react as it would to a bacterial infection. This diet made the mice's immune systems more aggressive over the long run, and even after the animals were put on a healthy eating plan, their bodies responded with greater inflammation—a response that may be linked to the development of type 2 diabetes and clogged arteries.[15] All this research can provide motivation for us to make over our attitudes and develop a positive mind-set toward healthy eating.

Strategy #2: Learn the Feel Better Fast food rules.

There are nine rules, or guidelines, that will help you start to eat healthier. You may already be following some of these guidelines—if so, good for you! The more of them you adopt, the better off your brain and body will be.

CONCENTRATE ON CONSUMING BRAIN-SMART CALORIES

Calories do matter. If you eat more of them than you burn, you will definitely gain weight, and as discussed in the introduction (see page xxv), as your weight goes up, the size and function of your brain go down. Yet *the quality of your calories matters more than the amount.* Contrast a 582-calorie meal of a large soda and a slice of pizza, which promotes inflammation, brain fog, and illness, with a 540-calorie meal of wild salmon, Swiss chard, sweet potato, and dark chocolate, which promotes good health. Your brain will be sick on the first regimen and healthier on the second. If you struggle with your weight, focusing on quality, not quantity, may also lead you to consume fewer calories and shed pounds: A recent study of 600 people led by the Stanford Prevention Research Center found that those who focused on eating healthier foods without worrying about cutting calories lost significant amounts of weight and improved on a number of health measures, including waist size and blood sugar and blood pressure levels.[16]

I am a value spender. Even though I have enough money, I hate wasting it. I think of calories like money and hate wasting them as well. Focus on foods that are nutritious, delicious, and calorie smart.

MAKE (ZERO-CALORIE) WATER YOUR BEVERAGE OF CHOICE

Your brain is 80 percent water. Being dehydrated by just 2 percent impairs your ability to carry out tasks that require attention, memory, and physical performance.[17] I recommend drinking about eight 10-ounce glasses of water a day. If you drink a glass of water 30 minutes before meals or snacks, you're likely to eat less and still feel satiated. However, avoid drinking water *with* your meal, as it slows down digestion by diluting stomach acid. And try to limit consumption of anything that dehydrates you, including caffeine, alcohol, and other diuretics.

Just as critical is that you avoid drinking your calories. Replace sodas (including diet sodas—see the section on artificial sweeteners on page 214), fruit juices, and other sugary drinks with water. *Drinking just one can of sweetened soda or fruit punch a day can result in a weight gain of up to five pounds in one year! No wonder so many Americans are always on a diet.*

EAT SMALL AMOUNTS OF PROTEIN SEVERAL TIMES A DAY

Think of protein the way you do medicine—that it should be taken in small doses with every meal and snack. Protein helps to balance blood sugar levels, decrease cravings, and burn more calories than eating high-carb, sugar-filled foods. Protein also provides your body with the amino acids it requires. Nuts, seeds, legumes, some grains, and vegetables contain *some* of the 20 essential amino acids you need. Fish, poultry, and most meats contain *all* of them. To the degree your budget allows, shop for animal protein that is free of hormones and antibiotics, free-range, and grass fed. It is more expensive than industrial, farm-raised animal protein, but it is a good investment in your health. Be careful not to overdo it on protein, as that can put an increased strain on your kidneys and promote inflammation. Somewhere in the range of 15 to 25 percent of your total daily calories is a healthy amount.

MAKE FRIENDS WITH FAT

Fat continues to get a bad rap, despite the fact that good fats are essential to the health of your brain and do not raise your cholesterol. In fact, low-fat diets are bad for the brain. A Mayo Clinic study found that people who ate either a fat-based or a protein-based diet had a 42 percent or a 21 percent lower risk, respectively, of developing mild cognitive impairment and dementia, but those who ate a diet based on simple carbohydrates (think bread, pasta, potatoes, rice, and sugar) had a 400 percent *increased* risk of developing these conditions.[18] Fat is not the problem—sugar is.

In a powerful new study from multiple highly regarded institutions around the world, researchers followed more than 135,000 people from 18 countries for an average of 7.4 years. They found that those who consumed the highest amount of dietary fat, including saturated fat, had a 23 percent reduced risk of death, while those who ate the highest amount of carbohydrates had a 28 percent increased risk of death. Higher consumption of saturated fat was surprisingly associated with a lower risk of stroke. The researchers concluded, "High carbohydrate intake was associated with higher risk of total mortality, whereas total fat and individual types of fat were related to lower total mortality. Total fat and types of fat were not associated with cardiovascular disease, myocardial infarction, or cardiovascular disease mortality."[19]

While it's smart to avoid fried fats, trans fats, and some saturated fats, cutting way back on healthy fats is harmful, because your body needs them for many crucial functions. Here's a brief look at how different kinds of fats impact health:

- **Unsaturated fats.** These are good fats because they contribute to heart and brain health. There are two kinds of unsaturated fats: *polyunsaturated* and *monounsaturated*. Two important polyunsaturated fats are

    - **Omega-3 fatty acids.** EPA and DHA, two omega-3s, are crucial for optimal brain health and are found in cold-water fish, such as salmon, tuna, and sardines. Deficiencies in these fatty acids have been associated with cognitive decline, depression, and many other illnesses. Higher levels of the omega-3 fatty acids EPA and DHA have been associated with a lower incidence of Alzheimer's disease and slower cognitive decline.[20]

- **Omega-6 fatty acids.** These are also necessary for good health, but they can be harmful when eaten in excess. Omega-6 fatty acids are found in most vegetable oils (soybean, sunflower, safflower, corn, and canola), as well as many fried foods, cereals, whole-grain breads, and processed foods—all common in what we call the standard American diet. Most people who eat this diet have an unhealthy ratio of omega-6 to omega-3 fatty acids—20 to 1 or higher—which is pro-inflammatory and increases the risk of heart disease, cancer, diabetes, and a host of other health problems. The optimal omega-6 to omega-3 ratio in your blood is likely under 4 to 1.

The best way to balance your omega-6 to omega-3 ratio is to eat fewer foods that contain omega-6s and more that contain omega-3 EPA and DHA. Certain plant foods, including flaxseeds and green leafy vegetables, contain alpha-linoleic acid (ALA), an omega-3 fatty acid that some people can convert in small amounts to EPA/DHA. However, you can't rely on it as your only source of omega-3s; taking fish-oil supplements can help ensure healthy levels.

- **Saturated fats.** Saturated fats tend to be less healthy than unsaturated fats, but they differ depending on their chemical makeup. Short- to medium-chain saturated fats (those with 4–12 carbons) are healthier than longer-chain ones, according to cardiologist Mark Houston of Vanderbilt University.[21] Here are a few examples of potentially healthier and unhealthier saturated fats; check food labels for them:

  - **Butyric (4-carbon) acid** is found in fiber-rich foods (sweet potatoes, vegetables, beans, nuts, and fruit), butter, and ghee.
  - **Caprylic (8-carbon), capric (10-carbon), and lauric (12-carbon) acids** are medium-chain fatty acids found in coconut.
  - **Myristic acid** is a **14-carbon** saturated fat found in most animal fats and some vegetable oils. There is some evidence that this fatty acid can be detrimental to heart health and should be consumed only in small amounts.
  - **Palmitic acid** is a **16-carbon**, long-chain saturated fat that creates the marbling in corn-fed beef. It has a negative impact on cholesterol and heart health.

- **Stearic acid** is an **18-carbon**, long-chain fatty acid found in grain-fed meats, sausage, bacon, cold cuts, peanuts, peanut butter, margarines, fried potatoes, whole milk, cheeses, and vegetable oils (sunflower oil has the most). Chocolate is high in stearic acid but also high in antioxidants and flavonoids, which help to balance its health benefit.

The healthiest dietary strategy is to cut back on certain types of saturated fats (especially myristic, palmitic, and stearic acids) and increase consumption of polyunsaturated fatty acids found in fish oil, nuts, and seeds.

- **Trans fats.** These synthetic fats are found in partially hydrogenated vegetable oils, and they have no place in anyone's diet.[22] They decrease healthy blood flow and increase the likelihood of blood clots, which can cause strokes and heart disease. They are found in shortening and many processed foods, margarines, commercially prepared fried foods, and packaged baked goods, including donuts, crackers, and snack foods. When a packaged-food label reads "trans fat–free," it may be a lie. Regulations do not require that trans fats be listed on a food label if the level is below the legal limit of 0.5 grams per serving. For many baked goods and pastries that are in excess of five ounces— a single pastry is often labeled as several servings, even though most people eat it as one serving—that can translate to two or three grams of trans fat. Even small amounts of these very unhealthy fats should be avoided. Fortunately, the FDA has banned trans fats in processed foods; the ban went into effect in June 2018 for the great majority of foods.

CHOOSE HEALTHY (HIGH-FIBER, BLOOD-SUGAR-STEADYING) CARBOHYDRATES

So-called "smart" carbohydrates are essential to life because they are loaded with nutrients, help to balance your blood sugar, and decrease cravings. Most vegetables, legumes, and fruits, such as apples, pears, and berries, that are low glycemic (unlikely to raise blood sugar) are smart carbs. High-glycemic, low-fiber carbohydrates steal your health because they promote inflammation, diabetes, and depression.[23] Examples include sugar and foods that quickly turn to sugar, such as bread, rice, pasta, and white potatoes.

Fiber is a special type of carbohydrate that enhances digestion, reduces the risk of colon cancer, and helps to balance blood pressure and blood sugar. The average American consumes far too little—less than 15 grams of fiber daily.

Women should consume 25–30 grams of fiber every day; men, 30–38 grams. High-fiber foods, such as broccoli, berries, onions, flaxseeds, nuts, green beans, cauliflower, celery, and sweet potatoes (the skin of one sweet potato has more fiber than a bowl of oatmeal!) have the added benefit of making you feel full faster and longer.

FILL YOUR PLATE WITH COLORFUL VEGETABLES AND FRUITS

Colorful vegetables and fruits have tremendous health benefits. They provide an enormous array of the plant nutrients, vitamins, minerals, and antioxidants that are necessary for good health. Plant foods also help prevent cancer and reduce inflammation, which contributes to Alzheimer's disease, heart disease, arthritis, gastrointestinal disorders, high blood pressure, and many other illnesses. A 2016 study found a linear correlation between the number of fruits and vegetables you eat and your level of happiness.[24] *The more colorful fruits and vegetables you eat—up to eight servings a day—the happier you become, and it happens almost immediately.* No antidepressant works this fast! Just stick with a two-to-one ratio of vegetables to fruits to limit sugar.

ADD BRAIN-HEALTHY FLAVOR WITH HERBS AND SPICES

Food seasonings contain so many health-promoting substances that it almost makes sense to store them in the medicine cabinet rather than the spice cupboard! Here are some of the most powerful of these herb and spice brain boosters.

- Basil
- Black pepper
- Cayenne pepper
- Cinnamon
- Cloves
- Garlic
- Ginger
- Marjoram
- Mint
- Nutmeg
- Oregano
- Parsley
- Rosemary
- Saffron
- Sage
- Thyme
- Turmeric (curcumins)

AVOID OR ELIMINATE FOODS THAT CAN POTENTIALLY HURT YOU

Some foods are not worth the downsides that come along with them. The following are several to limit or avoid altogether if you want to keep your brain healthy. If you struggle with mood issues, anxiety, temper problems, or learning challenges, eliminate all of the foods listed for at least a month.

Then, once all of them are out of your system, add back one each week and see which, if any, may be causing you trouble. This process may make an amazing difference in your health. While I believe everyone would benefit from eliminating these foods permanently, I know not everyone may choose to do that. Most people are willing to start with the elimination diet. When they see how much better they feel off these foods, many will make permanent changes.

- **Sugar.** Americans eat about 140 pounds of sugar a year. Refined sugar is 99.4 to 99.7 percent pure calories, with no vitamins or minerals—just carbohydrates. Sugar is addictive, interferes with the actions of calcium and magnesium, increases inflammation and erratic brain-cell firing, and has been implicated in aggression. Sugar consumption has been associated with brain fog, depression, ADHD, increased triglycerides and "bad" LDL cholesterol, and lower "good" HDL cholesterol. In brain imaging studies, sugar increases slow brain waves (associated with memory problems), and a study at UCLA showed that sugar negatively alters learning and memory.[25] Avoid agave, too, because of its high fructose content.

- **Artificial sweeteners.** Consuming sugar alternatives can contribute to chronically high insulin levels, which increases your risk for Alzheimer's disease, heart disease, diabetes, metabolic syndrome, and other health problems. Artificial sweeteners do not help you lose weight. In fact, they may lower metabolism, leading to weight gain. Avoid aspartame (NutraSweet, Equal), saccharin (Sweet'N Low), and sucralose (Splenda). If you want something sweet, use small amounts of erythritol or stevia.

- **Gluten.** This sticky substance is found in wheat, barley, rye, kamut, bulgur, and spelt, and in most commercially made breads, cakes, cookies, cereals, and pasta. It is also hidden in everything from salad dressings and sauces to processed foods and cosmetics. Gluten-related health issues are on the rise, including celiac disease, type 1 diabetes, and Hashimoto's thyroid disease—all of which are autoimmune conditions. Gluten can also trigger psychological disturbances, skin rashes, acne, inflammation, alopecia (baldness), arthritis, and food addiction. In one study, putting celiac patients on a gluten-free diet significantly decreased anxiety.[26] Gluten can also reduce brain blood flow.[27] There's no healthy reason to eat it.

- **Soy.** Soy (found in tofu, edamame, and soy sauce and also added to a huge range of foods) contains large amounts of omega-6 fatty acids, phytoestrogens (which may contribute to the development of cancer, early puberty in girls, and impotence in men), and phytic acid, which is thought to reduce the absorption of vital minerals.

- **Corn.** Why do farmers feed animals corn, soy, and potatoes? To make them fat! Corn is high in omega-6s and very low in omega-3s, making it pro-inflammatory. Corn has been shown to damage the intestinal lining and create leaky gut. Most of the corn in the US is sprayed with the glyphosate pesticide Roundup, which has been associated with cancer, depression, Parkinson's disease, MS, hypothyroidism, and liver disease.[28]

- **Dairy.** Cow's milk is perfect for calves but unnecessary for humans. After the age of two, fewer than 35 percent of humans produce the enzyme lactase, which is needed to break down lactose (milk sugar) and digest milk. Lactose is converted to galactose and glucose, which elevates blood sugar and can cause inflammation. Casein, one of the proteins in dairy, is an excitotoxin. Left unchecked, excitotoxins lead to brain inflammation and neurodegenerative diseases. In several studies, a link has been suggested between milk drinking and Parkinson's disease.[29] Most dairy cattle are given antibiotics and hormones, which can also end up in your body. Unsweetened almond milk is a good substitute for cow's milk.

CHOOSE ORGANIC, TOXIN-FREE FOODS WHENEVER POSSIBLE

Fast food, sugar, simple carbohydrates, dairy products, trans fats, excess omega-6 fatty acids, and foods that are processed, engineered, or refined promote chronic inflammation. These are the foods that the standard American or Western diet is built upon. That's why it's so important, whenever possible, to shop for organically grown or raised foods, which are free of hormones, antibiotics, and chemicals. Try to eliminate food additives and artificial preservatives, dyes, and sweeteners, too, and look for meat that is grass fed.

Fish is a great source of healthy protein and fat, but some varieties tend to have more toxins. The larger the fish, the more mercury it may contain, so it's best to eat mostly smaller varieties and have the larger ones (like tuna) less frequently. Eat a fairly wide variety of fish, preferably those highest in omega-3s, like wild Alaskan salmon, sardines, anchovies, hake, and haddock. Learn more at www.seafoodwatch.org.

I understand that many people cannot afford to buy only organic and sustainably raised food. That is why I recommend consulting the Environmental

Working Group's annual lists of produce with the highest and lowest levels of pesticide residues to help inform your choices. (Stay updated at www.ewg.org.)

Strategy #3: Time your meals to get healthier.

If you have symptoms of low blood sugar, getting your diet right can make an immediate positive difference for you. I had a patient who was arrested multiple times for angry outbursts, but in my office, he was typically one of our sweetest patients. One day he came to see me, sweating profusely, and he was angry and inappropriate with our office staff. Suspecting low blood sugar, I ordered a glucose tolerance test. We measured his blood glucose level at baseline and again 30 minutes and two hours after he drank the equivalent of sugar water. His two-hour blood glucose level was dangerously low. When the brain does not get enough glucose, watch out!

Symptoms of Hypoglycemia (Low Blood Glucose)

- Feeling sleepy/drugged
- Mental confusion
- Inability to concentrate
- Impaired memory
- Dizziness, light-headedness
- Nervousness
- Depression
- Irritability
- Blurred vision
- Overwhelming fatigue

- Anxiety/panic attacks
- Palpitations
- Shaky hands
- "Butterflies" in stomach
- Flushing/sweating
- Faintness/fainting
- Head pressure
- Frontal headache
- Insomnia
- Abdominal pain/diarrhea

If you suspect you suffer from low blood sugar levels, make a practice of eating four to five meals a day that combine protein, fat, and smart carbohydrates to help steady your blood sugar.

If you do not have hypoglycemia, "intermittent fasting" or "time-restricted feeding" can significantly improve memory,[30] mood,[31] fat loss,[32] weight, blood pressure, and inflammatory markers.[33] Nightly 12-to-16-hour fasts turn on a process called autophagy, which helps your brain take out the trash it accumulates during the day.[34] This can help you think more clearly and feel more energetic, and it's simple—if you eat dinner at 6 p.m., don't eat again until 6–10 a.m. the next day. Your brain will have the time it needs to cleanse itself.

Not eating within two to three hours of bedtime also reduces your risk of heart attack and stroke.[35] In healthy people, blood pressure drops by at least 10 percent when they go to sleep, but blood pressure in late-night eaters stays high, increasing the risk of vascular problems. Also, new research suggests that if you have more calories at lunch and then eat a light dinner, you are more likely to lose weight than the other way around.[36]

Strategy #4: Choose 20 foods you love that love you back.

To be successful at optimizing your diet, you must find foods you love that love you back. As I detailed in chapter 4 (see page 69), we are creatures of habit and change can be hard. That is why you have to set yourself up to win. Do this by finding 20 high-quality, delicious foods and beverages, based on the rules outlined above. If you can find 20 foods, odds are you will be able to find 40, 80, 100, or more. To give you a head start, here is a list of 162 of my favorite Feel Better Fast Brain-Healthy Foods and Beverages that comply with our food rules. Some of these items may be new to you, but you can research them more online or ask your grocer where to find them.

FEEL BETTER FAST BRAIN-HEALTHY FOODS AND BEVERAGES

Beverages

1. Water
2. Beet juice (to increase blood flow)
3. Cherry juice (to help sleep)
4. Coconut water
5. Herbal tea
6. Lightly flavored waters, such as Hint
7. Spa water (sparkling water with berries, a sprig of mint, or a slice of lemon, orange, peach, or melon)
8. Sparkling water (add a splash of chocolate or orange stevia [brand: SweetLeaf] for a refreshing, calorie- and toxin-free "soda")

9. Unsweetened almond milk (for amazing taste, add a few drops of flavored stevia)
10. Vegetable juice or green drinks (without added fruit juice)
11. Water with cayenne pepper to boost metabolism

Nuts, Seeds, Nut and Seed Butters, and Meal

12. Almonds, raw
13. Almond butter
14. Almond flour
15. Brazil nuts
16. Cacao, raw
17. Cashews
18. Cashew butter
19. Chia seeds
20. Coconut
21. Flax meal
22. Flaxseeds
23. Hemp seeds
24. Pistachios
25. Pumpkin seeds
26. Quinoa
27. Sesame seeds
28. Walnuts

Legumes (small amounts, all high in fiber and protein, help balance blood sugar[37])

29. Black beans
30. Chickpeas
31. Green peas
32. Hummus
33. Kidney beans
34. Lentils
35. Navy beans
36. Pinto beans

Fruits—choose low-glycemic, high-fiber varieties

37. Acai berries
38. Apples
39. Apricots
40. Avocados
41. Blackberries
42. Blueberries
43. Cantaloupe
44. Cherries
45. Cranberries
46. Figs
47. Goji berries
48. Goldenberries
49. Grapefruit
50. Grapes (red and green)
51. Honeydew melon
52. Kiwis
53. Kumquats
54. Lemons
55. Lychees
56. Mangosteens
57. Nectarines
58. Olives
59. Oranges

60. Passion fruit
61. Peaches
62. Pears
63. Plums
64. Pomegranates

65. Pumpkin
66. Raspberries
67. Strawberries
68. Tangerines
69. Tomatoes

Vegetables

70. Artichokes
71. Arugula
72. Asparagus
73. Beets and
    beet greens
74. Bell peppers
75. Broccoli
76. Brussels sprouts
77. Butter lettuce
78. Butternut squash
79. Cabbage
80. Carrots
81. Cauliflower
82. Celery
83. Celery root
84. Chicory
85. Collard greens
86. Cucumbers
87. Green beans
88. Horseradish
89. Jicama

90. Kale
91. Leeks
92. Maca root
93. Mustard greens
94. Okra
95. Onions
96. Parsnips
97. Red or green
    leaf lettuce
98. Romaine lettuce
99. Scallions
100. Seaweed
101. Spinach
102. Summer squash
103. Sweet potatoes
104. Swiss chard
105. Turnips
106. Watercress
107. Wheatgrass juice
108. Zucchini

Prebiotic Foods (nondigestible substances that promote the growth of healthy bacteria in the gut)

109. Dandelion greens
110. Psyllium

(Several foods already listed are also prebiotics: artichokes, asparagus, chia seeds, beans, cabbage, raw garlic, onions, leeks, and root vegetables, including beets, carrots, jicama, squash, sweet potatoes, turnips, and yams.)

Probiotic Foods

111. Brined vegetables (not vinegar, as some people have negative reactions to it)
112. Chlorella
113. Kefir
114. Kimchi
115. Kombucha
116. Miso soup
117. Pickles
118. Sauerkraut
119. Spirulina

Mushrooms[38]

120. Black truffles
121. Chaga
122. Chanterelles
123. Maitake
124. Oyster
125. Porcini
126. Reishi
127. Shiitake
128. Shimeji
129. White button

Oils

130. Avocado oil
131. Coconut oil (good for high-temperature cooking)
132. Macadamia nut oil
133. Olive oil (avoid for high-temperature cooking)

Eggs/Meat/Poultry/Fish

134. Arctic char
135. Chicken or turkey
136. Eggs
137. King crab
138. Lamb (high in omega-3s)
139. Rainbow trout
140. Salmon, wild caught
141. Sardines, wild caught
142. Scallops
143. Shrimp

Brain-Healthy Herbs and Spices

144. Basil
145. Black pepper
146. Cayenne pepper
147. Cinnamon
148. Cloves
149. Garlic
150. Ginger
151. Marjoram
152. Mint
153. Nutmeg
154. Oregano
155. Parsley
156. Peppermint
157. Rosemary
158. Saffron
159. Sage
160. Thyme
161. Turmeric (curcumins)

Special Category

> 162. Shirataki noodles (made from the root of a wild yam plant [brand: Miracle Noodles] to replace pasta noodles)

I don't know about you, but I've been in bad relationships in the past. I'm so thankful now that I have a partner and wife who is good for me and loves me in return for my love. Choosing healthy food is so much easier than finding the right life partner! I am committed to only eating and loving food that is good for me and loves me back.

Strategy #5: Know which foods to lose and which to choose to help attention, energy, mood, memory, anxiety, pain, and sleep.

When you are feeling low, there are nutrients you should lose and others you should choose that will help you feel better fast. Following the general "Foods to Lose" list are diagrams and lists of food choices that will improve your attention and energy, moods, memory, and sleep and will reduce anxiety and pain.

FOODS TO LOSE: THESE MAKE YOU FEEL GOOD NOW BUT *NOT* LATER

- Pro-inflammatory foods, such as fast food (pizza, donuts, French fries, ice cream), sugar, simple carbohydrates, refined grains, wheat flour, dairy products, and omega-6 fatty acids (found in grain-fed meats, corn, soybeans, and vegetable oils—corn, safflower, sunflower, soybean, canola, and cottonseed)
- Trans fats—avoid anything with "partially hydrogenated" or "vegetable shortening" on the label
- Processed meats—sodium nitrites can combine with amines to form nitrosamines, which are carcinogenic
- Food additives, such as MSG and aspartame
- Anything that disrupts the gut lining, such as gluten
- Alcohol[39]
- Aspartame[40]
- Caffeine[41]

Why Do Restaurants Offer Bread and Alcohol before Meals?

It's a great question. After all, restaurants could instead offer you cheese, almonds, or fresh-cut veggies with a little mashed avocado. The answer is that bread and alcohol reduce the function of your prefrontal cortex (PFC) and make you both hungrier and more likely to order additional food and drinks. Without the PFC supervising your decisions, you are apt to spend more money at the restaurant on alcohol and dessert.

Bread—especially white bread made from bleached and processed flour—spikes blood sugar, which pushes trypto-phan, the amino acid building block for the neurotransmitter serotonin, into the brain. Serotonin helps you feel happier and less anxious, which is why many people, especially females, fall in love with bread, cupcakes, cookies, and the like. One study showed that males produced about 52 per-cent more serotonin than females, which makes females more susceptible to depression.[42] On SPECT, I've seen anti-depressants called SSRIs (selective serotonin reuptake inhibitors, which raise serotonin levels) lower function in the PFC. Many of my patients who have taken SSRIs report that they feel less depressed, anxious, or worried, but they also tend to be more impulsive and less motivated. One of my patients, who owned a group of restaurants, told me that he had to stop taking Zoloft, a commonly prescribed SSRI, because although he was less depressed, he wasn't get-ting his paperwork done. He just wasn't motivated or able to focus, which is bad if you own a business. Anything that lowers PFC function makes you more impulsive and less worried about long-term consequences. Starting a meal with bread or simple carbohydrates helps you feel better, but it also makes you more impulsive when the dessert tray comes by toward the end of the meal.

Alcohol also reduces PFC function, making it more likely

you will order extra food, make a stupid comment, or do something you later regret. We've long heard that alcohol in moderation can be healthy, but after looking at thousands of brains of moderate to heavy drinkers, I've just never believed it. A study at Johns Hopkins found that people who drink every day have smaller brains,[43] and when it comes to the brain, size does matter. Plus, alcohol is related to seven different types of cancer, including those involving the mouth, throat, esophagus, liver, colon, rectum, and breast.[44] Alcohol is used to clean your skin of bacteria before you receive an injection and as a preservative for scientific specimens. It's hard to imagine that it can be good for the 100 trillion bugs living in your gut that are essential to your life.

That's not all. Alcohol can decrease judgment and decision-making skills, increase cravings, and make you less coordinated. Excessive alcohol is related to high blood pressure, stroke, irregular heartbeat, heart disease, and a weaker immune system. According to a recent study, heavy drinking and alcohol use disorders are the biggest preventable risk factors for dementia, especially early-onset dementia, which starts before age 65.[45] To detoxify alcohol, your liver uses glutathione and other essential antioxidants. This can make you more vulnerable to the buildup of toxins. Alcohol intake is associated with a fatty liver, damaged neurons, and decreased blood flow to the cerebellum, an amazing part of the brain that is associated with physical and thought coordination. Alcohol interferes with the absorption of vitamin B1 and is a common cause of nerve pain. It is listed as the seventh leading preventable cause of death, and excessive use can cause untold suffering, divorce, incarceration, and financial problems. For people who want a better brain but also want to drink, I recommend no more than two to four standard-size drinks a week—*not* a day.

Hold the bread and alcohol, wait for your meal, and you will be happier with the end result.

FOODS TO CHOOSE: THESE MAKE YOU FEEL GOOD NOW *AND* LATER

To Boost Attention/Energy: A higher-protein, lower-carbohydrate diet, especially consumed around the times you need to focus, can be helpful. Consider this diagram:

PROTEIN-DOMINANT MEAL

You consume a protein-rich meal (think steak and seafood)

Raises blood levels
of all amino acids

You feel more energetic and focused
but may also be more worried and rigid

All amino acids compete
to enter the brain

Tryptophan (building block for serotonin) loses;
tyrosine (building block for dopamine) wins

- Dopamine-rich foods—for focus and motivation: turmeric,[46] green tea (for theanine),[47] lentils, fish, lamb, chicken, turkey, beef, eggs, nuts and seeds (pumpkin and sesame), high-protein veggies (such as broccoli and spinach), and protein powders
- Beets—increase blood flow to the brain
- Celery[48]
- Flavonoid-containing foods—blueberries, strawberries, raspberries, cocoa[49]
- Green tea[50]
- Green leafy vegetables
- Omega-3-rich foods—flaxseeds, walnuts, salmon, sardines, beef, shrimp, walnut oil, chia seeds, avocados, and avocado oil
- Spices—peppermint,[51] cinnamon,[52] and rosemary
- Water

To Boost Mood: Foods that raise serotonin can be helpful. Consider this diagram:

CARBOHYDRATE-DOMINANT MEAL

You consume a carbohydrate-rich meal
(e.g., pears, sweet potatoes, quinoa, zucchini, black beans)

Pancreas releases insulin

All amino acid blood levels,
except tryptophan, drop as
they enter muscles

You feel happier and less worried
but may also feel unfocused
and less motivated

Tryptophan enters the brain and is converted to serotonin;
dopamine levels become lower

- Serotonin-rich foods—combine tryptophan-containing foods, such as eggs, turkey, seafood, chickpeas, nuts, and seeds (building block for serotonin), with healthy carbohydrates, such as sweet potatoes and quinoa, to elicit a short-term insulin response that drives tryptophan into the brain. Dark chocolate[53] also increases serotonin.
- Limit simple carbohydrates, such as bread, pasta, potatoes, and rice, as they may help you feel good in the short run but increase inflammation and illness in the long run.
- Prebiotic-rich foods—see "Feel Better Fast Brain-Healthy Foods and Beverages," on page 219.
- Probiotic-rich foods[54]—see "Feel Better Fast Brain-Healthy Foods and Beverages," on page 220.
- Spices—saffron,[55] turmeric (curcumins),[56] and saffron plus curcumins[57]
- Fruits and vegetables—eat up to eight servings a day[58] to feel happier.
- Maca—this root vegetable and medicinal plant, native to Peru, has been shown to reduce depression.[59]
- Omega-3-rich foods—see "To Boost Attention/Energy" on page 224.

To Boost Memory: The Western, pro-inflammatory diet is associated with a smaller hippocampus and cognitive impairment.[60] A new way of eating for Americans is essential if we want to keep our brains healthy. Consider this diagram:

CHOLINE-RICH MEAL

You consume choline sources (eggs, shrimp, scallops, etc.)

Blood choline levels increase

Your thinking and memory improve

Brain choline increases and brain makes acetylcholine

- Antioxidant-rich foods—acai fruit, parsley, cocoa powder, raspberries, walnuts, blueberries, artichokes, cranberries, kidney beans, blackberries, pomegranates, chocolate, olive and hemp oils (not for cooking at high temperatures), dandelion greens, and green tea
- Chocolate (cocoa flavonols)[61]
- Choline-rich foods—to support acetylcholine and memory:[62] shrimp, eggs, tofu, scallops, chicken, turkey, beef, cod, salmon, shiitake mushrooms, chickpeas, lentils, and collard greens
- Omega-3-rich foods—see "To Boost Attention/Energy" on page 224.

To Reduce Anxiety: Low blood sugar states are often associated with anxiety. Being "hangry" (irritable from extended periods without eating) and being anxious often go together.

- Gamma-aminobutyric acid (GABA)–rich foods—for antianxiety: broccoli, almonds, walnuts, lentils, bananas, beef liver, brown rice, halibut, gluten-free whole oats, oranges, rice bran, and spinach
- Green tea, which contains L-theanine, an ingredient that helps you feel happier, more relaxed, and more focused[63]

- Magnesium-rich foods—pumpkin and sunflower seeds, almonds, spinach, Swiss chard, sesame seeds, beet greens, summer squash, quinoa, black beans, and cashews
- Omega-3-rich foods[64]—see "To Boost Attention/Energy" on page 224.
- Probiotic-rich foods—see "To Boost Mood" on page 225.

To Reduce Pain:

- Omega-3-rich foods—see "To Boost Attention/Energy" on page 224.
- Serotonin-rich foods—see "To Boost Mood" on page 225.

To Boost Sleep:

- Magnesium-rich foods—see "To Reduce Anxiety" on page 226.
- Serotonin-rich foods—see "To Boost Mood" on page 225.

THE FEEL BETTER FAST DIET: FIVE SIMPLE STRATEGIES

1. Give yourself an attitude makeover.

2. Learn the Feel Better Fast food rules:

   - Concentrate on consuming brain-smart calories.
   - Make (zero-calorie) water your beverage of choice.
   - Eat small amounts of protein several times a day.
   - Make friends with fat.
   - Choose healthy (high-fiber, blood-sugar-steadying) carbohydrates.
   - Fill your plate with colorful vegetables and fruits.
   - Add brain-healthy flavor with herbs and spices.
   - Avoid or eliminate foods that can potentially hurt you: sugar, artificial sweeteners, gluten, soy, corn, and dairy.
   - Choose organic, toxin-free foods whenever possible.

3. Time your meals to get healthier.

4. Choose 20 foods you love that love you back.

5. Know which foods to lose and which to choose to help attention, energy, mood, memory, anxiety, pain, and sleep.

TINY HABITS THAT CAN HELP YOU FEEL BETTER FAST—AND LEAD TO BIG CHANGES

10 -: 15
SECONDS MINUTES

Each of these habits takes just a few minutes. They are anchored to something you do (or think or feel) so that they are more likely to become automatic. Once you do the behaviors you want, find a way to make yourself feel good about them—draw a happy face, pump your fist, or do whatever feels natural. Emotion helps the brain to remember.

1. When I am tempted by French fries, sugary treats, or soda, I will resist and say to myself, "I only love foods that love me back."

2. Before I leave the house, I will put a full water bottle inside my purse or computer bag.

3. When I prepare my food shopping list, I will include fish and vegetables.

4. When I finish dinner, I will note the time and make plans to eat my next meal at least 12 hours later to give my brain time for waste removal.

5. When I pick up a new item at the grocery store, I will read the food label.

6. When I'm in a low mood, I will eat a piece of low-sugar or sugar-free dark chocolate to boost my serotonin level.

7. When I eat a food I love that loves me back, I will note it down in my "favorite healthy foods" list.

8. When the waiter comes for my order at a restaurant, I will say, "Please don't bring bread to the table." Making that one decision will help me make healthier choices throughout the meal.

9. When I go food shopping, I will look for organic fruits and vegetables first.

CHAPTER 10

ADVANCED AND BRAIN-TYPE NUTRACEUTICALS

A PERSONALIZED, TARGETED APPROACH TO GETTING THE NUTRIENTS YOU NEED

If people "eat wild, fresh, organic, local, nongenetically modified food grown in virgin mineral- and nutrient-rich soils that has not been transported across vast distances and stored for months before being eaten . . . and work and live outside, breathe only fresh unpolluted air, drink only pure, clean water, sleep nine hours a night, move their bodies every day, and are free from chronic stressors and exposure to environmental toxins," then it is possible that they might not need supplements. However, because people live in a fast-paced society where they pick up food on the fly, skip meals, eat sugar-laden treats, buy processed foods, and eat foods that have been chemically treated, most people could use a little help from a multiple vitamin/mineral supplement.

MARK HYMAN, MD, AS QUOTED IN *THE BRAIN WARRIOR'S WAY*

When I'm treating people, one question I always ask myself is *What would I prescribe if this were my mother, my wife, or my child?* More and more, after 35 years as a psychiatrist, I find myself recommending natural treatments. I am not opposed to medications and I have prescribed them for a long time, but I want you to use all of the tools available, especially if they are effective, less expensive, and have fewer side effects than medications.

My interest in nutraceuticals started after I began using brain SPECT imaging to help understand and treat my patients. One of the early lessons SPECT taught me was that some medications, especially those often prescribed for anxiety and pain, had a negative effect we could see on the scans. Later I learned some research suggested that a number of these medications increased the risk of dementia and strokes.[1] In medical school I was taught,

"First, do no harm. Use the least toxic, most effective treatments." As I looked for alternatives to these treatments to help the children and adults I was serving, I discovered that many natural supplements had strong scientific evidence behind them, with fewer side effects than prescription medications.

JENNIFER: MEDS MADE HER WORSE

One of the cases that got me interested in natural treatments involved my own niece. When Jennifer was seven, my sister brought her to see me for problems with moodiness and temper. I tried a number of medications for her without any success. My sister was calling me upset three times a week, and I kept using stronger and stronger medicines. But medications are not without risks and side effects, and when my niece started to gain weight, I took her off all of them and decided to try her on a group of natural supplements I had heard about from a colleague.

One day about four months later, I realized I hadn't heard anything from my sister in a long time. I called her and said, "Hey, don't you love me anymore? How's my niece?"

She said, "Danny, you cannot believe the difference in her. She is so much better. She is calmer, more compliant, and she is getting straight As in school. Of course I love you." The supplements have had long-term benefits for her without any side effects. Last year Jennifer graduated from law school.

WHAT YOU NEED TO KNOW ABOUT NUTRACEUTICALS

Supplements with medicine-like health benefits. That's a simple way to think of *nutraceuticals*, a term that's a combination of the words *nutrient* and *pharmaceutical*. Many of these natural products have been studied extensively and found to be effective. Other advantages: They can be less expensive than drugs, and insurance companies don't need to be informed that you have taken them. This last point is key, since taking prescription medications may affect your insurability. I know many people who have been denied coverage or made to pay higher rates for health, life, disability, and long-term-care insurance because they have taken certain medications. If there are effective natural alternatives, it is worth considering them.

At Amen Clinics we have had success using combinations of nutraceuticals on patients with very damaged brains. In 2009, we started the world's first and largest brain imaging study on active and retired NFL players. Many of them complained of problems with memory, mood, and focus and scored very poorly on the cognitive tests we gave them. As a group, their SPECT scans looked awful. For the treatment arm of the study, we used brain health education and targeted supplements, including a multivitamin/mineral complex, high-dose omega-3 fatty acids, ginkgo and vinpocetine for blood flow support, acetyl-L-carnitine for energy support, alpha-lipoic acid as an antioxidant and for blood sugar support, N-acetylcysteine as an antioxidant, huperzine A to support acetylcholine and memory, and phosphatidylserine for memory support. Our protocol demonstrated increased blood flow to multiple brain areas, including the prefrontal cortex and hippocampus, and improvements in memory, attention, and processing speed.[2]

BEFORE:
12 YEARS IN THE NFL

AFTER 6 MONTHS ON
NUTRACEUTICALS

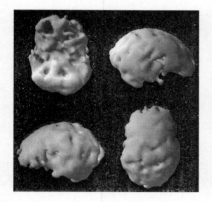 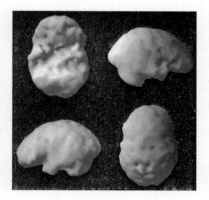

Severe overall decreased blood flow

Marked overall improvement

Nutraceuticals do have drawbacks. Although they tend to be less expensive than medications, you may pay more for them because insurance usually doesn't cover their cost. What's more, they are not completely without side effects, and they can interact with medications. "Natural" is not synonymous with "harmless"; both mercury and asbestos are natural, but both are dangerous to your health. St. John's wort, one of my favorite natural antidepressants, can cause sun sensitivity, and it can also decrease the effectiveness of a number of medications, including birth control pills. (Just imagine: St. John's wort has lifted your depression, but you also discover you are pregnant. You may not think this is the best timing.)

Quality control is an ongoing issue. Studies have shown that supplements don't always contain what the label claims, which means they may not work or, alternatively, could be harmful. Don't rely on the expertise of a health food store clerk for your supplement information. Instead, research brands online and develop a relationship with one or more, communicating your questions and issues to their technical and quality control staff.

Notwithstanding these issues, the benefits of nutraceuticals (and their relatively low risks compared to medications) make them worth considering, especially if you can get thoughtful, research-based information. I have witnessed targeted nutraceuticals make a positive difference in the lives of my patients, my family, and myself, which is why I take them every day and recommend them.

THREE NUTRACEUTICALS EVERYONE SHOULD TAKE

I typically recommend three nutraceuticals to all of my patients because they are critical to optimal brain function: a multivitamin/mineral, omega-3 fatty acids, and vitamin D.

1. A Multivitamin/Mineral

To feel better fast now and later, you need to give your brain the nutrition it requires. But there is evidence that many people are not getting it: More than 90 percent of Americans do not eat at least five servings of fruits and vegetables a day, the minimum required to get the nutrients you need, according to the Centers for Disease Control and Prevention (CDC).[3] An editorial in the *Journal of the American Medical Association* also asserted that most adults don't get all the vitamins they need through diet alone and recommended a daily vitamin supplement for everyone because it helps prevent chronic illness.[4]

In the past 15 years, there have been more than 25 reports of mental health benefits from multivitamin/mineral formulas consisting of more than 20 minerals and vitamins.[5] In addition, studies show that multivitamin/mineral complexes can help with attentional issues,[6] mood,[7] and even aggression.[8] Two randomized, controlled trials were conducted after the 6.3-magnitude earthquake in February 2011 in Christchurch, New Zealand,[9] and the devastating flooding in southern Alberta, Canada, in June 2013.[10] Both trials showed reduced acute stress and anxiety scores in those taking a multivitamin/mineral. In the New Zealand earthquake study, the incidence of posttraumatic stress disorder (PTSD) decreased from 65 percent to 19 percent after one month of treatment, while the control group showed little improvement. These two trials suggest that multivitamin/mineral complexes could be an inexpensive public health intervention for normal populations following natural disasters.

A 2010 study tested the effects of taking a multivitamin versus a placebo on 215 men ages 30 to 55. After a month, the multivitamin group reported improved moods and showed better mental performance, as well as having a greater sense of vigor, less stress, and less mental fatigue after completing mental tasks—essentially making them both happier and smarter.[11] Another placebo-controlled study looked at the effects of multivitamins on 81 healthy children and found that those who took multivitamins performed better on two out of three attention tasks.[12]

2. Omega-3 Fatty Acids

Omega-3 fatty acids are essential to well-being, as we touched on in chapter 9. Low levels are one of the leading preventable causes of death, according to researchers at the Harvard School of Public Health.[13] Studies have shown that 95 percent of Americans do not get enough dietary omega-3 fatty acids. Low levels of EPA and DHA, two of the most important omega-3s, are associated with

- Inflammation[14]
- Heart disease[15]
- Depression and bipolar disorder[16]
- Suicidal behavior[17]
- ADHD[18]
- Cognitive impairment and dementia[19]
- Obesity[20]

Unfortunately, most people are low in EPA and DHA unless they are focused on eating fish (which can be high in mercury and other toxins) or they are taking an omega-3 supplement. We tested the omega-3 fatty acid levels of 50 consecutive patients not taking fish oil (the most commonly used source of EPA and DHA) who came into Amen Clinics and found that 49 had suboptimal levels. In another study, our research team correlated the SPECT scans of 166 patients with their EPA and DHA levels and found that those with the lowest levels had lower blood flow, the number one predictor of future brain problems, in the right hippocampus and posterior cingulate (one of the first areas to die in Alzheimer's disease), among other areas.[21] On cognitive testing, we also found low omega-3s correlated with decreased scores in mood. Most adults should take between 1,000 and 2,000 milligrams of high-quality fish oil per day, balanced between EPA and DHA.

Are Your Medications Depleting Your Nutrients?

Many medications can cause nutrient depletions. While you shouldn't stop taking necessary medicines without checking with your doctor, it is important to be aware of potential nutritional pitfalls so you can replace vital nutrients. Some (or all) of the following types of medications may cause problems:

- Antacids: Decrease stomach acid, calcium, phosphorus, folic acid, and potassium. Also can contribute to dysbiosis, or small bowel overgrowth of unhealthy bacteria, which can cause vitamin K deficiency and low mineral absorption
- Antibiotics: Decrease vitamins B and K
- Antidiabetics: Decrease coenzyme Q10 (CoQ10) and vitamin B12
- Antihypertensive medications: Decrease vitamins B6 and K, CoQ10, magnesium, and zinc
- Anti-inflammatories (NSAIDs): Decrease vitamins B6, C, D, and K, folic acid, calcium, zinc, and iron
- Cholesterol-lowering medications (especially statins): Decrease CoQ10, omega-3 fatty acids, and carnitine
- Female hormones: Decrease folic acid, magnesium, B vitamins, vitamin C, zinc, selenium, and CoQ10
- Oral contraceptives: Decrease B vitamins, magnesium, folic acid, selenium, zinc, tyrosine, and serotonin. Roughly 16 to 52 percent of women taking oral contraceptives experience depression. Antidepressants are typically the first-line treatment; nutritional deficiencies are rarely considered. A recent study found that oral contraceptives can double the risk of suicide in teenage girls and significantly increase the risk in adult women.[22]

3. Vitamin D: Optimize Your Level

Its best-known roles may be in building bones and boosting the immune system, but vitamin D is also an essential vitamin for brain health, mood, and memory. Low levels have been associated with depression, autism, psychosis,

Alzheimer's disease, multiple sclerosis, heart disease, diabetes, cancer, and obesity. Seventy percent of the population is low in vitamin D because we are spending more time indoors and using more sunscreen (the vitamin is absorbed through the skin). It is easy to remedy a low level; get a blood test to check it, and if it is low (below 30 ng/mL), take between 2,000 and 10,000 IU a day. Recheck after two months to make sure your level is in the healthy range.

30
SECONDS Take a daily multivitamin/mineral complex, 1,000–2,000 mg of fish oil balanced between EPA and DHA, and, if needed, vitamin D.

SUPPORT FOR YOUR MEMORY

Chapter 2 contains a discussion of the 11 risk factors that steal brain cells and contribute to memory loss, which I wrote about in my recent book, *Memory Rescue*. The risk factors are summarized in the words BRIGHT MINDS; each letter stands for one of the risks, from blood flow to toxins, mental health problems to sleep issues. *Memory Rescue* provides dozens of strategies to address each risk factor so that you can prevent cognitive impairment or get your memory back (see pages 38–44 for more). One of the strategies is to take specific nutraceuticals that address your BRIGHT MINDS issues. Here are some of those recommendations.

- **Blood flow**: ginkgo biloba, vinpocetine, green tea catechins, cocoa flavonols, resveratrol
- **Retirement/Aging**: phosphatidylserine, acetyl-L-carnitine, huperzine A
- **Inflammation**: omega-3 fatty acids, curcumins,[23] probiotics
- **Genetics**: curcumins, resveratrol, blueberry extract, green tea extract, vitamin D
- **Head trauma support**: omega-3 fatty acids
- **Toxins**: n-acetylcysteine, vitamin C, magnesium, pre- and probiotics
- **Mental health**: omega-3 fatty acids; also see the brain types, below
- **Immunity/infections**: vitamins C and D, aged garlic, Lion's mane mushrooms, zinc
- **Neurohormone deficiencies**: zinc (testosterone), l-tyrosine (thyroid), DHEA, probiotics, ashwagandha (cortisol)
- **Diabesity**: chromium picolinate, berberine, cinnamon, alpha-lipoic acid
- **Sleep**: melatonin, magnesium, gamma-aminobutyric acid (GABA), 5-hydroxytryptophan (5-HTP) (if a worrier)

KNOW YOUR BRAIN TYPE AND SUPPORT IT WITH SUPPLEMENTS

Not all brains, even healthy ones, are the same. That's a key lesson we have learned from our brain imaging work at Amen Clinics. When we first started to do SPECT scans in 1991, we were looking for the one pattern that was associated with anxiety, depression, addictions, bipolar disorder, obsessive-compulsive disorder, autism, or ADD/ADHD. But we soon discovered that no single brain pattern was associated with these illnesses; each one has multiple types that require their own unique treatments. It made sense that there would never be just one pattern for depression, for example, as not all depressed people are the same. Some are withdrawn, others are angry, and still others are anxious or obsessive. Taking a one-size-fits-all approach invites failure and frustration. Another lesson we learned is that symptom-guided treatment is often ineffective and harmful.

The scans helped us understand the type of anxiety, depression, ADHD, obesity, or addiction a person had, so we could better target treatment to individual brains. This one idea led to a dramatic breakthrough in our own personal effectiveness with patients, and it opened up a new world of understanding and hope for the tens of thousands of people who have come to see us and the millions of people who have read our books or seen our shows. In previously published books, I've written about seven types of ADHD, seven types of anxiety and depression, six types of addictions, and five types of overeaters. Understanding these types is critical to getting the right help. Here is a summary of five of the common brain types, along with recommended supplements for each one.

Brain Type 1: Balanced

People with this brain type tend to have healthy brains overall and be

- Focused
- Flexible
- Positive
- Relaxed

The SPECT scans of a balanced brain show full, even, symmetrical activity with no holes. The basic supplements just mentioned are the foundation for this type.

HEALTHY BRAIN SPECT SCAN

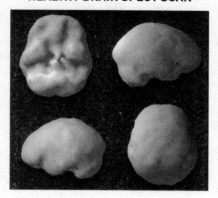

Full, even, symmetrical activity

Brain Type 2: Spontaneous

People with this brain type tend to be

- Spontaneous
- Risk-taking
- Creative, "out-of-the-box" thinkers
- Restless
- Easily distracted
- Unable to focus unless they are interested

The SPECT scans of this type typically show lower activity in the front of the brain in the PFC. The PFC functions as the brain's brake (see chapter 3, page 53). It is the little voice in our heads that helps us decide between the banana and the banana split. The PFC stops us from saying or doing things that are not in our best interest, but it can also stop creative, out-of-the-box thinking. The Spontaneous Brain Type tends to be associated with lower dopamine levels in the brain and may cause people to be more restless, take more risks, and struggle to stay focused on something unless they are very interested in it. Our research team has published several studies showing that when people with this brain type try to concentrate, they actually have less activity in the PFC, which causes them to need excitement or stimulation in order to focus (think of firefighters and race car drivers).[24] Smokers and heavy coffee drinkers also tend to fit this type, as they use these substances to turn their brains on.

SPONTANEOUS BRAIN TYPE

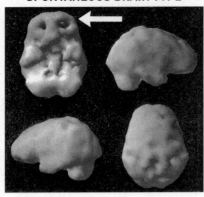

Low PFC activity at the front of the brain

Any supplement or medicine that calms the brain, such as 5-HTP or SSRIs (selective serotonin reuptake inhibitors), may make the Spontaneous Brain Type worse, as it will lower the already low PFC function, which can then take the brakes off your behavior. We have treated many people who had done things they later regretted, such as becoming hypersexual or spending money they did not have, when they were put on SSRIs. It turned out they had low activity in the PFC, and the serotonin-boosting medications diminished their judgment.

This brain type is best optimized by boosting dopamine levels to strengthen the PFC. Higher-protein, lower-carbohydrate diets tend to help, as do physical exercise and certain stimulating supplements, such as rhodiola, green tea extract, L-theanine, ashwagandha, panax ginseng, ginkgo biloba, and phosphatidylserine. Try them in the order listed here for a few days each to see which work best for you. If one or more overstimulates or upsets you, stop taking it and move on to the next in the list.

- *Rhodiola*, an herb that is grown at high altitudes in Asia and Europe, has been traditionally used to fight fatigue, improve memory, and increase attention span. It is called an adaptogen because it helps the body adapt to stress and assists in bringing our body processes back to normal. In an Amen Clinics study we conducted with scientist Mahtab Jafari, PhD, from the University of California, Irvine, we found that rhodiola helped to increase blood flow to the brain, especially the prefrontal cortex. Our study group also reported better mood and energy. Look for *Rhodiola rosea* root standardized to contain 3 percent rosavins and a minimum of one percent salidrosides. The typical adult dose is 170–200 mg twice a day.

- *Green tea extract* is made from the dried leaves of *Camellia sinensis*, an evergreen shrub. It has been used to improve focus; as a remedy for many ailments, including anxiety; and to assist with weight loss. The green tea component epigallocatechin gallate (EGCG) is a potent free-radical scavenger. The typical daily adult dose is 200–300 mg. Up to three cups of green tea can be consumed daily instead of a supplement, but pregnant women should use caution as green tea contains caffeine.

- *L-theanine* is an amino acid uniquely found in green tea. It crosses the blood brain barrier and can increase dopamine. It also increases GABA and serotonin, so it tends to have a balancing effect on the brain. It helps with focus as well as mental and physical stress. The typical dose is 100–200 mg two to three times a day.

- *Ashwagandha* (*Withania somnifera*, Indian ginseng, Indian winter cherry) is a shrub found in India, Nepal, and Pakistan that is commonly used to help focus and relaxation. The plant itself is an adaptogen, with properties that enable the body to better handle stress, anxiety, and fatigue. It helps to rejuvenate and energize the nervous system and increase physical endurance. It also has antioxidant, anti-inflammatory, and antiaging effects. It is well tolerated; few adverse effects have been reported. Those who take medications for thyroid issues, hypertension, or diabetes should exercise caution, as ashwagandha may stimulate thyroid function, cause a decrease in blood pressure, or lower blood sugar. The recommended dose is 125 mg twice a day.

- *Panax ginseng* is a plant with fleshy roots that typically grows in cooler climates, including the northern regions of eastern Asia, Korea, and Russia. Ginseng is most widely known as a stimulant that promotes energy, improves circulation, and increases blood supply. For these reasons it has been used to improve cognitive and physical performance during endurance exercise. The typical adult dose is 200 mg twice a day.

- *Ginkgo biloba* is a powerful nutraceutical from the Chinese ginkgo tree that enhances circulation, memory, and concentration. The most studied form of ginkgo biloba is an extract called EGb 761, which has been studied in blood-vessel disease, clotting disorders, depression, and Alzheimer's disease. In a 2003 double-blind, placebo-controlled study using SPECT, Brazilian researchers studied 48 men between the ages of 60 and 70 for eight months and found significant improvements in blood flow and global cognitive functioning among those taking gingko. The placebo group showed the opposite, with decreased brain blood flow and poorer scores on cognitive testing.[25] Consider taking ginkgo if you suffer from low energy or have trouble concentrating. There is a small risk of internal bleeding, so if you are taking any other blood-thinning agents, the dosages may need to be reduced. The typical adult dose is 60–120 mg twice daily.

- *Phosphatidylserine* (PS) is a naturally occurring nutrient found in foods such as fish, green leafy vegetables, soy products, and rice. PS is a component of cell membranes, which change in composition as we age. It is essential to brain health, as it maintains neurons and neuronal networks so that the brain can continue to form and retain memories. Reportedly, taking PS may help improve age-related declines in memory, learning, verbal skills, and concentration. Research done with positron emission tomography (PET) studies, similar to SPECT, on patients who have taken PS show that it produces a general increase in metabolic activity in the brain.[26] The typical adult dose is 100–300 mg a day.

Brain Type 3: Persistent

People with this brain type tend to

- Be persistent
- Be relentless or strong-willed
- Like things a certain way
- Get "stuck" on thoughts
- Hold on to hurts
- See what is wrong in themselves or others

Take-charge people who won't take no for an answer are likely to have this brain type. They tend to be tenacious and stubborn. In addition, they may worry, have trouble sleeping, be argumentative and oppositional, and hold grudges from the past. The Persistent Brain Type often has increased activity in the front part of the brain, in an area called the anterior cingulate gyrus (ACG)—what I have described previously as the brain's gear shifter. It helps people go from thought to thought or move from action to action, and it is involved with being mentally flexible and going with the flow. When the ACG is overactive, usually due to low levels of serotonin, people can have problems shifting attention, which can make them persist—even when it may not be a good idea for them to do so. Caffeine and diet pills tend to make this brain type worse because they stimulate brains that do not need more stimulation. Indeed, people who have a Persistent Brain Type may feel as though they need a glass of wine at night, or two or three, to calm their worries.

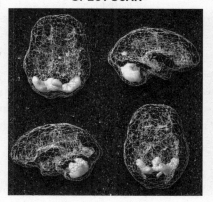

NORMAL "ACTIVE" BRAIN SPECT SCAN

Most active areas in the cerebellum at the back of the brain

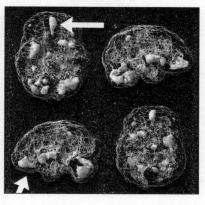

PERSISTENT BRAIN TYPE

High ACG activity at the front of the brain

High-glycemic carbohydrates like bread, pasta, and sweets turn to sugar quickly and increase serotonin, which is calming to the brain. That's why Persistent Brain Types can become addicted to these simple carbohydrates. They often use carbs as "mood foods" to self-medicate an underlying mood issue. It is best to avoid these quick fixes because they can cause long-term health problems. (See chapter 9, "To Boost Mood," page 225, for healthy food choices that will drive serotonin into the brain.) Instead, use physical exercise to boost serotonin, and consider taking supplements such as L-tryptophan, 5-HTP, and saffron.

- *L-tryptophan* is a naturally occurring amino acid and building block for serotonin that is particularly abundant in milk, meat, and eggs. With my patients, I have found that it helps to decrease stress[27] and aggressiveness;[28] improve sleep, cognitive flexibility, and mood;[29] and foster a positive mind-set in females.[30] One of the problems with dietary L-tryptophan is that a significant portion of it does not enter the brain. Instead, much of what we consume is used to make proteins and vitamin B3. This necessitates taking large amounts of L-tryptophan—I recommend a dose of 1,000–3,000 mg a day for adults. Take it on an empty stomach because other amino acids in proteins can block its absorption and its entry into the brain.

• *5-HTP*, another amino acid, is a step further along in the serotonin production pathway. It is more widely available than L-tryptophan and more easily taken up in the brain—70 percent versus 3 percent of L-tryptophan. About 5 to 10 times more powerful than L-tryptophan, 5-HTP boosts serotonin levels in the brain and helps to calm ACG hyperactivity (greasing the cingulate, if you will, to improve shifting one's attention). A number of double-blind studies have shown that it is also an effective mood enhancer[31] and appetite suppressor.[32] The recommended adult dose of 5-HTP is 50–300 mg a day. Children should start with a half dose. As with L-tryptophan, it is best to take 5-HTP on an empty stomach to help with absorption. The most common side effect is an upset stomach, which is usually very mild. Start with a low dose and work your way up slowly.

• *Saffron*, one of the world's most expensive spices, is grown mostly in Iran, Greece, Spain, and Italy and traditionally has been consumed to help digest spicy food and soothe an irritated stomach. It also has been used for hundreds of years as a folk medicine for a variety of health problems. In recent years there has been significant research showing that saffron can help boost serotonin and benefit mood,[33] memory,[34] and sexual function;[35] decrease the symptoms of PMS;[36] and, when combined with methadone, help alleviate withdrawal symptoms in patients undergoing treatment for opioid addiction.[37] The recommended adult dosage is 15 mg twice a day.

Brain Type 4: Sensitive

People with this brain type tend to

• Be sensitive
• Feel deeply
• Be empathic
• Struggle with moods
• Be more pessimistic
• Struggle with negative thoughts

The SPECT scans of the Sensitive Brain Type tend to show increased activity in the limbic or emotional centers of the brain, making these people empathic and deeply feeling but also subject to issues with their moods. They may also struggle with being more pessimistic and having negative thoughts.

NORMAL "ACTIVE" BRAIN SPECT SCAN

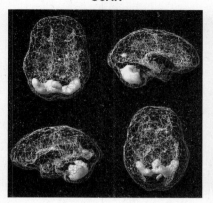

Most active areas in the cerebellum at the back of the brain

SENSITIVE BRAIN TYPE

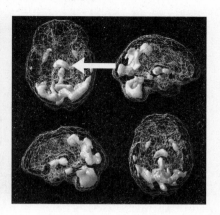

High deep limbic activity (arrow)

Exercise, omega-3 fatty acids (1,000–2,000 mg a day), vitamin D, and a nutraceutical known as s-adenosyl-methionine (SAMe) may help the Sensitive Brain Type. If someone with this type is also a Persistent Brain Type (yes, it's possible to be a combination of types), the supplements or medications that boost serotonin may help the most.

- *SAMe* is crucial for the production of several neurotransmitters (dopamine, epinephrine, and serotonin)[38] and in gene regulation, and it has additional, very important actions that allow the brain to function properly. The brain normally manufactures all the SAMe it needs from the amino acid methionine. When someone is depressed, the synthesis of SAMe from methionine is impaired; taking SAMe has been shown to have antidepressant qualities. A 2017 comprehensive review by the American Psychiatric Association Council on Research Work Group found SAMe a promising treatment for depression.[39] SAMe has also been found to reduce joint inflammation and pain. People who have a tendency toward bipolar disorder should check with their doctor before trying this supplement. The typical adult dose is 200–400 mg two to four times a day. Usually it is best taken early in the day as it may be more stimulating for some. SAMe has been found to enhance mood more effectively if taken with 250 or 375 mg a day of trimethylglycine (TMG, betaine).[40]

Brain Type 5: Cautious

People with this brain type tend to be

- Cautious
- Prepared
- Motivated
- Reserved
- Busy-minded
- Restless

On SPECT images, we often see heightened activity in the anxiety centers of the brain, such as the basal ganglia, insular cortex, or amygdala. The neurotransmitter GABA helps calm overfiring in the brain, and low levels of GABA frequently cause people with this brain type to struggle more with anxiety and subsequently be more cautious and reserved. On the flip side, they also tend to be more prepared.

**NORMAL "ACTIVE" BRAIN
SPECT SCAN**

**CAUTIOUS
BRAIN TYPE**

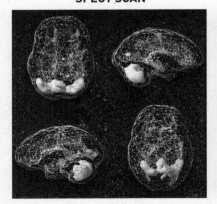
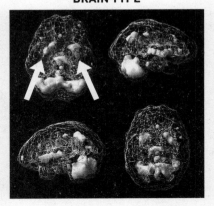

Most active areas in the cerebellum
at the back of the brain

High basal ganglia activity (arrows)

Meditation and hypnosis can help soothe this brain type (see chapter 1, pages 11–20), as can a combination of vitamin B6 (25 mg); magnesium glycinate, magnesium malate, or magnesium citrate (the forms of magnesium that are best absorbed by the body; take 150–300 mg two to three times a day); and GABA, the calming neurotransmitter (250–750 mg two to three times a day).

It is common to have more than one brain type, and when we look at all of the potential combinations, it adds up to 16 types, such as Spontaneous-Persistent-Sensitive or Sensitive-Cautious. Many years ago we realized that not everyone can come to one of our clinics to get scanned, so based on thousands of scans, we've developed a questionnaire that helps predict what yours might look like. The questionnaire is not as effective as actually looking at the brain, but it is still helpful and used by thousands of medical and mental health professionals around the world.

:05-06 You can find out your brain type as part of our free Brain Health
MINUTES   Assessment on www.brainhealthassessment.com, where we also have specific suggestions to help each type.

Nutraceuticals can have a powerful effect on your brain health, often without the side effects that medications can have. Start with a multivitamin/mineral, omega-3 fatty acid supplement, and vitamin D if needed. Then try adding one supplement at a time, based on your primary symptoms and brain type, and see what helps you to feel better.

FOUR STRATEGIES TO USE NUTRACEUTICALS TO FEEL BETTER FAST

1. Take a multivitamin/mineral, omega-3 fatty acids, and vitamin D if your levels are low.

2. Find out if any medications you are taking might be depleting your body of essential nutrients and, if so, consider supplementing the shortfall.

3. Know your risks of memory loss and supplement to prevent cognitive impairment.

4. Find out which of the five basic brain types you have at www.brainhealthassessment.com, and try different supplements to improve your brain's healthy function.

TINY HABITS THAT CAN HELP YOU FEEL BETTER FAST—AND LEAD TO BIG CHANGES

:05-06 MINUTES Each of these habits takes just a few minutes. They are anchored to something you do (or think or feel) so that they are more likely to become automatic. Once you do the behaviors you want, find a way to make yourself feel good about them—draw a happy face, pump your fist, or do whatever feels natural. Emotion helps the brain to remember.

1. When I eat my breakfast, I will take a multivitamin/mineral and omega-3 fatty acid supplement. I will also know my vitamin D level and take extra if needed.

2. If I take medication, I will also take specific supplements to replenish any essential nutrients the prescription may be depleting (see chart on page 234).

3. On Sunday mornings I will refill my supplement organizer.

PART 6

X IS FOR THE X FACTOR

The X factor is a variable in a given situation that could have the most significant impact on the outcome. Over the past 30 years, brain imaging changed everything for my patients, my family, and me. By looking at the brain in people who had complex problems or who were treatment resistant, I gained new knowledge that made the difference between success and failure, healing and maintaining illness, even life and death. This chapter provides the top 10 lessons that we and the patients at Amen Clinics have learned from our collaborative work with brain SPECT imaging, which will help you determine when you or a loved one should consider a scan.

CHAPTER 11

THINK DIFFERENT

10 PRACTICAL LESSONS FROM 150,000 BRAIN SCANS

No one really wants to see a psychiatrist. No one really wants to be labeled as defective or abnormal. But everyone wants a better brain. What if mental health was really brain health?

DANIEL AMEN

Apple's iconic "Think Different" commercial is my all-time favorite. The slogan was widely considered a response to IBM's slogan "Think." The Apple advertisement ran from 1997 to 2002, at the height of the criticism of the brain imaging work we do at Amen Clinics. It was a stressful time for us. Whenever the "Think Different" commercial would air, I would become emotional, as it described my professional journey and made me feel that I wasn't the only crazy person trying to change a small part of the world. I can still hear Richard Dreyfuss's smooth voice saying,

Here's to the crazy ones.
The misfits.
The rebels.
The troublemakers.
The round pegs in the square holes.
The ones who see things differently.
They're not fond of rules.
And they have no respect for the status quo.
You can quote them, disagree with them, glorify or vilify them.

About the only thing you can't do is ignore them.
Because they change things.
They push the human race forward.
And while some may see them as the crazy ones, we see genius.
Because the people who are crazy enough to think they can change the
     world, are the ones who do.

Now, nearly 30 years after we first began our brain imaging work, we have built the world's largest database of functional brain imaging scans related to behavior. The SPECT scans have taught us and our patients so many important lessons. In this chapter I will provide you with our top 10 lessons, which can help you feel better fast and dramatically change your life.

TOP 10 LESSONS FROM SPECT SCANS

Lesson #1: Current psychiatric diagnostic models are outdated because they don't assess the brain.

It's much harder to fix something if you don't know what is going wrong.

THOMAS INSEL, MD, FORMER DIRECTOR OF THE NATIONAL INSTITUTE OF MENTAL HEALTH

Today, the typical way most people are diagnosed and treated for mental health issues is by going to a professional and telling him or her their symptoms. The doctor or therapist listens, examines them, looks for symptom clusters, and then diagnoses and treats them. Patients may say, "I'm depressed," for example, and the doctor will look at them and then give them a diagnosis with the same name—depression. Treatment is typically an antidepressant medication.

If you are anxious, you usually get an "anxiety disorder" diagnosis and end up with a prescription for an antianxiety medication. Many people with attentional problems end up with a diagnosis called attention deficit disorder or attention deficit hyperactivity disorder and are prescribed a stimulant medication, such as Ritalin or Adderall. My favorite example of this phenomenon is the diagnosis for people who have temper problems and explode intermittently. They often get a diagnosis called intermittent explosive disorder, or IED. The acronym is ironic, calling to mind an improvised explosive device, and these patients often wind up in anger management classes or on any number of medications.

CURRENT PSYCHIATRIC DIAGNOSTIC MODEL

SYMPTOMS	DIAGNOSIS	TREATMENT
Depression	Depression	Antidepressants
Anxiety	Anxiety disorder	Anti-anxiety medications
Attentional problems	ADD or ADHD	Stimulants
Intermittent explosions, anger	Intermittent explosive disorder (IED)	Anger management classes or medications

This is very similar to the way Abraham Lincoln was diagnosed with melancholy (depression) back in 1840. He told his physician, Anson Henry, his symptoms, which were consistent with depression; Dr. Henry listened to Lincoln recounting his symptoms, examined him, looked for symptom clusters, and then diagnosed Lincoln and started treatment. That was 178 years ago, but it remains the mainstay of diagnosis today—identifying symptom clusters without any information on how the brain works. Psychiatrists are the only medical specialists who virtually never look at the organ they treat. Cardiologists look, neurologists look, gastroenterologists look, orthopedists look. Psychiatrists guess.

There is a better way.

Lesson #2: Psychiatric diagnoses are not single or simple disorders; they all have multiple types, and each requires its own treatment.

This was one of the earliest lessons SPECT taught us. Giving someone the diagnosis of depression is like giving him or her the diagnosis of chest pain. No doctor would do that because it doesn't identify the cause of the pain or what to do for it. Consider with me: What can cause chest pain? Heart attacks, heart arrhythmias, pneumonia, grief, anxiety, chest-wall trauma, gas, and ulcers, just to name a few. Likewise, what can cause depression? Loss, grief, low thyroid, brain infections, brain trauma, a brain that works too hard, or a brain that does not work hard enough. Do you think all of these will respond to the same treatment? Of course not.

In my past writings I have described seven brain types associated with anxiety and depression, seven types of ADD, six types of addicts, five types of overeaters, and even three types associated with violence. No one treatment will work for everyone who is depressed, anxious, inattentive, addicted, over-weight, or aggressive. They all have different brain types. Looking at the brain helps us develop a more complete understanding of our patients' problems and more personalized, targeted treatment.

Often when psychiatrists or psychologists come to our office for a tour, I will start by showing them a set of healthy SPECT scans. Then I will show them scans from two 15-year-old multiple murderers.

In May 1998, Kip shot and killed his father and mother. The next day he went to his high school and shot 27 more people, killing 2. Kip had seen several psychiatrists and had taken psychiatric medications that were not helpful. As part of his trial, he had been scanned, and his scan showed overall severely decreased blood flow to his brain, especially in his prefrontal cortex (PFC) and temporal lobes. It was one of the worst scans of a 15-year-old I have ever seen. The damage on his scan was likely from a brain infection, loss of oxygen, or some form of toxic exposure in the past.

Compare Kip to Peter, who killed his mother and eight-year-old sister with a baseball bat for no apparent reason. His scan showed overall increased activity, especially in the area of the anterior cingulate gyrus (ACG), which caused him to get stuck on negative thoughts.

Here are two boys who have the same clinical presentation—multiple murders—but radically different brain patterns. One shows overall low activity; the other overall high activity. Do you think they will respond to the same treatment? Of course not. But how would you know what to do unless you actually looked at their brains? Kip needed a psychiatrist or other physician to find the cause of his damaged brain, then rehabilitate it; Peter needed his doctor to help calm his brain so it did not hijack his behavior.

KIP (SURFACE)　　　　　　**PETER (SURFACE)**

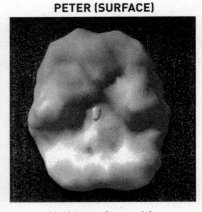

Overall low surface activity　　　　　Healthy surface activity

KIP (ACTIVE)

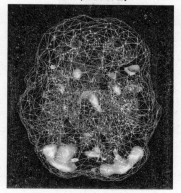

Overall low activity

PETER (ACTIVE)

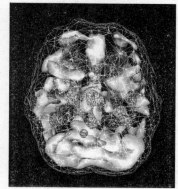

Overall high activity

Lesson #3: Looking at the brain decreases stigma, increases compliance with treatment, and completely changes the discussion around mental health.

In 1980 when I told my father I wanted to be a psychiatrist, he asked me why I didn't want to be a real doctor. Why did I want to be a nut doctor and hang out with nuts all day long? It hurt my feelings then, but 38 years later I understand why he had that reaction. When psychiatrists don't have hard biological data to help them make their diagnoses, many people do not take them seriously. Unfortunately, that leaves a huge emotional hole for patients, who often feel belittled or defective if they have to seek help for a "mental" illness.

Imaging completely changes the discussion around mental health. Quite frankly, few people really want to see a psychiatrist. My wife almost canceled her first date with me when she found out I was a psychiatrist. No one wants to be labeled as defective, crazy, or abnormal, but everyone wants a better brain. What if mental health were really brain health? Scans have taught our patients that lesson over and over.

One of the reasons I fell in love with SPECT was that it immediately decreased stigma for patients. After seeing their scans, they viewed their problems as medical, not moral. This decreased the sense of shame and guilt that is often associated with having a mental health issue. The brain scan images also helped families become more supportive of the person who was struggling, similar to the way they would if a family member had diabetes or cancer. There was an increased sense of compassion and forgiveness.

Lesson #4: If what you're doing is not working, look at the brain.

Aaron, 52, was a highly successful business owner who was married and enjoying life at all levels. Out of the blue, he woke up one morning in a panic with a terrible sense of impending doom. He was sweating profusely; his heart was racing; and he and his wife had no idea what was wrong. His family physician ran tests and then prescribed Lexapro, an antidepressant medication, for stress. Within a few days the panic attacks worsened, and Aaron was also put on Xanax, a benzodiazepine antianxiety medicine. A week later he woke up with the thought of putting a gun in his mouth and pulling the trigger. Horrified, he came to our clinic after seeing me on television.

Sudden changes in behavior are usually associated with brain trauma, toxins, infections, or a defined emotional trauma. Aaron's brain SPECT scan showed damage to his PFC and his left temporal lobe, a pattern that looked consistent with a traumatic brain injury. When I asked him about it, he didn't remember any injuries until I asked him specifically about falls or accidents. At that, he hit his forehead with his hand and told me that two weeks before the first panic attack, he had taken a hard fall off his mountain bike. The front tire hit a jagged rock as he was riding down a steep hill, which sent him flying over the handlebars onto his head. He did not lose consciousness, which is why he didn't think the injury was important, but he struck the ground so hard his helmet broke.

With this information, Aaron's clinical presentation made sense. To deal with his anxiety, his physician had given him two medications that decrease brain activity—an SSRI (Lexapro) and a benzodiazepine. But because he already had low activity from the injury, the medications were making him worse, even to the point of suicidal thoughts. We needed to activate and rehabilitate his brain, not put a toxic bandage on it. When you damage your brain, you can clearly damage your life. Fortunately, the brain is mendable. On a program that included eliminating the medications that were harmful to him (I am not opposed to medications; these were just the wrong ones for Aaron), adding supplements to nourish his brain, and using hyperbaric oxygen to encourage healing, within eight days he began to feel much better. Six months later he was symptom-free, and his follow-up scan showed significant improvement.

HEALTHY SPECT SCAN

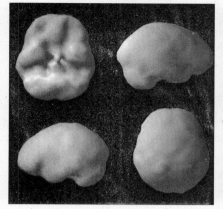

Full, even, symmetrical activity

AARON'S INITIAL SPECT SCAN

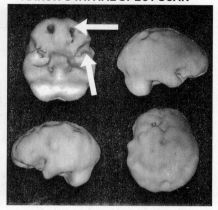

Holes indicate severely decreased blood flow in the PFC and left temporal lobe.

AARON'S AFTER TREATMENT SPECT SCAN

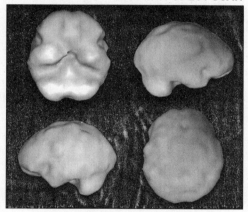

Marked overall improvement

Lesson #5: Looking at the brain improves outcomes, and people get better faster.

The most important reason to look at the brain is to improve outcomes. That was my clinical experience when we first started scanning patients, but to find out what the data showed, we started a formal outcome study in 2011 on many of the patients we saw. To date we have six-month outcome results on more than 7,000 patients. The study made it crystal clear that in general, we see people with complex issues who have been unsuccessfully treated by multiple health care providers. On average, our patients have 4.2 diagnoses (such as a combination of ADHD, depression, anxiety, and addictions), they have seen 3.3 medical or mental health providers before coming to us, and they have tried an average of five different medications. After six months, 77 percent of our patients reported they were better. The number went up to 84 percent if they maintained treatment at Amen Clinics. Eighty-five percent reported an improved quality of life. (Our study was published in the peer-reviewed medical journal *Advances in Mind-Body Medicine*.[1]) In a 2014 Canadian study, non-Amen clinicians and researchers using our method found that psychiatric patients who underwent SPECT-guided treatment improved significantly more than patients who did not.[2]

In another study we published, we found that SPECT changed how the doctor would diagnose or treat patients more than three-quarters of the time. A group of seven psychiatrists evaluated the charts of more than 100 consecutive patients who came to one of our clinics. In stage one, the psychiatrists reviewed the clinical histories and diagnostic checklists, but not the results of SPECT studies, and then gave each patient a diagnosis and treatment plan. (As we've discussed, this is how mental health diagnoses and treatment plans are typically done.) In stage two, the evaluators were given access to the SPECT studies for each patient. Having the scans changed the diagnosis or treatment plan in 79 percent of cases. The most clinically significant diagnostic changes were undetected brain trauma (23 percent) and toxicity patterns (23 percent); changes in the treatment arena involved medications or nutraceuticals (60 percent).[3]

Lesson #6: Looking at the brain completely changes the discussion about good and evil.

A picture may be worth a thousand words, but a map is priceless. A map tells you where you are and gives you directions on how to get where you want to go. Without an accurate map you are lost, and that may cost you precious time in getting the help you need—or it may even cost your life. SPECT is a map to help guide people to better brains and better lives.

As our brain imaging work became more widely known across California, we began to receive requests from judges and defense attorneys who were trying to understand difficult behavior and wanted our help. As of today, we have scanned hundreds of convicted felons and more than 100 murderers, including several mass murderers, two of whom I mentioned in Lesson #2. We have learned that people who struggle or do bad things often have troubled brains. That's to be expected. But what's more surprising is that many of those brains could be rehabilitated.

As I wrote in *Change Your Brain, Change Your Life,*

> Here is a radical idea. . . . What if we evaluated and treated
> troubled brains, rather than simply warehousing them in toxic,
> stressful environments? In my experience we could potentially save
> tremendous amounts of money by making a significant percentage
> of these people more functional, so that when they got out of prison
> they could work, support their families, and pay taxes. Dostoyevsky
> once said, "A society should be judged not by how it treats its
> outstanding citizens, but by how it treats its criminals."[4]

Our brain imaging work has taught us that instead of just meting out punishment for crimes, we must ask why people do bad things and then find ways to help them if they'll let us. We will be better as a society. The current approach to judgment and punishment in our country seems more about vengeance and retribution than rehabilitation. This is a costly mistake and diminishes the soul of our society. Behavior, at least in part, is related to the actual physical functioning of the brain, which can be improved when put in a healing environment.

If you're not personally paying attention to your brain, your life can go seriously off track. It's like the lyrics from the old Phil Ochs folksong "There but for Fortune," which tell of a prisoner in jail being

> *a young man with so many reasons why*
> *And there but for fortune, may go you or I*

Only I'd argue it should be rewritten: "There but for *a healthier brain* may go you or I." And it is not just about criminal behavior. It's about any troubled behavior, such as suicide attempts, marital affairs, domestic violence, mishandling money, misbehaving at school or work, or acting inappropriately as one ages.

JASON: AFTERMATH OF A BIKE ACCIDENT

Jason was 19 years old and madly in love with Jessica, who loved him back. One day, he got into a bicycle accident where his front tire hit a curb and he flew over the handlebars and landed on the left side of his head. He had a brief loss of consciousness. The emergency room doctor was too busy to say much, except to tell Jason and his parents that he had a mild concussion and should be watched closely for the next few days.

Within a month, Jason's behavior changed. No one related it to the concussion. Jason became negative, angry, and obsessively jealous, unlike any behavior he displayed before. Jessica became afraid and broke up with him, which made Jason worse. He couldn't stop thinking of her.

Three months later, Jessica had a new boyfriend. When Jason found out, he went over to her house, tied up the boyfriend, and raped Jessica. The police were called, and there was a standoff, where Jason threatened to kill himself. (He had started having serious suicidal thoughts after the accident.) Jason eventually was taken into custody.

When his defense attorney learned about the bicycle accident, he called a neuropsychologist, who tested Jason, found evidence of potential brain damage, and recommended a brain SPECT scan and my involvement in the case.

Jason's scan was very abnormal, indicating trauma to his left temporal lobe (often associated with brain trauma, violence, paranoia, and sometimes suicidal thoughts), excessive activation of his ACG (the gear shifter mechanism in his brain was stuck, and he could not let go of bad thoughts), and low PFC activity (leading to poor impulse control). This pattern is one we often see in cases of violence and obsession.

In jail, Jason was still suicidal. Based on his scans, I recommended a combination of medications to rebalance his brain, an antiseizure medication to help his temporal lobes, and the antidepressant venlafaxine, which helps to calm the ACG and boost the PFC. The medication was helpful; his mood improved and the suicidal thoughts went away. He told me he had not felt that well since before his accident, which was saying something given that he was about to go to trial for several felonies.

The judge in Jason's trial was running for reelection on a "tough on crime" platform. He was not interested in hearing any of this "new neuroscience nonsense" (his words), and he sentenced Jason to 11 years in prison. When Jason arrived, the overworked prison psychiatrist was also uninterested in hearing about Jason's brain scans and improvement on medication. He diagnosed Jason with antisocial personality disorder and took him off his medication. Four months later, Jason hanged himself. I am still furious and cry when I think about him. Yes, what he did was horrible. Yes, he should have been punished. People with troubled brains are still accountable for their choices. But to ignore, deny, and withhold treatment for the problems stemming from Jason's concussion is unconscionable and heartbreaking. We must do better, but it takes the ability to think differently.

JASON'S SPECT SCAN

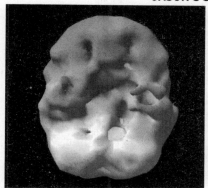 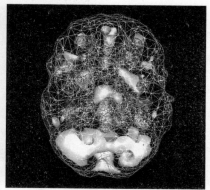

Surface scan
Damage to left temporal lobe

Active scan
Increased ACG activity

Of course, neuroscience alone will never completely help us understand the puzzle of troubled behavior; many people who have significant brain dysfunction never commit a crime or seriously hurt others. Behavior is typically driven by a combination of biological, psychological, social, and spiritual forces. However, if you ignore the brain, you'll never truly understand why people do what they do, and you will never be able to fully help them.

Lesson #7: Looking at the brain helps to prevent mistakes.

Imaging has helped us prevent errors, such as stimulating an overactive brain, calming one that is underactive, or labeling behavior as willful when it was clearly brain-based. Avoiding mistakes saves patients the frustration of unsuccessful treatments, allows us to help them faster, and gives them more hope for the future.

COTI: AN EVIL CYST

When I first met Coti, a 17-year-old, he told me he wanted to cut his mother up into little pieces. His dark, evil thoughts were out of control. He had been through treatment with six psychiatrists and had tried both a 15-month residential treatment program and a 30-day drug treatment program. When we scanned him, I discovered he had the largest cyst I've seen, the size of a tennis ball, occupying the space of his left frontal and temporal lobes. His behavior improved when the cyst was removed, although he still had leftover issues because of the damage the cyst had caused.

Over the years I have heard many people complain about the cost of scans, yet for people like Coti, untreated brain problems are dramatically more expensive in terms of money, family stress, and lack of freedom.

COTI'S SPECT SCAN

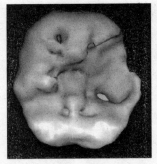

Damage to the left frontal and temporal lobes from a large cyst

RICHARD: OUTBURSTS OF A TROUBLED BRAIN

Richard ran a large business in Southern California. He was very bright, but over time his business suffered from excessive turnover because he had cruel temper outbursts toward his employees and his wife. He was often apologetic after an incident, but many people refused to work under the stress he caused. His board of directors forced him to see me. Richard's SPECT scan showed low overall activity in his PFC and both temporal lobes. He also had a cyst in his left temporal lobe. When it was drained and Richard went on a brain rehabilitation program that included supplementation and hyperbaric oxygen therapy, his behavior improved and he was able to keep his job. Two months after the brain surgery, he told me he was doing much better emotionally and had not lost his temper at all, which was a miracle. He was able to step back more easily from stressful situations and be more strategic. He said, "I am amazed that my troubled brain had hijacked so many relationships."

RICHARD'S SPECT SCAN

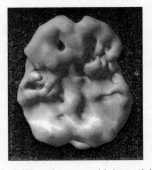

Low PFC and temporal lobe activity

Lesson #8: Looking at the brain provides hope.

Over the years, I have signed thousands of the books I have written for appreciative supporters who have bought them. Ever since we started our brain imaging work, I have signed nearly all of them with the words *with hope*. The images provide hope that there is a better way, and there is hope for healing.

DENNY: A SOLDIER'S STORY

Security is a primary value for my wife, Tana. She grew up in an unsafe, chaotic environment, and even though we live in a very safe neighborhood, she loves training in martial arts (she has two black belts—one in kempo karate and another in tae kwon do) and taking survival courses. She recently took our daughter Chloe on a survival weekend and met Denny, one of her instructors. Her heart broke when she heard his story. He is a former United States Marine who had three traumatic brain injuries, including one in Fallujah, Iraq, in 2007 when he and several of his friends were riding in a truck that was hit by an improvised explosive device (IED). He was knocked unconscious, and when he awoke he was bleeding from multiple places and two of his friends were dead. He was rushed into surgery and was later diagnosed with the chronic effects of multiple traumatic brain injuries and posttraumatic stress disorder. His healing journey involved one medication after another without much relief. He became so hopeless that he tried to end his own life. He finally found a program at Stanford University that was helpful, but it only dealt with the emotional trauma. No one had performed a functional brain imaging study on him, so Tana invited him to the clinic.

Denny's SPECT scan showed severe damage affecting his PFC in the front of his brain (focus, forethought, judgment, and impulse control), left temporal lobe (memory, learning, and dark thoughts), and occipital lobes in the back (visual processing). The good news was that it was clear that his brain could be dramatically improved with the right treatments.

DENNY'S SPECT SCAN

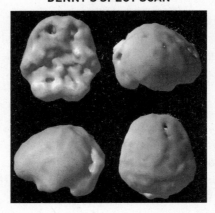

Holes indicate areas of severely decreased blood flow.

After looking at his scan, Denny was actually grateful his brain didn't look worse and that he had a "physical" reason for feeling as awful as he did. He was now motivated to make his brain much better.

A week later he wrote to Tana, "It's only been a week, and I can already feel a difference. Since the scan I have increased my activity level (fitness), modified my diet, and maintained the supplement regimen. I'm doing great! My energy level and attention span have increased, allowing me to focus more. My daughter and I have been outdoors every day. Since I started adjusting my habits, I am happier and more positive. I really want for my brain to have an improvement that can be visible in my scan. That motivation is what has gotten me back to normal."

Lesson #9: Alzheimer's and other forms of dementia start years, even decades, before people have any symptoms.

One of the most profound lessons from our brain imaging work is that Alzheimer's disease and other forms of dementia can be seen on SPECT scans years before people have any symptoms. SPECT is a leading indicator of problems, meaning it shows evidence of the disease process years before people show signs of it. Anatomical studies, such as CT and MRI, are lagging indicators. They show problems later in the course of the illness, when interventions tend to be less effective.

This lesson led us to advocate for doing scans and implementing prevention techniques as early in a person's life as possible. If you consider the fact that 50 percent of the population will get Alzheimer's disease by the age of 85, prevention should really take center stage in anyone who wants to live to 85 or beyond.

Chalene Johnson is a bestselling author, motivational speaker, and mother of two. Despite all her success, when she first came to see us she struggled with memory, focus, distractibility, procrastination, and always being late to appointments. To give you an idea of how bad it was, she had to shut herself in the basement closet just to get work done because any noise seemed to distract and irritate her. To make things worse, Chalene had a family history of Alzheimer's disease.

Her SPECT scan looked terrible. It showed evidence of ADHD with low activity in her frontal lobes, as well as low activity in areas vulnerable to Alzheimer's. The scan really got her attention. Over the next two years, she did everything we asked. Her follow-up scan showed dramatic improvement, decreasing her risk of future problems. More important, she told me that her performance at work, at home, and in her relationships all improved. Plus, she was finally able to get out of the basement!

CHALENE'S "BEFORE" SPECT SCAN

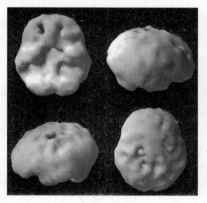

Low PFC activity (consistent with ADHD)
Low activity indicating vulnerability
to later Alzheimer's

AFTER TREATMENT SPECT SCAN

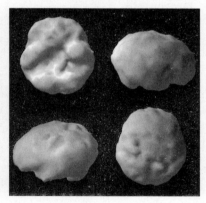

Marked overall improvement

Lesson #10: The most important lesson from 150,000 scans is that you can change your brain, and it will change your life.

This is the biggest and most exciting lesson our patients have learned from our work. And it is personal.

ANDREW: MY NEPHEW'S BRUSH WITH DISASTER

I got a call late one night in April 1995 that my nine-year-old godson Andrew, who's also my nephew, had attacked a little girl on the baseball field that day for no particular reason. I was on the phone with Sherrie, my sister-in-law, feeling shocked, and I said, "Excuse me?"

She said, "Danny, he's different. He's mean. He never smiles anymore. I went into his room today, and I found two pictures that he had drawn. In one of them, he was hanging from a tree. In the other picture, he was shooting other children." In retrospect, *Andrew was Columbine, Sandy Hook, Aurora, and Parkland waiting to happen.*

I told Sherrie I wanted to see Andrew the next day. They drove from Southern California to Northern California, where we had our first clinic. When I walked into my office and saw Andrew sitting on the couch, my heart melted. I loved this child and was terribly worried about him. I said, "Honey, what's going on?"

He said, "Uncle Danny, I'm mad all the time, and I don't know why."

I asked, "Is anybody hurting you?"

He said, "No."

"Is anybody teasing you?"

And he said, "No."

"Is anybody touching you in places they shouldn't touch you?" I was searching for answers to his senseless behavior.

And he said, "No."

My first thought was *You have to scan him.* My next thought, because you know we're always talking to ourselves, was *You want to scan everybody. You know, maybe it's because he's the second son in a Lebanese family. You're the second son in a Lebanese family.* Then all of a sudden, the rational voice in my head said, *Stop it! Nine-year-old children do not attack people for no reason. Scan him. If his scan is normal, then you can explore other reasons for his behavior.*

I went with Andrew to the imaging center and held his hand while he held his teddy bear and got scanned. When his brain scan came up on the computer screen, I could see that Andrew was missing the function of his left temporal lobe. I looked at Dr. Jack Paldi, my mentor, and said, "Why doesn't he have a left temporal lobe?"

To make sure Sherrie and my brother Jim wouldn't hear, Dr. Paldi wrote on a piece of paper, "It's a cyst, a stroke, or a tumor." I was sad, because something was clearly wrong, yet also relieved that something was wrong—there was a possible explanation for Andrew's unusual behavior. Andrew had an MRI that day, which showed he had a cyst (a fluid-filled sac) the size of a golf ball occupying the space where his left temporal lobe should have been. By that time in 1995, we had already correlated left temporal lobe issues with violence. I called Andrew's pediatrician in Southern California and asked him to find someone to drain the cyst.

ANDREW AND HIS MISSING LEFT TEMPORAL LOBE ON SPECT

ANDREW (AGE 9)   ANDREW'S SPECT SCAN

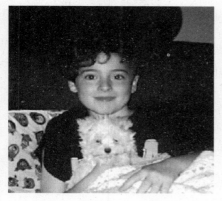

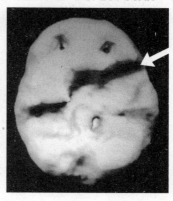

Andrew and his dog, Buster   Missing function of the left temporal lobe

Two weeks later, the pediatrician called me back and said he had talked to three neurologists. None of them recommended we do anything about the cyst, and they thought it probably had nothing to do with Andrew's behavior problems. He told me, "They wouldn't operate on him unless he had real symptoms."

Furious, I said, "Let me get this right. I have a homicidal, suicidal boy. What do you mean by real symptoms?"

"I think they mean seizures, or he loses consciousness, or he has speech problems," he replied defensively.

"This is insanity," I replied and hung up.

I then called a friend of mine at Harvard, who is a pediatric neurologist, and she told me the same thing. Frustrated, I thought to myself, *Neurologists . . . neurologists . . . neurosurgeons. Neurosurgeons operate.* I called the pediatric neurosurgery department at UCLA and talked to Dr. Jorge Lazareff, who later became famous for separating the Guatemalan twins who were connected at their heads. He was famous to me before then because when I told him about Andrew, he said, "When cysts are symptomatic, we drain them. Obviously, he has serious symptoms."

No kidding, I thought to myself.

After surgery, I received two phone calls. One was from Sherrie, who was so excited. She told me the surgery went really well, and when Andrew woke up afterward, he smiled at her. She said, "Danny, he hasn't smiled for a year."

The second call was from Dr. Lazareff, who said, "Dr. Amen, that cyst was so aggressive and put so much pressure on Andrew's brain that it actually thinned the bone over his left temporal lobe. His temporal bone was eggshell thin. If he had been hit in the head with a ball, it would have killed him instantly. Either way, Andrew would have been dead in six months if you hadn't persisted."

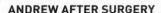

ANDREW AFTER SURGERY

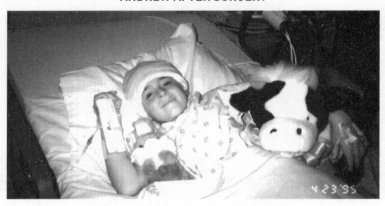

It's a day I'll never forget—the day I lost my anxiety about our brain imaging work and the criticism I had endured. Nine hundred ninety-nine psychiatrists out of a thousand would have medicated Andrew or put him in psychotherapy. I became even more passionate than ever about our work. Andrew was blessed in the sense that he had someone who loved him paying attention to his brain when his behavior was off. Now, 23 years later, Andrew is married, employed, owns his own home, and pays taxes. Because someone looked at his brain, he has been a wonderful son and husband and will be a better father and grandfather.

How do you know unless you look? If you don't look, you hurt people, and that's not fair. That's not science. That's not medicine. It's stupidity. We can do better. When I think of the single most important lesson I've learned from the 150,000 scans we've done, it is this: *You can literally change people's brains, and when you do, you change their lives.*

In November 2017, unbeknownst to me, someone posted on Facebook a six-minute clip of me telling Andrew's story during a lecture I gave at Saddleback Church in Southern California.[5] The post went viral, and within a few weeks it had 38 million views, more than 700,000 shares, and more than 25,000 comments. Many of the comments made me cry. Here are a few that touched my soul.

From JG:

I hadn't seen my brother in 10 years since we were afraid of his behavior.

When he was young, he was invited to every major college because he was brilliant, yet over the years, especially after he was in the military, he began to decline mentally. He had several head injuries in his life, one major one while in the service. My brother had been aggressive with erratic behavior for years, and was diagnosed with schizophrenia, as was our mother. It seemed logical at the time 20 years ago.

My brother became homeless, an alcoholic, and addicted to painkillers from being hit by a drunk driver and ended up in a VA group home. He was robbed and attacked during that time. His injuries caused him to need two brain surgeries last year.

Out of the blue my other brother and I got a call from a young psychiatrist from the VA hospital telling us that our older brother had a severe infection, pressure, and scarring in his left temporal lobe. His brain scan showed several injuries and infection; and he wanted the hospital to clean out the scar tissue, but the head surgeon didn't want to perform the surgery, believing our brother was a "homeless drunk." The hospital was keeping our brother in the psychiatric ward for aggressive behavior, where we went to visit him—one of the saddest days of my life to see him there. The young psychiatrist had seen my brother's brain scan and thought much of his behavior was due to his injuries and pressure on his brain. He convinced another neurosurgeon to do my brother's brain surgery. . . .

One year later, my brother has returned to us, like a new person, it's an absolute miracle. It's very sad to think he lived being considered schizophrenic for all those years. I asked the young psychiatrist why he pushed so hard to help my brother, and he said he could tell by talking to him that he seemed far too brilliant and knew he must have a family somewhere so he went looking for us. He told me he had another case very similar to our brother's injuries and that the other patient had become aggressive after a car accident, so he decided to search for family and push for my brother to have surgery. God bless such a brilliant man for practicing medicine.

From SC:

> Starting at age seven, I was severely depressed. That's not normal.
> Finally, at age 35, I found a psychiatrist who demanded a brain
> MRI. What did they find? Mesio temporal sclerosis (scarring of the
> temporal lobe), a form of epilepsy that caused horrible symptoms.
> I'm on medication and have a whole new life.

From JP:

> I spent years suffering from anxiety, depression, a changed
> personality. I would have "episodes" where words, written or
> spoken, made no sense to me. I told my psychologist and my
> doctor about these episodes. They just said they didn't know what
> it was. Finally, I changed psychiatrists and she sent me for an EEG.
> Something wasn't right so I was sent for an MRI where they found
> a tumor (meningioma). They immediately sent me to the hospital
> and three days later removed it. Five years later I have no anxiety,
> no depression, no weird episodes. I am off all medications. And I
> am myself again. Thank God my psychiatrist got things moving
> for me.

20 LESSONS FROM OUR PATIENTS

As I was writing this chapter, I asked our patients to tell me the biggest lessons they learned from looking at their brains. Here are 20 answers, chosen from among many.

1. Prior to having my scan, I was misdiagnosed and thus mistreated.
    After having my scans, it is like I have a new life.

2. I would say that having my son scanned was what changed my life
    the most and made me a better mom. Seeing his brain made me
    realize he wasn't just being defiant, but that when he concentrated,
    his brain was extremely anxious. It made me realize that instead of
    yelling and fighting with him like I usually would, I needed to be
    more patient. He is now doing well in school and playing basketball
    like a rock star, and our relationship has never been better.

3. I learned as an adult that I still have lasting brain effects from heart surgery as an infant. It helped explain many of my struggles and gave me direction on how to get help.

4. If I didn't see the damage to my brain, I wouldn't have taken the actions needed to make it better.

5. The first scan helped me realize I wasn't crazy. It made total sense I had focus and anxiety issues, but I never admitted it to myself. The second scan three months later verified the supplements and diet changes had calmed my brain dramatically, which is why I was feeling so much better.

6. I never got a scan, but I use the images every day to help children understand the devastating effects of alcohol on the brain. I lost my sister to a DWI crash and she was the one drinking. Shortly thereafter, [when] I became a drug and alcohol prevention educator, I found Dr. Amen's book *Change Your Brain, Change Your Life*. I learned so much and now show his video, *Which Brain Do You Want?*—which shows brain scans of healthy teenagers versus drug-abusing teenagers—to both high school and middle school children. It totally changes the way the kids view drugs and their brains.

7. One of the things that I learned was how important it was to me to have a healthy brain. At the time, I didn't think about my brain health daily, because out of sight, out of mind (ironically).

8. I had no idea how I was hurting my brain, and my future, with alcohol and weed.

9. The SPECT scan made it real to me that the head trauma I had from a car accident and playing football had me headed for dementia. After seeing the scan, I know what to do to help my frontal cortex get bigger, rather than continue [to] shrink. Yes, size does matter!

10. My scan showed areas of overactivity that were contributing to my anxiety. I was put on the right medicine for my brain, and WOW, almost overnight I noticed the difference. Little things didn't bother me anymore.

11. I don't have to helplessly stand by and wait for my brain to deteriorate. It showed me that there are many options to keep my brain healthy.

12. My SPECT scan helped me (and my family!) better understand who I am and then taught me how to be the best version of myself! I went from feeling crazy and frustrated to feeling empowered and energized. Information + action = life change!

13. The SPECT scan allowed my doctors to tailor treatment to my specific brain. Finally, 10 years since my last concussion, I can work full-time again in my academic job.

14. I was once in denial that I had depression and anxiety, due to the lack of physical proof. With the SPECT scan, I was able to see with my own eyes the workings of my brain, which allowed me to accept the truth and move forward with the necessary treatment.

15. The most important lesson from my SPECT scan was that although my cognitive and visual issues are "all in my head," they are not a "figment of my imagination"! It's life-changing, real data that must be respected! And there is help available!

16. I oversaw care of my mother for 19 years, through her ever-worsening dementia. It was a horrible, draining experience. After my mother died, I felt concerned about my own brain, so, at 63, I had a SPECT scan. My scan came back clear, which gave me peace of mind for my future. I also used the opportunity to become my best version of brain health. Since my mother lived to 93, I figure I saved myself 30 years of worry and more. I am very, very grateful!

17. I had my brain scanned and the results were shocking. I have ADD. I'm 61 years old and have been searching for the missing piece of my brain since I quit high school at age 16 because I couldn't sit still or focus on schoolwork. Today it's possible to change my brain/change my body. I've lost weight, I feel better and have better relationships, work is better, and I'm happy.

18. I learned that the symptoms I was experiencing were due to over-activity in certain areas of my brain. Therefore, I learned self-compassion. It was a huge gift.

19. Getting the scan and learning where I was overactive and underactive was priceless. I could now have a more accurate game plan to address my specific needs, versus just a shotgun approach. Having more information allowed for a more accurate diagnosis and treatment

plan, which in the end led to a quicker and more permanent solution to the issues I was having. It's the closest thing to having a crystal ball that I have seen.

20. Your brain WANTS to heal itself, and given the right conditions, it CAN.

WHEN SHOULD YOU THINK ABOUT GETTING A FUNCTIONAL IMAGING STUDY, SUCH AS SPECT?

We order SPECT studies on most of our patients because they generally come to us after they have failed to get better with other specialists and therapies. Many patients tell us, "You are my last hope." In these cases, we need more detailed information to see if we can identify something that has been overlooked. In general, I think of SPECT as radar. If it is sunny outdoors, it is easy for pilots to land planes at the airport. So if you have a simple case, you don't need a scan. But if it is stormy out, with dark clouds, lightning, and thunder, radar can be lifesaving. Likewise, if your case is complicated and you have not gotten better with other providers or treatments, a scan could be lifesaving.

Here are answers to several common questions about SPECT.

Will the SPECT study give me an accurate diagnosis?

No. A SPECT study by itself will not provide a diagnosis. SPECT studies help the clinician understand more about the specific function of your brain. Each person's brain is unique, which may lead to unique responses to medicine or therapy. Diagnoses about specific conditions are made through a combination of clinical history, personal interviews, information from families, diagnostic checklists, SPECT studies, and other neuropsychological tests. No imaging study alone is a "doctor in a box" that can give accurate diagnoses on individual patients.

Why are SPECT studies ordered?

Some of the common reasons include

1. Evaluating seizure activity
2. Evaluating cerebral vascular disease
3. Evaluating cognitive impairment and dementia

4. Evaluating the effects of mild, moderate, and severe head trauma
5. Suspicion of an underlying organic brain condition, such as seizure activity contributing to behavioral disturbance, prenatal trauma, or exposure to toxins
6. Evaluating aggressive behavior that's atypical or unresponsive to treatment
7. Determining the extent of brain impairment caused by drug or alcohol abuse
8. Subtyping ADHD, anxiety, depression, addictions, and obesity
9. Evaluating treatment-resistant couples for underlying conditions that might be contributing to their relationship issues
10. General wellness screenings for people who are interested in brain optimization

Are there any side effects or risks from the study?

The study does not involve a dye, and people do not have allergic reactions to the study. The possibility exists, although in a very small percentage of patients, of a mild rash, facial redness and edema (swelling), fever, and a transient increase in blood pressure. The amount of radiation exposure from one brain SPECT study is approximately the same as from one head CT scan, or one-third of an abdominal CT scan. Pregnant women should not have a SPECT study.

How is the SPECT procedure done?

The patient is placed in a quiet room, and an intravenous (IV) line is started. The patient remains quiet for approximately 10 minutes with eyes open to allow his or her mental state to equilibrate to the environment. The imaging agent is then injected through the IV. After another short period of time, the patient lies on a table and the SPECT camera rotates around his or her head (the patient does not go into a tube). The time on the table is approximately 15 minutes. If a concentration study is ordered, the patient returns on another day to repeat the process; a concentration test is performed during the injection of the isotope.

Are there alternatives to having a SPECT study?

In our opinion, SPECT is the most clinically useful study of brain function. There are other studies, such as quantitative electroencephalograms

(QEEGs), positron emission tomography (PET) studies, and functional magnetic resonance imaging (fMRIs). PET studies and fMRIs tend to be more costly, and they are performed mostly in research settings. QEEGs can provide useful information, but they often do not give information on the deep areas of the brain.

Does insurance cover the cost of SPECT studies?

Reimbursement by insurance companies varies according to your plan. It is a good idea to check with the insurance company ahead of time to see if a SPECT study is a covered benefit.

Is the use of brain SPECT imaging accepted in the medical community?

Brain SPECT studies are widely recognized as an effective tool for evaluating brain function in seizures, strokes, dementia, and head trauma. There are literally thousands of research articles on these topics. In our clinic, based on our experience over 28 years, we have developed this technology further to evaluate aggression and nonresponsive psychiatric conditions. Unfortunately, many physicians do not fully understand the application of SPECT imaging and may tell you that the technology is experimental, but more than 6,000 medical and mental health professionals around the world have referred patients to us for scans.

We've learned so much from SPECT scans, and I'm proud of the difference we've made in the lives of thousands of patients. Whether or not you pursue a scan, the most important thing I want you to take away from this chapter is hope. You can change your brain, and that can change your life.

10 PRACTICAL LESSONS FROM 150,000 SCANS— HOW THEY HELP YOU FEEL BETTER FAST AND MAKE IT LAST

1. Current psychiatric diagnostic models are outdated because they don't assess the brain.

2. Psychiatric diagnoses are not single or simple disorders; they all have multiple types, and each requires its own treatment.

3. Looking at the brain decreases stigma, increases compliance with treatment, and completely changes the discussion around mental health.

4. If what you're doing is not working, look at the brain.

5. Looking at the brain improves outcomes, and people get better faster.

6. Looking at the brain completely changes the discussion about good and evil.

7. Looking at the brain helps to prevent mistakes.

8. Looking at the brain provides hope.

9. Alzheimer's and other forms of dementia start years, even decades, before people have any symptoms.

10. The most important lesson from 150,000 scans is that you can change your brain, and it will change your life.

TINY HABITS THAT CAN HELP YOU FEEL BETTER FAST—AND LEAD TO BIG CHANGES

10 SECONDS –:20 MINUTES Each of these habits takes just a few minutes. They are anchored to something you do (or think or feel) so that they are more likely to become automatic. Once you do the behaviors you want, find a way to make yourself feel good about them—draw a happy face, pump your fist, or do whatever feels natural. Emotion helps the brain to remember.

1. When I read about someone who has done something terrible, I will wonder what might have been going on in his or her brain.

2. When someone is being difficult with me, I will try not to overreact, knowing the other person may have issues I am unaware of.

3. If I have struggled with mental health issues and get down on myself, I will say to myself, "My brain can be better if I do the right things for it."

PART 7

L IS FOR LOVE

Doing the right thing for your brain health is the ultimate act of love for self and others. Love is the motivation that prompts us to put in the consistent effort and make the changes required to get healthy. Plus, love is the culmination of all the steps we've looked at so far. In this chapter I'll explore six different types of love (need-love, gift-love, family-love, friendship, erotic love, and *agape* or selfless love) and how each relates to your ability to get and stay well. Altruism, which is a combination of gift-love and agape, has been shown to significantly increase happiness in a short period of time.

CHAPTER 12

LOVE IS YOUR SECRET WEAPON

DOING THE RIGHT THING IS THE ULTIMATE ACT OF LOVE FOR SELF AND OTHERS

Love your neighbor as yourself.
JESUS, MARK 12:31

Focusing on getting and keeping your brain healthy is the most loving choice you can make for yourself and others. I try to do the right things for myself not because I should : . . yuck . . . but because I love myself, and I love my wife, children, grandchildren, parents, and siblings, and the mission of our work at Amen Clinics. In order for me to have the energy, mental clarity, and good decision-making ability to be an excellent husband, father, grandfather, physician, and leader of our business, I need to have a brain and body that work at their peak. If I ignored my health, as so many Americans do, then I would make poorer decisions, act in less helpful ways, and increase the risk of being a burden to my family rather than being the leader of my family. I see pursuing good health as the ultimate act of love.

One of my very close friends was obese when I nudged him to get healthy. He told me he didn't care if he lived a long time because he knew he was going to heaven when he died. When his wife heard what he said, she became furious and told him, "Because of the bad health decisions you make every day, you are much more likely to die early and abandon me, leaving me lonely, afraid, and unprotected. That's not love. That's selfish. It feels like you hate me." He got the message and got healthy over the next year. He did it out of love.

In order to feel better fast and make it last, it is critical to develop consistent habits and rituals over a long period of time that help build resilience. That way, when crises come, as they do for all of us, you are considerably better able to deal with them because you have the mental horsepower you need. Yes, getting healthy takes some work, as any love relationship does, but it is worth it.

When you really understand that getting healthy is about love, you stop saying things about getting healthy being hard, expensive, or boring, or about not wanting to deprive yourself. As I have seen many times throughout my career with my patients, being sick is hard, expensive, and boring, and you definitely deprive yourself of what you really want most, which is your health, energy, focus, happiness, and mental clarity. Ask anyone who's had a serious illness—your health is your greatest asset and your greatest desire when it is gone. I love my four children, but honestly, I never want to have to live with them. I never want to be a burden to them, and I don't want them telling me what to eat or what to wear, or trying to take my driver's license away from me. If you love your independence, you must start taking care of your brain and body.

When you model a brain-healthy life, others in your life, such as your spouse, children, and coworkers, are likely to follow. Children do what you do, not what you tell them to do. If you ignore your health, eat low-quality food, smoke, drink alcohol when stressed, or take medicines for chronic illnesses, such as diabetes or hypertension, without changing your lifestyle, they are likely to follow your example. Ask yourself, *Am I modeling health or illness?* In the United States we value our freedom. We don't want anyone telling us what to do or how to live. I don't either, but ultimately, our behavior is not just about us; it is about generations of us.

A new field of genetics, called epigenetics, has exploded onto the scientific scene over the past 20 years. *Epigenetic* means "above or on top of the gene." It refers to the recent discovery that your habits, emotions, and environment can turn on or off certain genes, making illness more or less likely in you as well as in your children, grandchildren, and even great-grandchildren. Your habits, emotions, and environment have such a strong impact on your biology that they alter the genes you pass on to future generations. It is these epigenetic "marks" that tell your genes to switch on or off or to manifest more strongly or weakly.

Diet, stress, toxins, prenatal nutrition, and other environmental factors, via epigenetics, can alter the activity of genes that you pass on to your children and your children's children. If a mom or dad eats poorly, even before they conceive, their child has an increased risk of cancer, heart disease, mental health issues, and addiction.[1] Studies have shown that boys who started smoking cigarettes before age 11 increased the risk of obesity in their children.[2] A dumb decision early in life can impact generations to come—and not just related to obesity. Some researchers believe that epigenetics holds the key to understanding certain cancers, heart disease, diabetes, schizophrenia, addictions, autism, and forms of dementia.

To stress how important epigenetics is, think of it this way: A baby girl is born with all of the eggs she will ever have. Her diet, habits, stresses, and environment turn on or turn off certain genes that make illness more or less likely in her, but also in her babies and grandbabies. Helping her do the right things is not just about her; it is about generations of her. This is a sobering message but one that must be addressed now, given that all of us are in a war for the health of our brains and bodies.

WHAT DO YOU LOVE THAT HOLDS YOU BACK?

I am often amazed at what people say they love. I hear people say they "love" bread, wine, sodas, fries, donuts, or sugar and cannot imagine their lives without them. They seem to put these substances in the same category as their spouses, children, and family members.

In 2010, Rick Warren, author of *The Purpose Driven Life* and senior pastor of Saddleback Church—one of the country's largest congregations—recruited Dr. Mark Hyman and me to develop a health program for churches. Called the Daniel Plan (no, not after me—after the Old Testament prophet Daniel), the program has been adopted by thousands of churches with great success. During its first week 15,000 people signed up, and over the first year they collectively lost 250,000 pounds (the weight of a space shuttle). They reported improvements in energy, focus, creativity, sleep, and mood, and reductions in stress, blood pressure, blood sugar, sexual dysfunction (always fun to talk about at church), and the use of medication. As in any change program, there was a fair amount of pushback from the church staff when we first started.

In one instance, a staff member came to my office for a consultation. We were both drinking tea while talking about her health background when she said something very strange: She asked me to put my tea down. I thought it was an odd request, but I politely did as she asked.

"I didn't want you to spit it at me," she said.

"Excuse me," I replied, feeling very curious, "I've never spit tea at anyone."

"Last night, after you spoke at church," she said, "I told my husband that I would rather get Alzheimer's disease than give up sugar . . . I didn't want you to spit the tea at me when you heard what I said."

I paused, smiled, and then asked, "Did you date the bad boys in high school?"

"No," she replied.

"Well, you are in love with something that hurts you. You are in a bad relationship with sugar. It beats you up, and you come back for more because you love it. Sugar increases erratic brain-cell firing, it is pro-inflammatory, it changes your brain so it needs sugar in order to feel normal, and it is addictive, just like a bad relationship. It has actually been found in animal studies to be more addictive than cocaine."

Eventually this staff member fell in love with herself, broke up with sugar, and helped her whole family get healthy. What things do you love that might be holding you back and keeping you from genuinely loving yourself?

SIX TYPES OF LOVE

Getting well starts with self-love. You do the right thing, not for momentary pleasure—that is a four-year-old's mind-set—but because it helps you feel good, increases your energy, and helps you stay on the path toward your goals in life.

C. S. Lewis, the British theologian and novelist who wrote The Chronicles of Narnia and *The Screwtape Letters*, among many other books, also wrote *The Four Loves*. Two types of love he described are "need-love" and "gift-love."[3] A baby needs love from her mother so she can be fed; and the mother gifts love to nurture and feed her child. Doing the right things for your brain's health is "need-love," for without it you will never be your best. But doing the right things for your brain health is also "gift-love," as you are giving to others by modeling good health for them.

The Greek language has four words for *love*:

- **Storge** (pronounced with a hard *g* sound)—affectionate love between family members, such as a mother for her child, or a child for his father
- **Phileo**—friendship, brotherly love (*Philadelphia* means "the city of brotherly love")

- **Eros**—passionate love
- **Agape**—selfless love, gift-love, the highest form of love

In the Greek New Testament, *agapeseis* (the verb form of *agape*) was the word used to translate what Jesus said when He exhorted His followers to love their neighbors as themselves. When we do this, we emulate God Himself, because Scripture says that He is love (1 John 4:8). We can love others "because he loved us first" (1 John 4:19, NLT). Allowing that love to guide our choices brings meaning into our lives.

Getting and staying healthy is good for you (self-love), good for your family (storge), good for your friends and coworkers (phileo), and good for our society at large (agape). Plus, when you really understand getting healthy, you realize it is also great for your blood vessels and sex life (eros). Erectile dysfunction is often a result of an unhealthy lifestyle, which can be improved by taking care of your brain and body. Making choices based on all these facets of love is good for other people *and* good for us.

Ray and Nancy: Improving Brain Health as a Couple

Ray played linebacker for the San Diego Chargers in the early 1970s, and he came to see us as part of our NFL study in 2010. Part of Ray's motivation for participating in the study was that his wife, Nancy, had been recently diagnosed with frontal temporal lobe dementia, and he wanted me to evaluate her. He was upset at the physician who diagnosed Nancy. The physician told Ray that he should find a "care" home for her because within a year she would not know his name, and he would be unable to care for her.

Ray's brain scan showed evidence of brain trauma, as did those of almost all of our retired players, plus he was overweight. Nancy's scan was a disaster. She had severe decreased activity in the front part of her brain, consistent with the diagnosis of frontal temporal lobe dementia. Sitting down to review their scans was very emotional for Ray and Nancy—and for me, too. From our clinical experience, we knew we could help Ray. But there is still no known effective treatment for frontal temporal lobe dementia.

I told Ray, "We have no proven treatment for Nancy. But if she were my wife, and I love my wife (this sort of makes a difference on what you are willing to do—only being brutally honest here), I would do all of the things I could for her." Our strategy with cases like Nancy's is to do everything possible to try to slow or reverse the dementia process. And while it does not work for everyone, it can help some. The treatment plan involved attacking all of the risk factors discussed in chapter 2 (see pages 33–37). We had her stop drinking alcohol; completely changed her diet; increased exercise and new learning (she took surfing and singing lessons); put her on a multivitamin/mineral, fish oil, and other brain-boosting supplements; and gave her hyperbaric oxygen and neurofeedback, which will be discussed in appendix A (page 289).

Ten weeks later I saw them back for their first follow-up visit. Ray had made sure that Nancy completely followed the plan, and her follow-up scan showed dramatic improvement. In addition to her improved scan, her memory and cognitive function were better. Ray joked that we had to slow down, because soon enough she would be smarter than he was. In addition, Ray had lost 30 pounds! Impressed, I asked him how he did it. He said his motivation was helping his wife get well. If he did everything I suggested, she would too. He would model a brain-healthy life, and they would get healthier as a couple. Sometimes motivation is about love. Ray loved Nancy.

NANCY: FRONTAL TEMPORAL LOBE DEMENTIA BEFORE AND AFTER

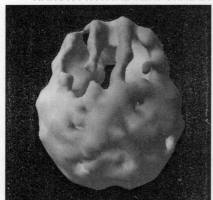 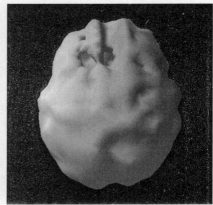

Before   After 10 weeks

Are you modeling health or illness for those you love? It matters.

When we do the right things for ourselves, we set up the people we love for success.

When we don't do the right things for ourselves, we set up the people we love for failure.

Yes, doing the right things for your health will irritate some of the people you love. In fact, based on a lot of personal experience, I think you'll find your friends and family may actively try to sabotage you. If they are not healthy, they will resent you for getting well. But over time, if you stay the course, they will eventually want what you have, and you will have the opportunity to create a revolution in your circle of family and friends.

Elly: Handing Down Brain Health

Elly came to see us from St. Petersburg, Russia. Before she started doing our program at home, Elly was obese, anxious, depressed, isolated, and in chronic back pain. Her mother had had dementia, which had been extremely hard on everyone in her family, and Elly was worried about developing it herself. After reading my book *Change Your Brain, Change Your Life*, she started incorporating one simple brain health strategy at a time. First she started taking brain-healthy supplements, which included a multivitamin/mineral, omega-3s, and extra vitamin D because her level tested low. Afterward, she noticed her energy was significantly better. Then she started drinking more water, which made a positive difference in her focus. As Elly began to feel better, she started exercising. She began walking and taking dancing lessons, which boosted her mood and decreased her isolation. Next, she took a big leap and changed her diet to the one discussed in chapter 9 (see page 203). Then she started taking Italian classes and learned to play the piano.

Over the next year, Elly lost 70 pounds. She told us she feels better than she has in decades and is pain-free. Elly then taught her children and grandchildren how to care for their brains. By teaching them about brain health, she was creating her own support group (both need-love and gift-love), making it more likely she'd stay on the program forever. Elly told me, "The best thing I can do for my children is keep my brain healthy for as long as I can and not be a burden to them."

Elly is the reason why we do what we do. I met Elly when she came to our California clinic to get scanned as a 90th birthday present to herself. Unlike scans of most 90-year-old brains, Elly's scan looked like that of someone in her sixties! Her brain was strong and healthy. When she saw her scan, she cried tears of joy. She said it would have looked much worse just a year earlier. By using these simple strategies, Elly changed the trajectory of the rest of her life, and her family's lives too. Elly loved herself and others and gave them one of the greatest gifts ever. Plus, she was thrilled she would not be a burden on her family (more agape gift-love).

GET OUTSIDE YOURSELF TO FEEL BETTER FAST

When Jesus told us to love each other as ourselves, He was giving us good health advice. Research suggests that whenever you feel down, anxious, or angry, it is best to get outside yourself to change your state of mind. In a new study, people who wrote about gratitude activated a part of their brains involved in happiness and altruism.[4] If you want to feel better fast, go to the aid of someone who needs help. According to a *New York Times* story, in the 1970s, former First Lady Barbara Bush became so depressed that she sometimes stopped her car on the side of the road for fear that she might deliberately crash the vehicle into a tree or an oncoming car. Mrs. Bush did not seek psychiatric help or medication for her depression, which she blamed on the hormonal changes of menopause and the stress of her husband's job as CIA director. Instead, she said she treated her depression by immersing herself in volunteer work and getting outside herself to help others.[5]

Being loving to strangers (agape)—or even to people you know (storge or phileo)—has the added benefit of making you feel happier, according to two studies. In one study, 86 participants were first asked about their life satisfaction and then divided into three groups. The first group was told to do an act of kindness every day for 10 days; the second group was told to do something new every day for 10 days; and the third group was given no instruction. When the 10 days had passed, the groups were retested on life satisfaction. Levels of happiness increased significantly and nearly equally among participants in the groups that had performed acts of kindness or novel activities, while happiness didn't change at all in the group that did neither.[6] Doing something for others for 10 days, especially if you vary the good deeds, is an effective way to make yourself feel better, the study suggests.

In another study, participants were divided into two groups and asked to recall either the last time they spent either $20 or $100 on themselves or the last time they had spent the same amount on someone else. After completing a scale measuring their levels of happiness, all of the participants were provided with a small sum of money and given the option of spending the money on themselves or on another person. The researchers found that study subjects were happier when they were asked to recall a time when they had purchased something for someone else, no matter the price of the gift. What's more, the happier they felt about being generous in the past, the greater the likelihood that they would spend money on someone besides themselves.[7] To feel better fast, it is better to give than to receive.

Turn toward Others

If you want to live a long life, focus on making contributions.
HANS SELYE

Research shows the happiest people are outward facing, focusing more on the people they serve than on themselves.[8] Even though the prayer attributed to St. Francis of Assisi was likely never written by him, it provides a research-based guide to happiness. When you feel stressed, consider repeating it or any other similar prayer or meditation, such as the Loving-Kindness Meditation (see chapter 1, pages 20–21).

PEACE PRAYER OF ST. FRANCIS
Lord, make me an instrument of your peace:
where there is hatred, let me sow love;
where there is injury, pardon;
where there is doubt, faith;
where there is despair, hope;
where there is darkness, light;
where there is sadness, joy.

O divine Master, grant that I may not so much seek
to be consoled as to console,
to be understood as to understand,
to be loved as to love.
For it is in giving that we receive,
it is in pardoning that we are pardoned,
and it is in dying that we are born to eternal life.
Amen.

As you conclude this book, may you find the courage to love yourself and others enough to make changes in your life, one strategy at a time. Your movement toward brain health will help you feel better fast and will leave a lasting legacy for those around you.

TINY HABITS THAT CAN HELP YOU FEEL BETTER FAST—AND LEAD TO BIG CHANGES

:03-30 MINUTES Each of these habits takes just a few minutes. They are anchored to something you do (or think or feel) so that they are more likely to become automatic. Once you do the behaviors you want, find a way to make yourself feel good about them—draw a happy face, pump your fist, or do whatever feels natural. Emotion helps the brain to remember.

1. When I approach any meal, I will ask myself if I am getting the nutrients I need to serve my health rather than steal from my health (need-love).

2. When I bring food to work, school, or an event, I will ask myself if it serves the health of those who will eat it, or if it steals from their health (gift-love).

3. When I shower in the morning, I will ask myself if I am doing what I can to be a healthy role model for my family (storge love).

4. Whenever I am around my friends, I will ask myself if I am modeling behavior that helps their health or makes it worse (phileo love).

5. When I hold my spouse's hand, I will gently squeeze it and remember that if our habits are healthy, our love life will be better and last longer throughout our lives (eros love).

6. When I watch the news, I will be on the lookout for ways to make a meaningful contribution to the health of my community (agape love).

SEVEN FEEL BETTER FAST BRAIN-XL SUMMARY QUESTIONS

Brain—Is the decision I'm about to make good for my brain or bad for it?

Rational Mind—Am I allowing untrue, negative thoughts to infect my brain and impact my happiness?

Attachments—Does my behavior today enhance or hurt my relationships?

Inspiration—Does this feeling or action have eternal value?

Nourishment—Do I eat and love mostly foods that love me back?

X Factor—If I looked at my brain, would it be healthy or not? If not, what am I going to do about it?

Love—Do I truly love myself so I can love others?

SEVEN FEEL BETTER FAST BRAIN-XL INTERVENTIONS

Brain—Know the BRIGHT MINDS risk factors and attack the ones that apply to you.

Rational Mind—Stop believing every stupid thought you have.

Attachments—Do something great today for someone you love.

Inspiration—Live in the center of your purpose today by doing something meaningful.

Nourishment—Start taking a multivitamin/mineral and omega-3 fatty acids, and know and optimize your vitamin D level. Aim to have eight servings of fruits and vegetables a day.

X Factor—If you are still struggling, look at your brain.

Love—Model a brain-healthy life for yourself and others.

Appendix A

ANSWERS TO COMMON QUESTIONS
ON FINDING MORE HELP

This appendix will answer common questions about seeking more help for resistant mental health issues:

- When is it time to seek professional help?
- What should I do when a loved one is in denial about needing help?
- How do I find a competent professional?
- Are there new and innovative treatments that can help me?

WHEN IS IT TIME TO SEEK PROFESSIONAL HELP?

This is relatively easy to determine. I recommend that people seek professional help when their attitudes, behaviors, feelings, or thoughts interfere with their ability to be successful in the world—whether in their relationships, in their work, or within themselves—and self-help techniques, such as the ones in this book, have not helped them fully alleviate the problem.

WHAT SHOULD I DO WHEN A LOVED ONE IS IN DENIAL ABOUT NEEDING HELP?

Unfortunately, the stigma associated with "psychiatric illness" prevents many people from getting help. People do not want to be seen as crazy, stupid, or defective, and they often don't seek support until they (or their loved one) can no longer tolerate the pain (on the job, in relationships, or inside themselves).

Here are several suggestions for people who are unaware that they would benefit from help or are unwilling to get the assistance they need:

1. *Try the straightforward approach first* (but with a new brain twist). Clearly tell the person what behaviors concern you. Tell him that the problems may be due to underlying brain patterns that can be tuned up. Explain that help may be available—not to cure a defect but rather to optimize how the brain functions. Tell the loved one that you know he is trying to do his best, but unproductive behavior, thoughts, or feelings may be getting in the way of his success. Emphasize access to help, not the person's defect.

2. *Give the loved one information.* Books, videos, and articles on the subjects you are concerned about can be of tremendous help. Many people come to see me because they read a book or article I wrote, or saw a video I produced. Good information can be very persuasive, especially if it is presented in a positive, life-enhancing way.

3. *Plant seeds.* When someone remains resistant to help, even after you have been straightforward and given him or her good information, plant seeds (ideas) about getting help and then water them regularly. Drop an idea, article, or other information about the topic from time to time. Be careful not to go overboard. If you talk too much about getting help, people will become resentful and won't pursue it, just to spite you.

4. *Protect your relationship with the other person.* People are more receptive to those they trust than to those who nag and belittle them. I do not let anyone tell me something bad about myself unless I trust him or her. Work on gaining the person's trust over the long run. It will make him or her more receptive to your suggestions. Do not make getting help the only thing that you talk about. Make sure you are interested in the person's whole life, not just in potential medical appointments.

5. *Give new hope.* Many people with mental health problems have tried to get help and found that it either didn't work or made them worse. Educate your loved one on new brain technology that helps professionals be more focused and effective in their treatment efforts.

6. *There comes a time when you have to say, "Enough is enough."* If, over time, the other person refuses to get help and his or her behavior has a negative impact on your life, you may have to separate yourself. Staying in a toxic relationship is harmful to your health, and it often

enables the other person to remain sick. Actually, I have seen that the threat or act of leaving can motivate a loved one to change, whether the problem area is drinking, drug use, or an underlying condition like attention deficit hyperactivity disorder (ADHD) or bipolar disorder. Threatening to leave is not the first tactic I would take, but after time it may be the best approach.

7. *Realize that you cannot force people into treatment* unless they are dangerous to themselves, dangerous to others, or unable to care for themselves. You can do only what you can do. Fortunately, today there is a lot more we can do than even 10 years ago.

HOW DO I FIND A COMPETENT PROFESSIONAL?

At Amen Clinics we get many e-mails, social media posts, and calls each week from people all over the world who are looking for competent professionals in their area whose mind-set is similar to mine and who utilize the principles outlined in this book. Because some of these principles are still on the edge of what is new in brain science, such professionals may be hard to locate. Still, finding the right person for evaluation and treatment is critical to the healing process. Choosing the wrong one can make things worse. There are a number of steps you can take to find the best person to assist you:

1. *Get the best person you can find.* Trying to save money up front may cost you a lot in the long run. The right help not only is cost-effective but saves unnecessary pain and suffering. Don't rely on a physician or therapist solely because he or she is on your managed care plan. That person may or may not be a good fit for you, and you shouldn't settle for someone who isn't a good fit. If he or she is on your insurance plan, that's great. Just don't let that be the primary criterion if you can help it.

2. *Use a specialist.* Brain science is expanding at a rapid pace. Specialists keep up with the latest developments in their fields, while generalists (family physicians) have to try to keep up with everything. If I had a heart arrhythmia, I would see a cardiologist rather than a general internist. I want to be treated by someone who has seen hundreds or even thousands of cases like mine.

3. *Get information about referrals from people who are highly knowledgeable about your problem.* Oftentimes well-meaning generalists give very bad

information. I have known many physicians and teachers who make light of diet, supplements, and lifestyle interventions. It may help to seek out a functional or integrative medicine doctor, who has specialized training and likely can refer you to other physicians as needed.

4. *Once you get the names of professionals, check their credentials.* State medical boards will have a public record of any legal or ethical trouble.

5. *Set up an interview with the professional to see whether or not you want to work with him or her.* Generally, you have to pay for a consultation, but it is worth spending time getting to know the people you will rely on for help. If you sense the fit isn't good, keep looking.

6. *Read professionals' writing or go hear them speak.* Many professionals write articles or books or speak at meetings or local groups. If you read their writings or hear them speak, you can often get a feel for the kind of people they are and their ability to help you.

7. *Look for a person who treats you with respect, who listens to your questions, and who responds to your needs.* Look for a relationship that is collaborative and trusting.

I know it is hard to find a professional who meets all of these criteria and who also has the right training in brain physiology, but it is possible. Be persistent. The right caregiver is essential to healing.

ARE THERE NEW AND INNOVATIVE TREATMENTS THAT CAN HELP ME?

Brain science is evolving quickly, and new treatments are being introduced at a rapid pace. At Amen Clinics we often recommend the following six innovative treatments to help our patients:

- hyperbaric oxygen therapy (HBOT)
- transcranial magnetic stimulation (TMS)
- ketamine infusions
- neurofeedback
- audiovisual entrainment (AVE)
- Irlen lenses

Hyperbaric Oxygen Therapy (HBOT): How "Air" Can Boost Healing

Healing cannot take place without healthy oxygen levels. HBOT relies on high-dose oxygen to speed up the healing process and reduce inflammation. Inside an HBOT chamber, where a patient sits or lies down for treatment, the air pressure is 1.3 to 2 times greater than normal. The increased air pressure helps the lungs gather more oxygen, allowing it to get into blood vessels and tissues, where it can increase production of growth factors and stem cells, promoting healing.

Normally, oxygen is carried throughout the body by red blood cells alone. With HBOT, oxygen dissolves into other bodily fluids, such as plasma, cerebral spinal fluid, and lymph and can be carried to regions where circulation is low or damaged. In vascular problems, strokes, and nonhealing wounds, for example, adequate oxygen cannot reach damaged areas and the body's natural healing ability is ineffective. When extra oxygen is able to reach those areas, it speeds the healing process. Researchers have found that increased oxygen strengthens the ability of white blood cells to kill bacteria, reduces swelling, and allows new blood vessels to grow into damaged tissues. It is a simple, noninvasive, and painless treatment with minimal side effects.

Research also suggests it can be helpful for

- head injuries[1]
- stroke[2]
- fibromyalgia[3]
- Lyme disease (as a helpful add-on treatment)[4]
- burns[5]
- diabetic ulcers and complications[6]
- wound healing[7]
- multiple sclerosis[8]
- irritable bowel disease[9]
- healing after surgery and radiation therapy[10]
- autism[11]
- cerebral palsy[12]

In 2011, Paul Harch, MD, and I and other colleagues published a study on 16 soldiers who had experienced blast-induced traumatic brain injuries. We did brain SPECT imaging and neuropsychological testing on the group before and after 40 sessions of HBOT. After treatment, our patients demonstrated significant improvement in their symptoms; full-scale IQ (a term for complete cognitive capacity; up 14.8 points); delayed and working memory scores; tests of impulsivity, mood, and anxiety; and quality of life scores. In addition, their SPECT scans showed remarkable overall improvement in blood flow.

Transcranial Magnetic Stimulation (TMS): An Alternative Way to Heal Mood

A form of "brain stimulation," TMS is used in the treatment of certain psychiatric and neurological disorders that have not improved with traditional approaches. TMS uses a noninvasive, highly focused, brief magnetic pulse to stimulate activity in the areas of the brain known to affect mood—without the troubling side effects people often experience when they take medication. TMS has been approved by the FDA for the treatment of resistant depression, but there is new evidence that it can enhance memory and potentially help improve a wide range of other brain-related issues, including

- depression[13]
- anxiety[14]
- addiction[15]
- smoking[16]
- posttraumatic stress disorder (PTSD)[17]
- obsessive-compulsive disorder (OCD)[18]
- cognitive problems, memory, and dementia[19]
- tinnitus (ringing in the ears)[20]
- stroke[21]

Electrical stimulation has been used for healing for centuries, starting more than 2,000 years ago when the Egyptians discovered that certain fish produce electrical impulses that could be used to treat pain and gout. The Greeks and Romans went on to practice these treatments too. Centuries later, in 1745, Altus Kratzstein, a German physician, wrote the first book on electrical therapy, which became the basis for Mary Shelley's *Frankenstein*. Toward the end of the 18th century, Italian physician and physicist Luigi Galvani discovered that passing an electrical current through the spine of a frog caused the amphibian's muscles to contract. He concluded that nerves were not water pipes, as Descartes had thought, but electrical conductors carrying information within the nervous system. Less than 50 years later, Michael Faraday discovered the fundamental principles of electromagnetic induction while attempting to stimulate nerves and the brain. His attempts were unsuccessful, but his advances led to the first successful transcranial magnetic stimulation in 1985. In 1997, TMS was approved for use in Canada, and in 2008 it was cleared by the FDA as a treatment for depression.

In a 2015 study, researchers from the University of São Paulo in Brazil studied the effect of TMS on memory in 34 elderly men and women with mild cognitive impairment (MCI). The scientists divided the participants into two groups. One group received 10 sessions of active TMS to stimulate the left front side of the brain, and the other group received sham (or fake) treatments. Cognitive testing before and after TMS showed the treatment group significantly improved on tests of everyday memory when compared to the sham group. Based on these findings, the researchers suggested that TMS might be effective as a treatment for MCI and "probably a tool to delay deterioration."[22]

TMS is a targeted treatment, and, unlike medication, it has no systemic side effects (because it doesn't get into your bloodstream). It is usually well-tolerated. Side effects are generally mild to moderate, and include headaches, scalp discomfort at the site of stimulation, tingling, spasms or twitching of facial muscles, and lightheadedness. These improve shortly after a session and decrease over time with additional sessions. Serious side effects are rare but may include seizures and mania, particularly in people with bipolar disorder. Treatment sessions last about 40 minutes, and you can resume your normal activities immediately afterward. After a full course of treatment, which ranges from 16 to 30 sessions, a high percentage of patients report a significant reduction in symptoms and experience improvement in their quality of life.

Ketamine Infusions: A Solution for Depression and Pain

When nothing else seems to work, I consider giving ketamine infusions.

Sixty-year-old Georgia had been in psychiatric care for decades. She struggled with anxiety and depression and had tried many different treatments, including multiple medications, multiple therapists, TMS, and nutritional supplements. When her depression worsened, she came to see me. She was having serious suicidal thoughts. We agreed she should try ketamine infusions.

Due to its hallucinogenic effects, ketamine has a reputation as a popular and illicit party drug, going by the nickname "Special K." It dulls pain, and users often feel detached or dissociated from their own bodies. It was first developed in the 1960s as an anesthetic and was given to soldiers during the Vietnam War. The drug has also been used in emergency rooms for curbing suicidal thoughts, making it a potential lifesaver. It's been put to use as an animal tranquilizer as well.

In 2000, researchers started studying ketamine as a treatment for depression and discovered that it improves mood much faster than traditional antidepressant medications and sometimes works when other drugs have failed. More than 100 studies have shown that ketamine has antidepressant effects.[23] Unlike antidepressants, which work by enhancing neurotransmitters like serotonin and dopamine, ketamine is thought to change the way brain cells talk to each other— similar to a computer reboot or hardware fix. It blocks a type of brain receptor thought to be involved with depression and pain, known as NMDA. Now, in a growing number of clinics, people with depression or pain for whom standard treatments haven't worked are being helped by a series of four to six infusions.

Georgia didn't like how she felt after the first treatment. Although ketamine made her feel weird, I encouraged her to go through the six-session course, as nothing else was working. After the second session everything changed. She called me and said she felt happy for the first time in decades. She felt energetic, clearheaded, and sexual. The depression lifted, but she still finished all six sessions and continued with monthly booster infusions. Two years later she remains improved.

Ketamine doesn't work for everyone, and the science of it is still emerging. But if you feel stuck, and nothing is working for serious depression or pain syndromes, it is worth considering. To learn more about ketamine treatments, visit the Ketamine Advocacy Network at www.ketamineadvocacynetwork.org.

Neurofeedback: Change Your Brain Waves to Get Healthier

Neurofeedback is a specialized form of biofeedback that gives people information about their brain waves, using sophisticated instruments to measure and change brain-wave patterns. More than 1,000 scientific studies show that neurofeedback can help a wide variety of mental health and brain-related conditions, such as

- memory in healthy people[24]
- memory poststroke[25]
- ADHD[26]
- obsessive-compulsive disorder[27]
- depression[28]
- traumatic brain injury[29]
- addiction[30]
- epilepsy[31]
- pain[32]
- balance in Parkinson's patients[33]

It can also help

- improve putting in golf[34]
- boost creativity in acting[35] and business[36]

Your brain produces a number of brain-wave patterns:

- *delta waves* (1–4 cycles per second)—very slow brain waves, seen mostly during sleep; high in traumatic brain injury and poor memory states

- *theta waves* (5–7 cycles per second)—slow brain waves, seen during creativity, daydreaming, and twilight states; higher in ADHD, impulsivity, poor memory, and brain fog states
- *alpha waves* (8–12 cycles per second)—brain waves seen during relaxed states
- *beta waves* (13–20 cycles per second)—fast brain waves seen during focused, thinking, analytic states; higher in anxiety states
- *high beta waves* (21–40 cycles per second)—fast brain waves seen during intense concentration or anxiety
- *gamma waves* (>40 cycles per second)—very fast brain waves, often seen during meditation and creative states

The basic neurofeedback technique uses behavioral reinforcement to help people change their brain-wave state. The more they can concentrate and produce fast beta brain waves, for example, the more rewards they can accrue. With Amen Clinics' neurofeedback equipment, a child or adult sits in front of a computer monitor with a biofeedback game. If he increases the beta activity or decreases the theta activity, the game continues. The game stops, however, when the player is unable to maintain the desired brain-wave state. People find the activity fun, and we gradually shape their brain-wave pattern to a healthier or more optimal one. This treatment technique is not an overnight cure. You often have to practice this form of biofeedback for 20 to 60 sessions to be able to recreate it on your own. But the results are worth it.

Audiovisual Entrainment (AVE): Better Your Brain with Sound and Light

Imagine sitting in a room at home with goggles and headphones on. Strobe lights flicker through the goggles and pulses come through the headphones, both designed to stimulate your mind. Our minds "think" in states of brain-wave frequency, and changes in frequencies are based on brain activity. When we stimulate the brain audiovisually with light and sound pulses, it begins to mimic or follow the same frequencies. This is called *entrainment*. In a sense, audiovisual entrainment (AVE) speaks to the mind in its own language—the language of rhythmic frequency—using a special machine that produces light and sound. The science of brain-wave entrainment, which means your brain picks up the rhythm in the environment, is one of the fastest-growing technologies in brain enhancement.

A review of 20 clinical studies concluded that AVE was helpful for people suffering from cognitive functioning deficits, stress, anxiety, PMS, and behavioral problems.[37] It has also been found to improve overall brain activity[38] and help with

- increasing brain blood flow[39]
- sleep[40]
- pain[41]
- alleviating stress[42]
- migraines[43]
- depression[44]

AVE can help improve your health on many levels: In studies, students showed an increase in GPA, concentration, and memory; seniors benefited from improved memory, cognition, and balance, which results in fewer falls;[45] and adults benefited from improved academic, corporate, and sports performance. Research publications show AVE efficacy with ADHD, seizure disorders, substance abuse, autistic spectrum disorders, mild traumatic brain injury, posttraumatic stress disorder, and depression.

The idea of using rhythm and frequency to facilitate shifts in our brain is nothing new. From music to sunlight, sound and light have long played a central role in shaping our human consciousness. When we listen to music, certain songs can make us happy, sad, or irritated. Fast beats tend to speed up our brain waves. Slow beats tend to slow down our brain waves. Through the amazing use of AVE, we are able to stimulate the brain with rhythmic pulses of light and sounds at specific frequencies to purposefully guide the brain into different brain-wave patterns. I like AVE because it is so easy to use and cost-efficient, and you can use it in the comfort of your own home, on your own time. If you are looking for a clinically proven, pharmaceutical-free way to improve your life and want to learn more about how AVE can help, go to www.mindalive.com.

Irlen Lenses: Brain-Calming Glasses

When I first heard about Irlen syndrome (also called scotopic sensitivity syndrome), I thought it was nonsense, mostly because I hadn't learned about it during my training. Sometimes I can be really narrow-minded. But when a friend who had severe, debilitating migraine headaches told me that being diagnosed with and treated for Irlen syndrome completely cured her headaches, I needed to know more.

Helen Irlen, PhD, is a school psychologist. Back in the early 1980s she was working under a federal research grant with college-educated adults who struggled with learning and reading difficulties. At that time she discovered that colored, filtered lenses could reduce stress on the brain and allow it to function better.

Irlen syndrome is a visual processing problem, where certain colors of the light spectrum tend to irritate the brain. It runs in families and is common after traumatic brain injuries. Anyone experiencing symptoms of anxiety, irritability, depression, or decreased concentration should be screened for Irlen syndrome. Common symptoms include

- light sensitivity; being bothered by glare, sunlight, headlights, or streetlights
- strain or fatigue with computer use
- fatigue, headaches, mood changes, restlessness, or an inability to stay focused when in a room with bright or fluorescent lights
- trouble reading words that are on white, glossy paper
- words or letters shifting, shaking, blurring, moving, running together, disappearing, or becoming difficult to perceive while reading
- difficulty reading music
- feeling tense, tired, or sleepy when reading, or even getting headaches when reading
- problems judging distance and difficulty with such things as escalators, stairs, ball sports, driving, or coordination
- migraine headaches

Heather, 42, had been in 10 car accidents when she came to see us for symptoms of ADHD, anxiety, and depression. During her history she told one of our physicians that she had trouble reading and fluorescent lights gave her headaches. Suspecting Irlen syndrome, he sent her for an evaluation.

When Heather was at the evaluation center, I got a call from one of my sisters, who had taken my nephew to be evaluated for Irlen syndrome at the same time. Several weeks earlier we had been together in Las Vegas for my birthday. We were on our way to an arcade on the second floor when halfway up the escalator I noticed my nephew was not next to me. He was still at the bottom of the escalator, having trouble getting on. He had depth-perception issues (common with Irlen syndrome), and rather than just walk onto the escalator like most people, he stood anxiously at the bottom before finally, very carefully, stepping on. He also was having trouble in school and was anxious and irritable. He needed to be evaluated.

I was with a patient when my sister called, so I didn't answer my phone. But when she called a second and third time, I thought my mother had died, and I answered, "What?"

"Danny," she said, "you can't believe what just happened with one of your patients. Heather is here from your clinic, and when she put the Irlen lenses on, the doorknob came out from the door. The bookcase came out from the wall. An overweight man walked by, and she blurted out, 'Potbelly.' It was like she saw in 3-D for the first time."

When we saw Heather two weeks later, she was beaming. With the Irlen lenses, her focus was better, her anxiety was reduced, and her mood had improved. Her prior brain scan had been remarkably overactive, but the Irlen lenses significantly calmed her brain.

HEATHER'S "ACTIVE" BRAIN SPECT BEFORE

WHILE WEARING IRLEN LENSES

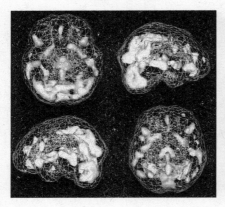
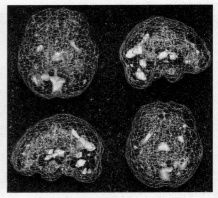

Excessive activity in many brain areas

Overall calming effect

We were all excited about Heather's progress until a few weeks later when her physician told me she was struggling with depression.

"What happened?" I asked.

"Like Paul Harvey always says," he replied, "here's the rest of the story. When Heather was a child, she was a prodigy guitar player. Apparently, she was amazing and gave performances around the area where she lived. But she could never learn to read music because the notes would move and dance on the page. At the age of 12, she took the guitar by its throat and smashed it, and she never played again. Now, 30 years later, she finds out that she has Irlen syndrome and is mourning the loss of what could have been."

Heather did not need Prozac to deal with the depression. She needed grief therapy, which we gave her. Within a few weeks she was back to feeling great and bought herself a new guitar. To learn more about Irlen syndrome, visit www.irlen.com.

Appendix B

WHERE DO YOU NEED HELP TO FEEL BETTER FAST?
A QUICK MENTAL HEALTH CHECKUP

> *Out of suffering have emerged the strongest souls;*
> *the most massive characters are seared with scars.*
> **KHALIL GIBRAN**

There are common reasons why people struggle with how they feel. Issues such as anxiety, depression, bipolar disorder, attention deficit hyperactivity disorder, addictions, posttraumatic stress disorder, and chronic stress are widespread among the population. According to the Centers for Disease Control and Prevention, almost 50 percent of the US population will suffer from a mental health issue at some point in their lives.[1] It is almost more normal to have a problem than not to have a problem. If you picked up this book, odds are that you (or someone you love) have struggled at some point with how you felt. Knowing your specific vulnerabilities is critical to getting the right help.

Only about one-third of people with depression or other mental health issues ever seek help. Asians, Hispanics, and African Americans are 30 percent less likely than whites to try to find assistance, and people age 60 and older are half as likely to seek treatment as those under 44.[2] This means that most people who suffer with mental health challenges never get the help they need and suffer unnecessarily when help is available.

On pages 302–304 are several questionnaires that will help you pinpoint where you might be struggling, followed by some simple suggestions to help you feel better fast. Please rate yourself on each of the symptoms listed below using the following 0–4 scale. If possible, have another person who knows you well (such as a spouse or parent) rate you too; this will give you the most complete picture. Having two or more symptoms with a score of 3 or 4 on any questionnaire may indicate a problem that needs to be taken seriously.

0	1	2	3	4	NA
Never	Rarely	Occasionally	Frequently	Very Frequently	Not Applicable/ Not Known

Anxiety Issues

____ 1. Anxious, tense, or nervous

____ 2. Panic attacks, which are periods of intense, unexpected fear or emotional discomfort

____ 3. Excessive tension, physical stress symptoms

____ 4. Fear of going crazy or doing something out of control

____ 5. Predict the worst

____ 6. Avoid conflict

____ 7. Freeze in anxious or upsetting situations

____ 8. Bite your fingernails or pick at your skin

____ 9. Need a lot of reassurance

____10. Avoid everyday places 1) for fear of having a panic attack, or 2) needing to go with other people in order to feel comfortable

____11. Cold or sweaty palms

Depression Issues

____ 1. Depressed or sad mood

____ 2. Decreased interest in things that are usually fun, including sex

____ 3. Significant weight gain or loss without trying, or appetite changes

____ 4. Recurrent thoughts of death or suicide

____ 5. Sleep changes, including lack of sleep or marked increase in sleep

____ 6. Physically agitated or "slowed down"

____ 7. Low energy or feelings of tiredness

____ 8. Feelings of worthlessness, helplessness, hopelessness, or guilt

____ 9. Decreased concentration or memory

Bipolar Disorder: Includes periods of depression (questions above) that tend to cycle with the manic symptoms below.

____ 1. Periods of an elevated, high, or irritable mood

____ 2. Periods of very high self-esteem or grandiose thinking

____ 3. Periods of decreased need for sleep without feeling tired

____ 4. More talkative than usual or feel pressure to keep talking

____ 5. Racing thoughts or frequent jumping from one subject to another

____ 6. Easily distracted by irrelevant things

___ 7. Marked increase in activity level

___ 8. Excessive involvement in pleasurable activities with painful consequences (affairs, gambling, etc.)

ADHD

___ 1. Trouble sustaining attention; easily distracted

___ 2. Difficulty completing projects

___ 3. Feeling overwhelmed by the tasks of everyday living

___ 4. Trouble maintaining an organized work or living area

___ 5. Inconsistent work performance

___ 6. Lack attention to detail

___ 7. Make decisions impulsively

___ 8. Have difficulty delaying what you want; must have your needs met immediately

___ 9. Restless, fidgety

___10. Make comments to others without considering their impact

___11. Impatient, easily frustrated

___12. Frequent traffic violations or near accidents

Addiction Issues

___ 1. Excessive use of substances (alcohol, drugs, food) or behaviors (gambling, sex, shopping, Internet, video games)

___ 2. Loss of control over substance use or behaviors

___ 3. Experienced negative consequences (relationships, money, health, law) because of substance use or behaviors, yet they did not cause you to stop

___ 4. Require more of a substance or behavior to make you feel good

___ 5. Experience withdrawal symptoms when you stop the substance use or behaviors

___ 6. Other people in your life complain about your substance use or repetitive behaviors

___ 7. Your substance use or repetitive behaviors distract you from your goals

___ 8. Feel guilty about your substance use or repetitive behaviors

Posttraumatic Stress Disorder (PTSD)

___ 1. Recurrent thoughts of a past traumatic event (e.g., sexual abuse, accident, fire)

____ 2. Recurrent distressing dreams of a past upsetting event

____ 3. A sense of reliving a past upsetting event

____ 4. A sense of panic or fear of events that resemble a past upsetting event

____ 5. Effort spent avoiding thoughts or feelings associated with a past trauma

____ 6. Persistent avoidance of activities/situations that cause remembrance of an upsetting event

____ 7. Inability to recall an important aspect of a past upsetting event

____ 8. Feeling detached or distant from others

____ 9. Feeling numb or restricted in your feelings

____10. Marked physical response to events that remind you of a past upsetting event, e.g., sweating when getting in a car if you have been in a car accident

Chronic Stress

____ 1. Family stress

____ 2. Work stress

____ 3. Health stress

____ 4. Financial stress

____ 5. Headaches

____ 6. Tension

____ 7. Irritability

____ 8. Insomnia

____ 9. Low frustration tolerance

____10. Trouble coping

ONCE YOU'VE IDENTIFIED YOUR MENTAL HEALTH ISSUES

1. **Get help.** Early treatment is essential to stave off the ravages of mental health issues. Treatment does not necessarily mean psychiatric medicines. At Amen Clinics, we prefer natural treatments whenever possible, such as those discussed throughout the book, including a healthy diet, exercise, omega-3 fatty acids EPA and DHA and other supplements, meditation, and cognitive behavioral therapy. All have a strong research basis showing they are effective. But if

these strategies don't work, or faster results are needed, medications are important to consider. Here are research-based strategies to boost your mental health if you are struggling with

- **Anxiety**
  - Brain-healthy habits (see chapter 2)
  - Exercise[3] (see chapter 4)
  - Hypnosis (see chapter 1)
  - Diaphragmatic breathing (see chapter 1)
  - Hand warming (see chapter 1)
  - Meditation (see chapter 1)
  - Calming music (see chapter 1)
  - ANT therapy (cognitive behavioral therapy, or CBT; see chapter 5)
  - Supplements to boost GABA, such as GABA itself,[4] magnesium, and theanine from green tea[5] (see chapter 10)

- **Depression and Negativity**—See my book *Healing Anxiety and Depression* for more detailed information on the seven types of anxiety/depression
  - Brain-healthy habits (see chapter 2)
  - Exercise[6] (see chapter 4)
  - Antioxidant-[7] and tomato-rich diet[8] (see chapter 9)
  - Omega-3 fatty acids—higher in EPA than DHA[9] (see chapter 10)
  - SAMe (s-adenosyl methionine) for depression,[10] especially in males[11] (see chapter 10)
  - Saffron[12] (see chapter 9)
  - Optimize vitamin D levels[13] (see chapter 10)
  - ANT therapy (cognitive behavioral therapy, or CBT; see chapter 5)[14]
  - Acupuncture[15]
  - Medication, if necessary
  - Methylfolate (as an add-on treatment to antidepressant medication)[16]

- **Bipolar Disorder**
  - Brain-healthy habits (see chapter 2)
  - Exercise[17] (see chapter 4)
  - Omega-3 fatty acids EPA and DHA[18] (see chapter 10)
  - Medication, if necessary

- **ADHD**—See my book *Healing ADD* for more detailed information on the seven types of ADD/ADHD, and take our free online test at www.ADDTypeTest.com.
  - Brain-healthy habits (see chapter 2)
  - Exercise[19] (see chapter 4)
  - Omega-3 fatty acids—higher in EPA than DHA[20] (see chapter 10)
  - Zinc[21]
  - Magnesium[22]
  - Iron (if ferritin levels are low)[23]
  - Phosphatidylserine[24]
  - Work with an ADHD coach
  - Medication, if necessary

- **PTSD**
  - Brain-healthy habits (see chapter 2)
  - EMDR (eye movement desensitization and reprocessing;[25] visit www.emdria.org) (see chapter 7)
  - Loving-Kindness Meditation[26] (see chapter 1)

- **Stress Management**
  - Brain-healthy habits (see chapter 2)
  - Exercise[27] (see chapter 4)
  - Prayer[28] and mindfulness meditation[29] (see chapter 1)
  - If you struggle with worry, consider supplements to raise the neurotransmitter serotonin, such as 5-hydroxytryptophan (5-HTP) or saffron[30]

2. **Try these research-proven tips.** Use them to lower stress and boost your level of happiness and overall mental health.

   - Start every day with the words "Today is going to be a great day." Your mind makes happen what it visualizes. When you start the day by saying these words, your brain will find the reasons it will be a great day.
   - Write down three things you are grateful for every day. Researchers found that people who did this significantly increased their sense of happiness in just three weeks.[31]
   - Every day, write down the name of one person you appreciate. Then tell him or her. Appreciation is gratitude expressed outwardly, and it builds positive bridges between people.

- Limit screen time. Studies report a higher level of depression and obesity with increased time spent with technology.
- Exercise—it is the fastest way to feel better. Go for a walk or a run.
- Enjoy some dark chocolate. It can boost blood flow to your brain,[32] help improve your mood, and decrease anxiety. In one study, seniors who ate more of it had a lower incidence of dementia than those who ate less.
- Listen to music. Just 25 minutes of Mozart or Strauss has been shown to lower blood pressure and stress. Listening to ABBA has also been shown to lower stress hormones—Mamma Mia![33]
- Choose experiences that give you a sense of awe, such as looking at a sunset or something else beautiful in nature.[34]
- Drink green tea, which contains L-theanine, an ingredient that helps you feel happier, more relaxed, and more focused.[35]
- Read an inspiring, powerful novel.[36]
- Take a walk in nature,[37] which is also associated with reducing worry.[38]
- Go barefoot outside. It decreases anxiety and depression by 62 percent, according to one study.[39]
- Listen to a sad song. Really. It was found to increase positive emotion.[40] Listening to lullabies and soothing music also decreased stress and improved sleep.[41]
- Stop complaining! It rewires your brain to see the negative in way too many places.[42]
- Spend time with positive people if you want to feel happy.[43] People's moods are contagious. (If you want to feel depressed, hang out with gloomy people.)
- Do something you love that brings you joy. For me, it is playing table tennis or spending time with my wife, kids, or grandkids.
- Write down your five happiest experiences, and then imagine reliving them.
- Engage in activities that make you feel competent.[44]
- Be patient. People tend to be happier with age, especially if they take care of their brains.[45]
- Learn to forgive; it can help reduce negative feelings.[46]
- Help someone else or volunteer; people in one study who did felt happier.[47] And make time for friends.[48]

- Get intimate with your spouse. Making love with a partner increased overall happiness and decreased stress hormones. In mice, it helped boost the hippocampus.[49]
- Journal your feelings. It helps to get them out of your head and allows you to gain perspective.[50]
- Learn to kill the ANTs (automatic negative thoughts). Whenever you feel sad, mad, nervous, or out of control, write down your negative thoughts. Next, ask yourself if they are really true or if they are a bit distorted, making you feel worse. Focusing your mind on positive, rational thoughts will help you feel much better.

Appendix C

KNOW YOUR IMPORTANT HEALTH NUMBERS

To feel better fast, you must know if your brain is working right, and then optimize it if it is not. To that end, it is critical to know your important health numbers. A fundamental business principle applies here: "You cannot change what you do not measure." You should check these numbers on an annual basis and whenever you feel out of sorts.

Body mass index (BMI). This measurement is the result of comparing weight to height. An optimal BMI is between 18.5 and 25; the overweight range falls between 25 and 30; more than 30 indicates obesity; and more than 40 indicates morbid obesity. To determine your BMI, google "BMI Calculator" and fill in your height and weight. Take this number seriously, because being overweight or obese is associated with having a smaller brain, and when it comes to your brain, size matters! Plus, obesity increases the risk for Alzheimer's disease and depression. In a new study, 40 percent of all cancers have been linked to excess weight.[1]

Blood pressure. Good blood pressure is critical for brain health. High blood pressure is associated with lower overall brain function, which means bad decision-making. The American Heart Association and the American College of Cardiology have revised their guidelines, which now means anyone with blood pressure of 130/80 millimeters of mercury will be diagnosed with stage 1 hypertension. Previously, a blood pressure of 140/90 was considered hypertension. (The category of "prehypertension" no longer exists.) That means more Americans than ever—half of all men and 38 percent of women, or

103 million people versus 72 million before this change—are now considered to have hypertension.[2] Here are the blood pressure numbers you should know:

Optimal
Systolic 90–120
Diastolic 60–80

Stage 1 Hypertension
Systolic 130–139
Diastolic 80–89

Stage 2 Hypertension
Systolic >/= 140
Diastolic >/= 90

Hypotension—blood pressure that is too low can also be a problem
Systolic < 90
Diastolic < 60

KEY LABORATORY TESTS

Laboratory tests provide another set of important numbers. Ask your health care professional to order them, or you can order them for yourself at websites like www.saveonlabs.com. If your numbers are abnormal, be sure to work with your health care professional to get them into optimal ranges. Here are the key lab tests that will provide insights into how well your body is functioning. All are blood tests unless otherwise indicated.

CBC (complete blood count). This blood test checks the health of your blood, including red and white blood cells. Low red blood cell count (anemia) can make you feel anxious and tired and can lead to memory problems. Enlarged red blood cells may mean you are drinking too much alcohol. A high level of white blood cells may indicate infection.

General metabolic panel with fasting blood sugar and lipid panel. This checks the health of your liver and kidneys, as well as your fasting blood sugar, cholesterol, and triglycerides.

Knowing your fasting blood sugar number is especially important.

- Normal is 70–100 milligrams per deciliter (mg/dL)
- Optimal is 70–89 mg/dL

- Prediabetes is 100–125 mg/dL
- Diabetes is 126 mg/dL or higher

Why is high fasting blood sugar a problem? Elevated blood sugar causes vascular (blood vessel) problems throughout your whole body, including your brain. Over time, blood vessels become brittle and vulnerable to breaking. High blood sugar leads not only to diabetes, but also to heart disease, stroke, visual impairment, impaired wound healing, wrinkled skin, and cognitive problems.

Cholesterol and triglycerides (fats) in the blood are also important, especially because they can negatively affect blood delivery to the brain. Cholesterol that is either too high or too low is bad for the brain. Higher cholesterol later in life has been associated with better cognitive performance,[3] longevity,[4] and a decreased risk of dementia. Normal levels are

- Total cholesterol: 135–200 mg/dL (below 160 has been associated with depression, suicide, homicide, and death from all causes, so 160–200mg/dL is optimal)
- HDL: >/= 60 mg/dL
- LDL: <100 mg/dL
- Triglycerides: <150 mg/dL

It is also important to know the particle size of your LDL cholesterol (ask your health care professional to order this test) because smaller particles are more toxic than larger ones. If your cholesterol numbers are not optimal and you wish to find out more, I recommend *The Great Cholesterol Myth* by Jonny Bowden, PhD, and Stephen Sinatra, MD.

Hemoglobin A1c, or HbA1c. This test, used to diagnose diabetes and prediabetes, is a measure of the average blood sugar levels for the prior two to three months. A result of 4–5.6 percent is normal for a nondiabetic; optimal is under 5.3 percent. A result in the 5.7–6.4 percent range indicates prediabetes. Higher numbers may signal diabetes.

Vitamin D. Low levels of vitamin D have been associated with obesity, depression, cognitive impairment, heart disease, reduced immunity, cancer, and all causes of mortality. The best blood test to get measures the 25-hydroxyvitamin D level. A normal vitamin D level is 30–100 nanograms (ng)/mL, with the most optimal range being 50–100 ng/mL.

Thyroid panel. Abnormal thyroid hormone levels are a common cause of anxiety, depression, forgetfulness, weight problems, and lethargy. Having low thyroid levels, or hypothyroidism, decreases overall brain activity, which can impair your thinking, judgment, and self-control. Low thyroid functioning can also make it nearly impossible to manage weight effectively. High levels (hyperthyroidism, less common than hypothyroidism) are associated with anxiety, insomnia, and feeling agitated. Healthy thyroid levels are

- TSH (thyroid-stimulating hormone): 0.4–3.0 IU/L
- Free T3: see normal ranges for the individual laboratory you use.
- Free T4: see normal range for the individual laboratory you use.
- Thyroid antibodies: thyroid peroxidase antibodies: < 9.0 IU/mL and thyroglobulin antibodies: < 4.0 IU/mL

Unfortunately, there is no single symptom or test result that will properly diagnose hypothyroidism. The key is to gather your symptoms and your blood test results and consult with your physician. Symptoms of low thyroid include fatigue, depression, mental fog, dry skin, hair loss (especially the outer third of your eyebrows), feeling cold when others feel normal, constipation, hoarse voice, and weight gain.

C-reactive protein (CRP). This test measures the inflammation in your body. *Inflammation* comes from the Latin word for "to set on fire" and describes a process associated with many chronic illnesses, including depression, dementia, and pain syndromes. A healthy CRP range is 0.0–1.0 mg/dL.

Homocysteine. Elevated homocysteine levels (>8 micromoles/liter) are associated with atherosclerosis (hardening and narrowing of the arteries) and an increased risk of heart attack, stroke, blood clot formation, and possibly Alzheimer's disease. Homocysteine is also a sensitive marker for a folate deficiency (folate is required for producing DNA and other genetic material).

Ferritin. This is a measure of iron stores. High levels are associated with inflammation and insulin resistance. Low levels are associated with anemia, restless leg syndrome, ADHD, and low motivation and energy. A level of 50–100 ng/mL is ideal. Women often have lower iron stores than men, due to blood loss from menstruation. Some theorize that this is one of the reasons that women tend to live longer than men. If your level is low, consider taking iron. If it is high, donating blood may help.

Free and total serum testosterone. For both men and women, low levels of testosterone have been associated with low energy, cardiovascular disease, obesity, low libido, depression, and Alzheimer's disease.

Normal levels for adult males are

- Total testosterone: 280–800 ng/dL; optimal is 500–800 ng/dL
- Free testosterone: 7.2–24 picograms (pg)/mL; optimal is 12–24 pg/mL

Normal levels for adult females are

- Total testosterone: 6–82 ng/dL; optimal is 40–82 ng/dL
- Free testosterone: 0.0–2.2 pg/mL; optimal 1.0–2.2 pg/mL

Estrogen and progesterone for women. Depending on the circumstances, these are measured in blood or saliva. Menstruating women are usually tested on day 21 of their cycle, while postmenopausal women can be measured anytime. Estrogen is responsible for vaginal lubrication and helps with libido and memory—and so much more. Progesterone calms emotions, contributes to a restful sleep, and acts as a diuretic. See the normal ranges for the individual laboratory you use.

Omega-3 Index. This measures the total amount of omega-3 fatty acids EPA and DHA in red blood cells and directly reflects their levels in the brain. The test is a clinically validated biomarker of the health of your brain. Your risk of cognitive decline rises by as much as 77 percent when your Omega-3 Index is low. Aim for a level above 8 percent.

Knowing and optimizing these numbers is critical to helping your brain work right. If any of them are abnormal, the function of your brain can be troubled too. Work with your health care provider to help get these numbers into the most optimal range possible.

Get in the habit of checking out your important health numbers on an annual basis.

About Daniel G. Amen, MD

The *Washington Post* has called Dr. Daniel G. Amen the most popular psychiatrist in America, and Sharecare, a digital health company designed to help people manage their health in one place, named him the web's most influential expert and advocate on mental health.

Dr. Amen is a physician, double board–certified psychiatrist, 10-time *New York Times* bestselling author, and international speaker. He is the founder of Amen Clinics in Costa Mesa, Los Angeles, and San Francisco, California; Bellevue, Washington; Reston, Virginia; Atlanta; New York; and Chicago. Amen Clinics have one of the highest published success rates treating complex psychiatric issues, and they have built the world's largest database of functional brain scans, totaling more than 135,000 scans on patients from 111 countries.

Dr. Amen is the lead researcher on the world's largest brain imaging and rehabilitation study of professional football players. His research has not only demonstrated high levels of brain damage in players, it has also shown the possibility of significant recovery for many with the principles that underlie his work.

Together with Pastor Rick Warren and Mark Hyman, MD, Dr. Amen is also one of the chief architects of Saddleback Church's Daniel Plan, a program to get the world healthy through religious organizations.

Dr. Amen is the author or coauthor of more than 70 professional articles, seven book chapters, and more than 30 books, including the #1 *New York Times* bestsellers *The Daniel Plan* and *Change Your Brain, Change Your Life*; as well as *Magnificent Mind at Any Age*; *Change Your Brain, Change Your*

Body; Use Your Brain to Change Your Age; Healing ADD; The Brain Warrior's Way; The Brain Warrior's Way Cookbook; Captain Snout and the Super Power Questions; and Memory Rescue.

Dr. Amen's published scientific articles have appeared in the prestigious journals *Brain Imaging and Behavior,* Nature's *Molecular Psychiatry, PLOS ONE,* Nature's *Translational Psychiatry,* Nature's *Obesity,* the *Journal of Neuropsychiatry and Clinical Neurosciences, Minerva Psichiatrica, Journal of Neurotrauma,* the *American Journal of Psychiatry, Nuclear Medicine Communications, Neurological Research, Journal of the American Academy of Child & Adolescent Psychiatry, Primary Psychiatry, Military Medicine,* and *General Hospital Psychiatry.* His research on posttraumatic stress disorder and traumatic brain injury was recognized by *Discover* magazine in its Year in Science issue as one of the "100 Top Stories of 2015."

Dr. Amen has written, produced, and hosted 12 popular shows about the brain on public television. He has appeared in movies, including *After the Last Round* and *The Crash Reel,* and in Emmy Award–winning television shows, such as *The Truth About Drinking* and *The Dr. Oz Show.* He was a consultant on the movie *Concussion,* starring Will Smith. He has also spoken for the National Security Agency (NSA), the National Science Foundation (NSF), Harvard's Learning & the Brain Conference, the Department of the Interior, the National Council of Juvenile and Family Court Judges, and the Supreme Courts of Delaware, Ohio, and Wyoming. Dr. Amen's work has been featured in *Newsweek, Time* magazine, the *Huffington Post,* the BBC, the *Guardian, Parade* magazine, the *New York Times,* the *New York Times Magazine,* the *Washington Post, Los Angeles Times, Men's Health,* and *Cosmopolitan.*

Dr. Amen is married to Tana. He is the father of four children and grandfather to Elias, Emmy, Liam, and Louie. He is also an avid table tennis player.

Gratitude and Appreciation

So many people have been involved in the process of creating *Feel Better Fast and Make It Last.* I am grateful to them all, especially the tens of thousands of patients and families who have come to Amen Clinics and allowed us to help them on their healing journey.

I am grateful to the amazing staff at Amen Clinics, who work hard every day serving our patients. Special appreciation to Jenny Cook, who helped me craft the book to make it easily accessible to our readers. I hope you agree. Also to our fearless leader, CEO Terry Weber, and my colleagues Dr. Parris Kidd, Dr. Rob Johnson, Lorenzo Sevilla, and Natalie Buchoz, who read every word of this book to be sure it makes sense.

I am grateful to Jan Long Harris at Tyndale, who saw the potential for this book to help many people, and my editor, Karin Buursma, who helped make this book the best it can be.

I remain grateful to my friends and colleagues at public television stations across the country, including my mentors and friends Alan Foster, BaBette Davidson, Maura Phinney, Jerry Liwanag, and countless others. Public television is a treasure, and we are grateful to be able to partner with stations to bring our message of hope and healing to millions.

Of course, I am grateful to my amazing wife, Tana, who is my partner in all I do, and to my family, including all who have tolerated my obsession with making brains better, especially my children, Antony, Breanne, Kaitlyn, and Chloe; grandchildren; and parents, Mary Meeks (Tana's mom) and Louis and Dorie Amen.

Resources

AMEN CLINICS

www.amenclinics.com

Amen Clinics, Inc., (ACI) was established in 1989 by Daniel G. Amen, MD. We specialize in innovative diagnosis and treatment planning for a wide variety of behavioral, learning, emotional, cognitive, and weight issues for children, teenagers, and adults. ACI has an international reputation for evaluating brain-behavior problems, such as ADD/ADHD, depression, anxiety, school failure, traumatic brain injury and concussions, obsessive-compulsive disorders, aggressiveness, marital conflict, cognitive decline, brain toxicity from drugs or alcohol, and obesity. In addition, we work with people to optimize brain function and decrease the risk for Alzheimer's disease and other age-related issues.

One of the primary diagnostic tools used at ACI is brain SPECT imaging. ACI has the world's largest database of brain scans for emotional, cognitive, and behavioral problems. We welcome referrals from physicians, psychologists, social workers, marriage and family therapists, drug and alcohol counselors, and individual patients and families.

Our toll-free number is (888) 288-9834.

Amen Clinics Orange County, California
3150 Bristol St., Suite 400
Costa Mesa, CA 92626

Amen Clinics Los Angeles
5363 Balboa Blvd., Suite 100
Encino, CA 91316

Amen Clinics Northern California
350 N. Wiget Ln., Suite 105
Walnut Creek, CA 94598

Amen Clinics Northwest
616 120th Ave. NE, Suite C100
Bellevue, WA 98005

Amen Clinics Washington, DC
10701 Parkridge Blvd., Suite 110
Reston, VA 20191

Amen Clinics New York
16 East 40th St., 9th Floor
New York, NY 10016

Amen Clinics Atlanta
5901 Peachtree-Dunwoody Road
NE, Suite C65
Atlanta, GA 30328

Amen Clinics Chicago
2333 Waukegan Rd., Suite 150
Bannockburn, IL 60015

Amenclinics.com is an educational, interactive website geared toward mental health and medical professionals, educators, students, and the public. It offers a wealth of information and resources to help you learn about optimizing your brain. The site contains more than 300 color brain SPECT images, thousands of scientific abstracts on brain SPECT imaging for psychiatry, a free brain health assessment, and much more.

BRAIN FIT LIFE

www.mybrainfitlife.com

Based on Dr. Amen's 35 years as a clinical psychiatrist, he and his wife, Tana, have developed a sophisticated online community to help you feel smarter, happier, and younger. It includes

- Detailed questionnaires to help you know your brain type and a personalized program targeted to your own needs
- WebNeuro, a sophisticated neuropsychological test that assesses your brain
- Fun brain games and tools to boost your motivation
- Exclusive, award-winning, 24-7 brain gym membership
- Physical exercises and tutorials led by Tana
- Hundreds of Tana's delicious, brain-healthy recipes
- Exercises to kill the ANTs (automatic negative thoughts)
- Meditation and hypnosis audios for sleep, anxiety relief, overcoming weight issues, pain management, and peak performance

- Amazing brain-enhancing music from Grammy Award winner Barry Goldstein
- Online forum for questions and answers, and a community of support
- Access to monthly live coaching calls with Daniel and Tana

BRAINMD HEALTH

www.brainmdhealth.com

For the highest-quality brain health supplements, courses, books, and information products

Notes

INTRODUCTION

1. T. R. Insel, "Disruptive Insights in Psychiatry: Transforming a Clinical Discipline," *Journal of Clinical Investigation* 119, no. 4 (2009): 700–705, doi: 10.1172/JCI38832.

2. M. F. Hoyt and M. Talmon, eds., *Capturing the Moment: Single Session Therapy and Walk-In Services* (New York: Crown House Publishing, 2014).

3. A. Akgul et al., "The Beneficial Effect of Hypnosis in Elective Cardiac Surgery: A Preliminary Study," *Thoracic and Cardiovascular Surgeon* 64, no. 7 (2016): 581–88, doi: 10.1055/s-0036-1580623.

4. R. Perkins and G. Scarlett, "The Effectiveness of Single Session Therapy in Child and Adolescent Mental Health. Part 2: An 18-Month Follow-Up Study," *Psychology and Psychotherapy* 81, part 2 (June 2008): 143–56, doi: 10.1348/147608308X280995.

5. BJ Fogg, "Tiny Habits Method," accessed April 23, 2018, http://tinyhabits.com/.

6. C. A. Raji et al., "Brain Structure and Obesity," *Human Brain Mapping* 31, no. 3 (March 2010): 353–64, doi: 10.1002/hbm.20870.

7. Fogg, "Tiny Habits Method."

CHAPTER 1: USE YOUR BRAIN TO RESCUE YOUR MIND AND BODY

1. R. Sapolsky, *Why Zebras Don't Get Ulcers*, 3rd ed. (New York: Holt Paperbacks), 2004.

2. H. Jiang et al., "Brain Activity and Functional Connectivity Associated with Hypnosis," *Cerebral Cortex* 27, no. 8 (August 1, 2017): 4083–93, doi: 10.1093/cercor/bhw220.

3. T. Tsitsi et al., "Effectiveness of a Relaxation Intervention (Progressive Muscle Relaxation and Guided Imagery Techniques) to Reduce Anxiety and Improve Mood of Parents of Hospitalized Children with Malignancies: A Randomized Controlled Trial in Republic of Cyprus and Greece," *European Journal of Oncology Nursing* 26 (February 2017): 9–18, doi: 10.1016/j.ejon.2016.10.007.

4. A. Charalambous et al., "Guided Imagery and Progressive Muscle Relaxation as a Cluster of Symptoms Management Intervention in Patients Receiving Chemotherapy: A Randomized Control Trial," *PLOS ONE* 11, no. 6 (June 24, 2016): e0156911, doi: 10.1371/journal.pone.0156911.

5. P. G. Nascimento Novais et al., "The Effects of Progressive Muscular Relaxation as a Nursing Procedure Used for Those Who Suffer from Stress Due to Multiple Sclerosis," *Revista Latino-Americana de Enfermagem* 24 (September 1, 2016): e2789, doi: 10.1590/1518-8345.1257.2789.

6. L. de Lorent et al., "Auricular Acupuncture versus Progressive Muscle Relaxation in Patients with Anxiety Disorders or Major Depressive Disorder: A Prospective Parallel Group Clinical Trial," *Journal of Acupuncture and Meridian Studies* 9, no. 4 (August 2016): 191–9, doi: 10.1016/j.jams.2016.03.008.

7. B. Meyer et al., "Progressive Muscle Relaxation Reduces Migraine Frequency and Normalizes Amplitudes of Contingent Negative Variation (CNV)," *Journal of Headache and Pain* 17, no. 1 (December 2016): 37, doi: 10.1186/s10194-016-0630-0.

8. A. B. Wallbaum et al., "Progressive Muscle Relaxation and Restricted Environmental Stimulation Therapy for Chronic Tension Headache: A Pilot Study," *International Journal of Psychosomatics* 38, nos. 1–4 (February 1991): 33–39.

9. T. Limsanon and R. Kalayasiri, "Preliminary Effects of Progressive Muscle Relaxation on Cigarette Craving and Withdrawal Symptoms in Experienced Smokers in Acute Cigarette Abstinence: A Randomized Controlled Trial," *Behavior Therapy*, 46, no. 2 (November 2014): 166–76, doi: 10.1016/j.beth.2014.10.002.

10. K. Golding et al., "Self-Help Relaxation for Post-Stroke Anxiety: A Randomised, Controlled Pilot Study," *Clinical Rehabilitation* 30, no. 2 (February 2016): 174–80, doi: 10.1177/0269215515575746.

11. S. Brunelli et al., "Efficacy of Progressive Muscle Relaxation, Mental Imagery, and Phantom Exercise Training on Phantom Limb: A Randomized Controlled Trial," *Archives of Physical Medicine and Rehabilitation* 96, no. 2 (February 2015): 181–87, doi: 10.1016/j.apmr.2014.09.035.

12. A. Hassanpour Dehkordi and A. Jalali, "Effect of Progressive Muscle Relaxation on the Fatigue and Quality of Life Among Iranian Aging Persons," *Acta Medica Iranica* 54, no. 7 (July 2016): 430–36; M. Shahriari et al., "Effects of Progressive Muscle Relaxation, Guided Imagery and Deep Diaphragmatic Breathing on Quality of Life in Elderly with Breast or Prostate Cancer," *Journal of Education and Health Promotion* 6 (April 19, 2017): 1, doi: 10.4103/jehp.jehp_147_14.

13. Y. K. Yildirim and C. Fadiloglu, "The Effect of Progressive Muscle Relaxation Training on Anxiety Levels and Quality of Life in Dialysis Patients," *EDTNA/ERCA Journal* 32, no. 2 (April–June 2006): 86–88.

14. A. K. Johnson et al., "Hypnotic Relaxation Therapy and Sexual Function in Postmenopausal Women: Results of a Randomized Clinical Trial," *International Journal of Clinical and Experimental Hypnosis* 64, no. 2 (2016): 213–24, doi: 10.1080/00207144.2016.1131590.

15. X. Ma et al., "The Effect of Diaphragmatic Breathing on Attention, Negative Affect and Stress in Healthy Adults," *Frontiers in Psychology* 8 (June 6, 2017): 874, doi: 10.3389/fpsyg.2017.00874; Y. F. Chen et al., "The Effectiveness of Diaphragmatic Breathing Relaxation Training for Reducing Anxiety," *Perspectives in Psychiatric Care* 53, no. 4 (October 2017): 329–36, doi: 10.1111/ppc.12184.

16. R. P. Brown and P. L. Gerbarg, "*Sudarshan Kriya* Yogic Breathing in the Treatment of Stress, Anxiety, and Depression. Part II—Clinical Applications and Guidelines," *Journal of Alternative and Complementary Medicine* 11, no. 4 (August 2005): 711–17.

17. L. C. Chiang et al., "Effect of Relaxation-Breathing Training on Anxiety and Asthma Signs/Symptoms of Children with Moderate-to-Severe Asthma: A Randomized Controlled Trial," *International Journal of Nursing Studies* 46, no. 8 (August 2009): 1061–70, doi: 10.1016/j.ijnurstu.2009.01.013.

18. S. Stavrou et al., "The Effectiveness of a Stress-Management Intervention Program in the Management of Overweight and Obesity in Childhood and Adolescence," *Journal of Molecular Biochemistry* 5, no. 2 (2016): 63–70.

19. T. D. Metikaridis et al., "Effect of a Stress Management Program on Subjects with Neck Pain: A Pilot Randomized Controlled Trial," *Journal of Back and Musculoskeletal Rehabilitation* 30, no. 1 (December 20, 2016): 23–33.

20. J. B. Ferreira et al., "Inspiratory Muscle Training Reduces Blood Pressure and Sympathetic Activity in Hypertensive Patients: A Randomized Controlled Trial,"

International Journal of Cardiology 166, no. 1 (June 5, 2013): 61–67, doi: 10.1016/j.ijcard .2011.09.069.

21. S. E. Stromberg et al., "Diaphragmatic Breathing and Its Effectiveness for the Management of Motion Sickness," *Aerospace Medicine and Human Performance* 86, no. 5 (May 2015): 452–57, doi: 10.3357/AMHP.4152.2015.

22. R. Fried et al., "Effect of Diaphragmatic Respiration with End-Tidal CO2 Biofeedback on Respiration, EEG, and Seizure Frequency in Idiopathic Epilepsy," *Annals of the New York Academy of Sciences* 602 (February 1990): 67–96.

23. P. R. Mello et al., "Inspiratory Muscle Training Reduces Sympathetic Nervous Activity and Improves Inspiratory Muscle Weakness and Quality of Life in Patients with Chronic Heart Failure: A Clinical Trial," *Journal of Cardiopulmonary Rehabilitation and Prevention* 32, no. 5 (September–October 2012): 255–61, doi: 10.1097/HCR.0b013e31825828da.

24. L. S. Wenck et al., "Evaluating the Efficacy of a Biofeedback Intervention to Reduce Children's Anxiety," *Journal of Clinical Psychology* 52, no. 4 (July 1996): 469–73; R. C. Hawkins et al., "Anxiety Reduction in Hospitalized Schizophrenics through Thermal Biofeedback and Relaxation Training," *Perceptual and Motor Skills* 51, no. 2 (October 1980): 475–82.

25. L. Scharff et al., "A Controlled Study of Minimal-Contact Thermal Biofeedback Treatment in Children with Migraine," *Journal of Pediatric Psychology* 27, no. 2 (March 2002): 109–19.

26. J. Gauthier et al., "The Role of Home Practice in the Thermal Biofeedback Treatment of Migraine Headache," *Journal of Consulting and Clinical Psychology* 62, no. 1 (February 1994): 180–4.

27. A. Musso et al., "Evaluation of Thermal Biofeedback Treatment of Hypertension Using 24-Hr Ambulatory Blood Pressure Monitoring," *Behaviour Research and Therapy* 29, no. 5 (1991): 469–78; E. B. Blanchard et al., "The USA-USSR Collaborative Cross-Cultural Comparison of Autogenic Training and Thermal Biofeedback in the Treatment of Mild Hypertension," *Health Psychology* 7 Supplement (February 1988): 175–92.

28. S. P. Schwarz et al., "Behaviorally Treated Irritable Bowel Syndrome Patients: A Four-Year Follow-Up," *Behaviour Research and Therapy* 28, no. 4 (1990): 331–35.

29. L. E. Williams and J. A. Bargh, "Experiencing Physical Warmth Promotes Interpersonal Warmth," *Science* 322, no. 5901 (October 24, 2008): 606–7, doi: 10.1126/science.1162548.

30. C. Wilbert, "Warm Hands, Warm Heart?" WebMD website, October 23, 2008, https://www .webmd.com/balance/news/20081023/warm-hands-warm-heart.

31. C. A. Lengacher et al., "Immune Responses to Guided Imagery During Breast Cancer Treatment," *Biological Research for Nursing* 9, no. 3 (January 2008): 205–14, doi:10.1177/1099800407309374; C. Maack and P. Nolan, "The Effects of Guided Imagery and Music Therapy on Reported Change in Normal Adults," *Journal of Music Therapy* 36, no. 1 (March 1, 1999): 39–55; Y. Y. Tang et al., "Improving Executive Function and Its Neurobiological Mechanisms through a Mindfulness-Based Intervention: Advances within the Field of Developmental Neuroscience," *Child Development Perspectives* 6, no. 4 (December 2012): 361–66, doi: 10.1111/j.1750-8606.2012.00250.x.

32. X. Zeng et al., "The Effect of Loving-Kindness Meditation on Positive Emotions: A Meta-Analytic Review," *Frontiers in Psychology* 6 (November 3, 2015): 1693, doi: 10.3389/fpsyg .2015.01693; B. L. Fredrickson et al., "Open Hearts Build Lives: Positive Emotions, Induced through Loving-Kindness Meditation, Build Consequential Personal Resources," *Journal of Personality and Social Psychology* 95, no. 5 (November 2008): 1045–62, doi: 10.1037/a0013262.

33. J. W. Carson et al., "Loving-Kindness Meditation for Chronic Low Back Pain: Results from a Pilot Trial," *Journal of Holistic Nursing* 23, no. 3 (September 2005): 287–304.

34. M. E. Tonelli and A. B. Wachholtz, "Meditation-Based Treatment Yielding Immediate Relief for Meditation-Naïve Migraineurs," *Pain Management Nursing* 15, no. 1 (March 2014): 36–40, doi: 10.1016/j.pmn.2012.04.002.

35. D. J. Kearney et al., "Loving-Kindness Meditation for Posttraumatic Stress Disorder: A Pilot Study," *Journal of Traumatic Stress* 26, no. 4 (August 2013): 426–34, doi: 10.1002 /jts.21832.

36. A. J. Stell and T. Farsides, "Brief Loving-Kindness Meditation Reduces Racial Bias, Mediated by Positive Other-Regarding Emotions," *Motivation and Emotion* 40, no. 1 (February 2016): 140–47, doi: 10.1007/s11031-015-9514-x.

37. M. K. Leung et al., "Increased Gray Matter Volume in the Right Angular and Posterior Parahippocampal Gyri in Loving-Kindness Meditators," *Social Cognitive and Affective Neuroscience* 8, no. 1 (January 2013): 34–39, doi: 10.1093/scan/nss076.

38. B. E. Kok et al., "How Positive Emotions Build Physical Health: Perceived Positive Social Connections Account for the Upward Spiral between Positive Emotions and Vagal Tone," *Psychological Science* 24, no. 7 (July 1, 2013): 1123–32, doi: 10.1177/0956797612470827.

39. R. J. Zatorre and I. Peretz, eds., *The Biological Foundations of Music* (New York: New York Academy of Sciences, 2001).

40. T. Schäfer et al., "The Psychological Functions of Music Listening," *Frontiers in Psychology* 4 (2013): 511.

41. J. Lieff, "Music Stimulates Emotions Through Specific Brain Circuits," *Searching for the Mind* (blog), March 2, 2014, http://jonlieffmd.com/blog/music-stimulates-emotions -through-specific-brain-circuits, as cited in B. Goldstein, *The Secret Language of the Heart* (San Antonio, TX: Hierophant Publishing, 2016), 29.

42. C. Grape et al., "Does Singing Promote Well-Being?: An Empirical Study of Professional and Amateur Singers During a Singing Lesson," *Integrative Physiological and Behavioral Science* 38, no. 1 (January–March 2003): 65–74, as cited in Goldstein, *The Secret Language of the Heart*, 29.

43. B. Goldstein, *The Secret Language of the Heart* (San Antonio, TX: Hierophant Publishing, 2016), 31.

44. R. H. Huang and Y. N. Shih, "Effects of Background Music on Concentration of Workers," *Work* 38, no. 4 (2011): 383–87, doi: 10.3233/WOR-2011-1141.

45. M. Hausmann et al., "Music-Induced Changes in Functional Cerebral Asymmetries," *Brain and Cognition* 104 (April 2016): 58–71, doi: 10.1016/j.bandc.2016.03.001.

46. Y. Ferguson and K. Sheldon, "Trying to Be Happier Really Can Work: Two Experimental Studies," *Journal of Positive Psychology* 8, no. 1 (January 2013): 23–33, doi: 10.1080 /17439760.2012.747000.

47. E. Brattico et al., "A Functional MRI Study of Happy and Sad Emotions in Music with and without Lyrics," *Frontiers in Psychology* 2 (December 1, 2011): 308, doi: 10.3389 /fpsyg.2011.00308.

48. R. Gillett, "The Best Music to Listen to for Optimal Productivity, According to Science," *Business Insider Australia*, July 25, 2015, https://www.businessinsider.com .au/the-best-music-for-productivity-2015-7.

49. A. G. DeLoach et al., "Tuning the Cognitive Environment: Sound Masking with 'Natural' Sounds in Open-Plan Offices," *Journal of the Acoustical Society of America* 137, no. 4 (April 2015): 2291, doi: 10.1121/1.4920363.

50. L. Lepron, "The Songs Scientifically Proven to Make Us Feel Good," Konbini (website), http://www.konbini.com/us/entertainment/songs-scientifically-proven-make-us -feel-good/.

51. Y. H. Li et al., "Massage Therapy for Fibromyalgia: A Systematic Review and Meta-Analysis of Randomized Controlled Trials," *PLOS ONE* 9, no. 2 (February 20, 2014): e89304, doi: 10.1371/journal.pone.0089304.

52. J. S. Kutner et al., "Massage Therapy vs. Simple Touch to Improve Pain and Mood in Patients with Advanced Cancer: A Randomized Trial," *Annals of Internal Medicine* 149, no. 6 (September 16, 2008): 369–79; S. H. Lee et al., "Meta-Analysis of Massage Therapy on Cancer Pain," *Integrative Cancer Therapies* 14, no. 4 (July 2015): 297–304, doi: 10.1177 /1534735415572885.

53. S. Babaee et al., "Effectiveness of Massage Therapy on the Mood of Patients after Open-Heart Surgery," *Iranian Journal of Nursing and Midwifery Research* 17, no. 2, supplement 1 (February 2012): S120–S124.

54. S. Khilnani et al., "Massage Therapy Improves Mood and Behavior of Students with Attention-Deficit/Hyperactivity Disorder," *Adolescence* 38, no. 152 (Winter 2003): 623–38.

55. F. Bazarganipour et al., "The Effect of Applying Pressure to the LIV3 and LI4 on the Symptoms of Premenstrual Syndrome: A Randomized Clinical Trial," *Complementary Therapies in Medicine* 31 (April 2017): 65–70, doi: 10.1016/j.ctim.2017.02.003.

56. Z. J. Zhang et al., "The Effectiveness and Safety of Acupuncture Therapy in Depressive Disorders: Systematic Review and Meta-Analysis," *Journal of Affective Disorders* 124, nos. 1–2 (July 2010): 9–21, doi: 10.1016/j.jad.2009.07.005; P. Bosch et al., "The Effect of Acupuncture on Mood and Working Memory in Patients with Depression and Schizophrenia," *Journal of Integrative Medicine* 13, no. 6 (November 2015): 380–90, doi: 10.1016/S2095-4964(15)60204-7.

57. L. de Lorent et al., "Auricular Acupuncture versus Progressive Muscle Relaxation in Patients with Anxiety Disorders or Major Depressive Disorder: A Prospective Parallel Group Clinical Trial," *Journal of Acupuncture and Meridian Studies* 9, no. 4 (August 2016): 191–99, doi: 10.1016/j.jams.2016.03.008

58. A. Xiang et al., "The Immediate Analgesic Effect of Acupuncture for Pain: A Systematic Review and Meta-Analysis," *Evidence-Based Complementary and Alternative Medicine* 3 (2017): 1–13, doi: 10.1155/2017/3837194.

59. C. W. Janssen et al., "Whole-Body Hyperthermia for the Treatment of Major Depressive Disorder: A Randomized Clinical Trial," *JAMA Psychiatry* 73, no. 8 (August 1, 2016): 789–95, doi: 10.1001/jamapsychiatry.2016.1031.

60. M. Lugavere, "6 Powerful Ways Saunas Can Boost Your Brain," Max Lugavere, https://www.maxlugavere.com/blog/5-incredible-things-that-happen-when-you-sit-in-a-sauna.

61. T. Laukkanen et al., "Sauna Bathing Is Inversely Associated with Dementia and Alzheimer's Disease in Middle-Aged Finnish Men," *Age and Ageing* 46, no. 2 (March 1, 2017): 245–49, doi: 10.1093/ageing/afw212.

62. S. Kasper et al., "Lavender Oil Preparation Silexan Is Effective in Generalized Anxiety Disorder—a Randomized, Double-Blind Comparison to Placebo and Paroxetine," *International Journal of Neuropsychopharmacology* 17, no. 6 (June 2014): 859–69, doi: 10.1017/S1461145714000017.

63. P. H. Koulivand et al., "Lavender and the Nervous System," *Evidence-Based Complementary and Alternative Medicine* 2013 (2013): 681304, doi: 10.1155/2013/681304.

64. S. Kasper et al., "Efficacy of Orally Administered Silexan in Patients with Anxiety-Related Restlessness and Disturbed Sleep—A Randomized, Placebo-Controlled Trial," *European Neuropsychopharmacology* 25, no. 11 (November 2015): 1960–67, doi: 10.1016/j.euroneuro.2015.07.024.

65. P. Sasannejad et al., "Lavender Essential Oil in the Treatment of Migraine Headache: A Placebo-Controlled Clinical Trial," *European Neurology* 67, no. 5 (2012): 288–91, doi: 10.1159/000335249.

66. M. Kheirkhah et al., "Comparing the Effects of Aromatherapy with Rose Oils and Warm Foot Bath on Anxiety in the First Stage of Labor in Nulliparous Women," *Iranian Red Crescent Medical Journal* 16, no. 9 (August 17, 2014): e14455, doi: 10.5812/ircmj.14455; T. Hongratanaworakit, "Relaxing Effect of Rose Oil on Humans," *Natural Product Communications* 4, no. 2 (February 2009): 291–96.

67. J. D. Amsterdam et al., "Chamomile (Matricaria recutita) May Provide Antidepressant Activity in Anxious, Depressed Humans: An Exploratory Study," *Alternative Therapies in Health and Medicine* 18, no. 5 (September–October 2012: 44–49.

68. C. Maller et al., "Healthy Nature Healthy People: 'Contact with Nature' as an Upstream Health Promotion Intervention for Populations," *Health Promotion International* 21, no. 1 (March 2006): 45–54.

69. P. Lambrou, "Fun with Fractals? Why Nature Can Be Calming," *Psychology Today* website, September 7, 2012, https://www.psychologytoday.com/blog/codes-joy/201209/fun-fractals.

70. C. J. Beukeboom et al., "Stress-Reducing Effects of Real and Artificial Nature in a Hospital Waiting Room," *Journal of Alternative and Complementary Medicine* 18, no. 4 (April 2012): 329–33, doi: 10.1089/acm.2011.0488.

71. H. Williams, "9 Ways to Improve Your Mood with Food: Herbs and Spices," AllWomensTalk website, http://health.allwomenstalk.com/ways-to-improve-your-mood-with-food/4.

CHAPTER 2: THE MISSING STRATEGY

1. J. Cepelewisz, "A Single Concussion May Triple the Long-Term Risk of Suicide," *Scientific American* (website), February 8, 2016, https://www.scientificamerican.com/article/a-single-concussion-may-triple-the-long-term-risk-of-suicide1/?utm_content=bufferb98ff&utm_medium=social&utm_source=linkedin.com&utm_campaign=buffer.

2. R. Douglas Fields, "Link between Adolescent Pot Smoking and Psychosis Strengthens," *Scientific American* website, October 20, 2017, https://www.scientificamerican.com/article/link-between-adolescent-pot-smoking-and-psychosis-strengthens/.

3. D. G. Amen et al., "Discriminative Properties of Hippocampal Hypoperfusion in Marijuana Users Compared to Healthy Controls: Implications for Marijuana Administration in Alzheimer's Dementia," *Journal of Alzheimer's Disease* 56, no. 1 (2017): 261–73, doi: 10.3233/JAD-160833.

4. M. A. Martinez et al., "Neurotransmitter Changes in Rat Brain Regions Following Glyphosate Exposure," *Environmental Research* 161 (February 2018): 212–19, doi: 10.1016/j.envres.2017.10.051.

5. T. Shakespeare and A. Whieldon, "Sing Your Heart Out: Community Singing as Part of Mental Health Recovery," *Medical Humanities*, published electronically November 25, 2017, doi: 10.1136/medhum-2017-011195.

6. K. Rehfeld et al., "Dancing or Fitness Sport? The Effects of Two Training Programs on Hippocampal Plasticity and Balance Abilities in Healthy Seniors," *Frontiers in Human Neuroscience* 11, no. 305 (June 15, 2017), doi: 10.3389/fnhum.2017.00305.

7. P. G. Harch et al., "A Phase I Study of Low-Pressure Hyperbaric Oxygen Therapy for Blast-Induced Post-Concussion Syndrome and Post-Traumatic Stress Disorder," *Journal of Neurotrauma* 29, no. 1 (January 1, 2012): 168–85, doi: 10.1089/neu.2011.1895.

8. T. Laukkanen et al., "Sauna Bathing Is Inversely Associated with Dementia and Alzheimer's Disease in Middle-Aged Finnish Men," 245–49.

9. K. C. Smolders et al., "A Higher Illuminance Induces Alertness Even during Office Hours: Findings on Subjective Measures, Task Performance and Heart Rate Measures," *Physiology and Behavior* 107, no. 1 (August 20, 2012): 7–16, doi: 10.1016/j.physbeh.2012.04.028.

10. R. A. Dienstbier, "The Impact of Humor on Energy, Tension, Task Choices, and Attributions: Exploring Hypotheses from Toughness Theory," *Motivation and Emotion* 19, no. 4 (1995): 255–67, http://digitalcommons.unl.edu/psychfacpub/111/.

11. A. P. Allen and A. P. Smith, "Effects of Chewing Gum and Time-on-Task on Alertness and Attention," *Nutritional Neuroscience* 15, no. 4 (July 2012): 176–85, doi: 10.1179/1476830512Y.0000000009; C. Lee, "How Chewing Gum Can Boost Your Brain Power," DailyMail.com, April 1, 2013, http://www.dailymail.co.uk/health/article-2302615/How-chewing-gum-boost-brain-power.html.

CHAPTER 3: CONTROL YOURSELF

1. H. S. Friedman and L. R. Martin, *The Longevity Project* (New York: Hudson Street Press, 2011).

2. P. Veliz et al., "Prevalence of Concussion Among US Adolescents and Correlated Factors," *JAMA* 318, no. 12 (September 26, 2017): 1180–82, doi: 10.1001/jama.2017.9087.

3. W. Mischel et al., "'Willpower' over the Lifespan: Decomposing Self-Regulation," *Social Cognitive and Affective Neuroscience* 6, no. 2 (April 2011): 252–56, doi: 10.1093/scan/nsq081.

4. J. Jaekel et al., "Preterm Toddlers' Inhibitory Control Abilities Predict Attention Regulation and Academic Achievement at Age 8 Years," *Journal of Pediatrics* 169 (February 2016): 87–92, doi: 10.1016/j.jpeds.2015.10.029.

5. Mischel et al., "'Willpower' over the Lifespan," 252–56.

6. J. Skorka-Brown et al., "Playing Tetris Decreases Drug and Other Cravings in Real World Settings," *Addictive Behaviors* 51 (December 2015): 165–70, doi: 10.1016/j.addbeh.2015 .07.020.

7. Jonathan Becher, "6 Quotes to Help You Understand Why It's Important to Say No," Forbes BrandVoice, August 12, 2015, https://www.forbes.com/sites/sap/2015/08/12 /quotes-on-saying-no/#19dda7fc5555.

8. C. Gallo, "Steve Jobs: Get Rid of the Crappy Stuff," *Forbes* website, May 16, 2011, https://www.forbes.com/sites/carminegallo/2011/05/16/steve-jobs-get-rid-of-the -crappy-stuff/#25b6fb271452.

9. "Kaiser Permanente Study Finds Keeping a Food Diary Doubles Diet Weight Loss," Kaiser Permanente website, July 8, 2008, https://share.kaiserpermanente.org/article /kaiser-permanente-study-finds-keeping-a-food-diary-doubles-weight-loss/; "Keeping a Food Diary Doubles Diet Weight Loss, Study Suggests," *ScienceDaily*, July 8, 2008, https://www.sciencedaily.com/releases/2008/07/080708080738.htm.

10. M. A. Scult et al., "Prefrontal Executive Control Rescues Risk for Anxiety Associated with High Threat and Low Reward Brain Function," *Cerebral Cortex* (November 17, 2017): doi: 10.1093/cercor/bhx304.

CHAPTER 4: CHANGE IS EASY—IF YOU KNOW HOW TO DO IT

1. *Oxford Living Dictionaries* online, s.v. "rut," accessed March 19, 2018, https://en.oxford dictionaries.com/definition/rut.

2. E. A. Evers et al., "Serotonin and Cognitive Flexibility: Neuroimaging Studies into the Effect of Acute Tryptophan Depletion in Healthy Volunteers," *Current Medicinal Chemistry* 14, no. 28 (2007): 2989–95.

3. R. L. Aupperle and M. P. Paulus, "Neural Systems Underlying Approach and Avoidance in Anxiety Disorders," *Dialogues in Clinical Neuroscience* 12, no. 4 (December 2010): 517–31.

4. M. J. Kim et al., "Intolerance of Uncertainty Predicts Increased Striatal Volume," *Emotion* 17, no. 6 (September 2017): 895–99, doi: 10.1037/emo0000331.

5. Aupperle and Paulus, "Neural Systems Underlying Approach and Avoidance in Anxiety Disorders," 517–31.

6. Evers et al., "Serotonin and Cognitive Flexibility," 2989–95.

7. S. N. Young, "How to Increase Serotonin in the Human Brain without Drugs," *Journal of Psychiatry and Neuroscience* 32, no. 6 (November 2007): 394–99.

8. P. Salmon, "Effects of Physical Exercise on Anxiety, Depression, and Sensitivity to Stress: A Unifying Theory," *Clinical Psychology Review* 21, no. 1 (February 2001): 33–61.

9. M. aan het Rot et al., "Bright Light Exposure During Acute Tryptophan Depletion Prevents a Lowering of Mood in Mildly Seasonal Women," *European Neuropsychopharmacology* 18, no. 1 (January 2008): 14–23, doi: 10.1016/j.euroneuro.2007.05.003.

10. K. Choi and H. J. Suk, "Dynamic Lighting System for the Learning Environment: Performance of Elementary Students," *Optics Express* 24, no. 10 (May 16, 2016): A907–A916, doi: 10.1364/OE.24.00A907; H. Slama et al., "Afternoon Nap and Bright Light Exposure Improve Cognitive Flexibility Post Lunch," *PLOS ONE* 10, no. 5 (May 27, 2015): e0125359, doi: 10.1371/journal.pone.0125359.

11. D. L. Walcutt, "Chocolate and Mood Disorders," *World of Psychology* (blog), Psych Central website, accessed March 19, 2018, http://psychcentral.com/blog/archives/2009/04/27 /chocolate-and-mood-disorders/; A. A. Sunni and R. Latif, "Effects of Chocolate Intake

on Perceived Stress; A Controlled Clinical Study," *International Journal of Health Sciences (Qassim)* 8, no. 4 (October 2014): 393–401.

12. A. Ghajar et al., "Crocus Sativus L. versus Citalopram in the Treatment of Major Depressive Disorder with Anxious Distress: A Double-Blind, Controlled Clinical Trial," *Pharmacopsychiatry* 50, no. 4 (July 2017): 152–60, doi: 10.1055/s-0042-116159; H. Fukui et al., "Psychological and Neuroendocrinological Effects of Odor of Saffron (Crocus sativus)," *Phytomedicine* 18, nos. 8–9 (June 15, 2011): 726–30, doi: 10.1016/j.phymed .2010.11.013.

13. W. Durant, *The Story of Philosophy* (New York: Pocket Books, 1953), 76.

14. Rahm Emanuel, interview with *Wall Street Journal*, November 19, 2008, https://www .youtube.com/watch?v=_mzcbXi1Tkk.

15. G. I. Schweiger and P. M. Gollwitzer, "Implementation Intentions: A Look Back at Fifteen Years of Progress," *Psicothema* 19, no. 1 (February 2007): 37–42.

16. P. Gollwitzer, "A Psychology Professor Reveals How to Break Bad Habits Once and for All," *Fortune*, January 26, 2017, http://fortune.com/2017/01/25/how-to-break-bad-habits-2/.

17. A. Achtziger et al., "Implementation Intentions and Shielding Goal Striving from Unwanted Thoughts and Feelings," *Personality and Social Psychology Bulletin* 34, no. 3 (March 2008): 381–93, doi: 10.1177/0146167207311201.

18. G. Stadler et al., "Physical Activity in Women: Effects of a Self-Regulation Intervention," *American Journal of Preventive Medicine* 36, no. 1 (January 2009): 29–34, doi: 10.1016 /j.amepre.2008.09.021.

19. G. Stadler et al., "Intervention Effects of Information and Self-Regulation on Eating Fruits and Vegetables over Two Years," *Health Psychology* 29, no. 3 (May 2010): 274–83, doi: 10.1037/a0018644.

20. I. S. Gallo et al., "Strategic Automation of Emotion Regulation," *Journal of Personality and Social Psychology* 96, no. 1 (January 2009): 11–31, doi: 10.1037/a0013460.

21. A. Achtziger et al., "Strategies of Intention Formation Are Reflected in Continuous MEG Activity," *Social Neuroscience* 4, no. 1 (2009): 11–27, doi: 10.1080/17470910801925350.

22. I. Paul et al., "If-Then Planning Modulates the P300 in Children with Attention Deficit Hyperactivity Disorder," *Neuroreport* 18, no. 7 (May 7, 2007): 653–57, doi: 10.1097/WNR .0b013e3280bef966.

23. P. M. Gollwitzer et al., "When Intentions Go Public: Does Social Reality Widen the Intention-Behavior Gap?" *Psychological Science* 20, no. 5 (May 2009): 612–18, doi: 10.1111/j.1467-9280.2009.02336.x.

24. Adapted from BJ Fogg's videos and other material on his website, www.bjfogg.com.

CHAPTER 5: MASTER YOUR RATIONAL MIND

1. Association for Psychological Science, "Believing the Future Will Be Favorable May Prevent Action," *ScienceDaily*, August 3, 2017, https://www.sciencedaily.com/releases /2017/08/170803145643.htm.

2. K. McSpadden, "You Now Have a Shorter Attention Span Than a Goldfish," *Time*, May 14, 2015, http://time.com/3858309/attention-spans-goldfish/.

3. J. Twenge, "What Might Explain the Unhappiness Epidemic?" The Conversation website, January 22, 2018, https://theconversation.com/what-might-explain-the-unhappiness -epidemic-90212.

4. R. F. Baumeister et al., "Bad Is Stronger Than Good," *Review of General Psychology* 5, no. 4 (December 2001): 323–370, doi: 10.1037/1089-2680.5.4.323.

5. J. McCoy, "New Outbrain Study Says Negative Headlines Do Better Than Positive," Business 2 Community website, March 15, 2014, https://www.business2community .com/blogging/new-outbrain-study-says-negative-headlines-better-positive-0810707.

6. R. Williams, "Are We Hardwired to Be Negative or Positive?" ICF website, June 30, 2014, https://coachfederation.org/are-we-hardwired-to-be-negative-or-positive/.

7. R. Hanson, "Confronting the Negativity Bias," *Rick Hanson* (blog), accessed March 25, 2018, http://www.rickhanson.net/how-your-brain-makes-you-easily-intimidated/.

8. C. A. Lengacher et al., "Immune Responses to Guided Imagery During Breast Cancer Treatment," *Biological Research for Nursing* 9, no. 3 (January 2008): 205–214, doi: 10.1177/1099800407309374; C. Maack and P. Nolan, "The Effects of Guided Imagery and Music Therapy on Reported Change in Normal Adults," *Journal of Music Therapy* 36, no. 1 (March 1, 1999): 39–55; A. G. Walton, "7 Ways Meditation Can Actually Change the Brain," *Forbes*, February 9, 2015, https://www.forbes.com/sites/alicegwalton/2015/02/09/7-ways-meditation-can-actually-change-the-brain/#84adaf414658.

9. H. Selye, *The Stress of Life* (New York: McGraw Hill, 1978), 418.

10. H H, "The 31 Benefits of Gratitude You Didn't Know About: How Gratitude Can Change Your Life," *Happier Human* (blog), accessed March 25, 2018, http://happierhuman.com/benefits-of-gratitude/.

11. C. Ackerman, "The Benefits of Gratitude: 28 Questions Answered Thanks to Gratitude Research," Positive Psychology Program website, April 12, 2017, https://positivepsychologyprogram.com/benefits-gratitude-research-questions/.

12. B. H. Brummett et al., "Prediction of All-Cause Mortality by the Minnesota Multiphasic Personality Inventory Optimism-Pessimism Scale Scores: Study of a College Sample during a 40-Year Follow-Up Period," *Mayo Clinic Proceedings* 81, no. 12 (December 2006): 1541–44, doi: 10.4065/81.12.1541.

13. L. S. Redwine et al., "Pilot Randomized Study of a Gratitude Journaling Intervention on Heart Rate Variability and Inflammatory Biomarkers in Patients with Stage B Heart Failure," *Psychosomatic Medicine* 78, no. 6 (July–August 2016): 667–76, doi: 10.1097/PSY.0000000000000316.

14. K. O'Leary and S. Dockray, "The Effects of Two Novel Gratitude and Mindfulness Interventions on Well-Being," *Journal of Alternative and Complementary Medicine* 21, no. 4 (April 2015): 243–45, doi: 10.1089/acm.2014.0119.

15. S. T. Cheng et al., "Improving Mental Health in Health Care Practitioners: Randomized Controlled Trial of a Gratitude Intervention," *Journal of Consulting and Clinical Psychology* 83, no. 1 (February 2015): 177–86, doi: 10.1037/a0037895.

16. E. Ramírez et al., "A Program of Positive Intervention in the Elderly: Memories, Gratitude and Forgiveness," *Aging and Mental Health* 18, no. 4 (May 2014): 463-70, doi: 10.1080/13607863.2013.856858.

17. S. M. Toepfer et al., "Letters of Gratitude: Further Evidence for Author Benefits," *Journal of Happiness Studies* 13, no. 1 (March 2012): 187–201.

18. T. K. Inagaki et al., "The Neurobiology of Giving Versus Receiving Support: The Role of Stress-Related and Social Reward-Related Neural Activity," *Psychosomatic Medicine* 78, no. 4 (May 2016): 443–53, doi: 10.1097/PSY.0000000000000302.

19. J. J. Froh et al., "Counting Blessings in Early Adolescents: An Experimental Study of Gratitude and Subjective Well-Being," *Journal of School Psychology* 46, no. 2 (April 2008): 213–33, doi: 10.1016/j.jsp.2007.03.005.

20. M. E. Seligman et al., "Positive Psychology Progress: Empirical Validation of Interventions," *American Psychologist* 60, no. 5 (July–August 2005): 410–21, doi: 10.1037/0003-066X.60.5.410.

21. K. Rippstein-Leuenberger et al., "A Qualitative Analysis of the Three Good Things Intervention in Healthcare Workers," *BMJ Open* 7, no. 5 (2017): e015826, doi: 10.1136/bmjopen-2017-015826.

22. M. Seligman, *Flourish: A Visionary New Understanding of Happiness and Well-Being* (New York: Free Press, 2011).

23. S. Wong, "Always Look on the Bright Side of Life," *Guardian*, August 11, 2009, https://www.theguardian.com/science/blog/2009/aug/11/optimism-health-heart-disease; H. A. Tindle et al., "Optimism, Cynical Hostility, and Incident Coronary Heart Disease and Mortality in the Women's Health Initiative," *Circulation* 120, no. 8 (August 25, 2009): 656–62, doi: 10.1161/CIRCULATIONAHA.108.827642; R. Hernandez et al., "Optimism and

Cardiovascular Health: Multi-Ethnic Study of Atherosclerosis (MESA)," *Health Behavior and Policy Review* 2, no. 1 (January 2015): 62–73, doi: 10.14485/HBPR.2.1.6.

24. Mayo Clinic, "Mayo Clinic Study Finds Optimists Report a Higher Quality of Life Than Pessimists," *ScienceDaily*, August 13, 2002, https://www.sciencedaily.com/releases /2002/08/020813071621.htm; C. Conversano et al., "Optimism and Its Impact on Mental and Physical Well-Being," *Clinical Practice and Epidemiology in Mental Health* 6 (2010): 25–29, doi: 10.2174/1745017901006010025; Harvard Men's Health Watch, "Optimism and Your Health," *Harvard Health Publishing*, May 2008, https://www.health.harvard .edu/heart-health/optimism-and-your-health.

25. E. S. Kim et al., "Dispositional Optimism Protects Older Adults from Stroke: The Health and Retirement Study," *Stroke* 42, no. 10 (October 2011): 2855–59, doi: 10.1161 /STROKEAHA.111.613448.

26. Association for Psychological Science, "Optimism Boosts the Immune System," *ScienceDaily*, March 24, 2010, www.sciencedaily.com/releases/2010/03/100323121757.htm.

27. B. R. Goodin and H. W. Bulls, "Optimism and the Experience of Pain: Benefits of Seeing the Glass as Half Full," *Current Pain and Headache Reports* 17, no. 5 (May 2013): 329, doi: 10.1007/s11916-013-0329-8.

28. International Association for the Study of Lung Cancer, "Lung Cancer Patients with Optimistic Attitudes Have Longer Survival, Study Finds," *ScienceDaily*, March 8, 2010, www.sciencedaily.com/releases/2010/03/100303131656.htm.

29. University of California, Riverside, "Keys to Long Life? Not What You Might Expect," *ScienceDaily*, March 12, 2011, https://www.sciencedaily.com/releases/2011/03 /110311153541.htm.

30. V. Venkatraman et al., "Sleep Deprivation Biases the Neural Mechanisms Underlying Economic Preferences," *Journal of Neuroscience* 31, no. 10 (March 9, 2011): 3712–18, doi: 10.1523/JNEUROSCI.4407-10.2011.

31. A. J. Dillard et al., "The Dark Side of Optimism: Unrealistic Optimism about Problems with Alcohol Predicts Subsequent Negative Event Experiences," *Personality and Social Psychology Bulletin* 35, no. 11 (November 2009): 1540–50, doi: 10.1177 /0146167209343124.

32. R. Ligneul et al., "Shifted Risk Preferences in Pathological Gambling," *Psychological Medicine* 43, no. 5 (May 2013): 1059–68, doi: 10.1017/S0033291712001900.

CHAPTER 6: HEALING CONNECTIONS

1. R. Waldinger, "What Makes a Good Life? Lessons from the Longest Study on Happiness," Tedx Talk, November 2015, https://www.ted.com/talks/robert_waldinger_what_makes _a_good_life_lessons_from_the_longest_study_on_happiness/transcript; R. Lund et al., "Stressful Social Relations and Mortality: A Prospective Cohort Study," *Journal of Epidemiology & Community Health* 68, no. 8 (2014): doi: 10.1136/jech-2013-203675.

2. Harvard Women's Health Watch, "The Health Benefits of Strong Relationships," Harvard Health Publishing website, December 2010, https://www.health.harvard.edu /newsletter_article/the-health-benefits-of-strong-relationships.

3. A. Sommerlad et al., "Marriage and Risk of Dementia: Systematic Review and Meta-Analysis of Observational Studies," *Journal of Neurology, Neurosurgery, and Psychiatry* online, November 28, 2017, doi: 10.1136/jnnp-2017-316274.

4. N. Donovan et al., "Loneliness, Depression and Cognitive Function in Older U. S. Adults," *Geriatric Psychiatry* 32, no. 5 (May 2017): 564–73, doi: 10.1002/gps.4495; University of Chicago, "Loneliness Is a Major Health Risk for Older Adults," *ScienceDaily*, February 16, 2014, https://www.sciencedaily.com/releases/2014/02/140216151411.htm.

5. N. I. Eisenberger and M. D. Lieberman, "Why Rejection Hurts: A Common Neural Alarm System for Physical and Social Pain," *Trends in Cognitive Sciences* 8, no. 7 (July 2004): 294–300, doi: 10.1016/j.tics.2004.05.010; N. I. Eisenberger, "The Neural Bases of Social Pain: Evidence for Shared Representations with Physical Pain," *Psychosomatic Medicine* 74, no. 2 (February 2012): 126–35, doi: 10.1097/PSY.0b013e3182464dd1.

6. M. R. Leary et al., "Teasing, Rejection, and Violence: Case Studies of the School Shootings," *Aggressive Behavior* 29, no. 3 (June 2003): 202–14, doi: 10.1002/ab.10061.

7. H. J. Markman and S. M. Stanley, *Fighting for Your Marriage: A Deluxe Revised Edition of the Classic Best-Seller for Enhancing Marriage and Preventing Divorce* (New York: Jossey-Bass, 2010).

8. P. Cuijpers et al., "Interpersonal Psychotherapy for Mental Health Problems: A Comprehensive Meta-Analysis," *American Journal of Psychiatry* 173, no. 7 (July 1, 2016): 680–87, doi: 10.1176/appi.ajp.2015.15091141; P. Cuijpers et al., "Interpersonal Psychotherapy for Depression: A Meta-Analysis," *American Journal of Psychiatry* 168, no. 6 (June 2011): 581–92, doi: 10.1176/appi.ajp.2010.10101411.

9. A. L. Brody et al., "Regional Brain Metabolic Changes in Patients with Major Depression Treated with Either Paroxetine or Interpersonal Therapy: Preliminary Findings," *Archives of General Psychiatry* 58, no. 7 (July 2001): 631–40.

10. L. Ngo et al., "Two Distinct Moral Mechanisms for Ascribing and Denying Intentionality," *Scientific Reports* 5 (December 2015): 17390, doi: 10.1038/srep17390.

11. G. Rizzolatti et al., "Premotor Cortex and the Recognition of Motor Actions," *Cognitive Brain Research* 3, no. 2 (March 1996): 131–41.

12. Sandra Blakeslee, "Cells That Read Minds," *The New York Times*, January 10, 2006, https://www.nytimes.com/2006/01/10/science/cells-that-read-minds.html.

13. P. Goldstein et al., "Brain-to-Brain Coupling during Handholding Is Associated with Pain Reduction," *Proceedings of the National Academy of Sciences* 115, no. 11 (March 13, 2018): E2528–E2537, doi: 10.1073/pnas.1703643115; University of Colorado at Boulder, "Holding Hands Can Sync Brainwaves, Ease Pain, Study Shows," *ScienceDaily*, March 1, 2018, https://www.sciencedaily.com/releases /2018/03/180301094822.htm.

14. S. L. Gable et al., "What Do You Do When Things Go Right? The Intrapersonal and Interpersonal Benefits of Sharing Positive Events," *Journal of Personality and Social Psychology* 87, no. 2 (August 2004): 228–45, doi: 10.1037/0022-3514.87.2.228.

15. M. E. P. Seligman, *Flourish: A Visionary New Understanding of Happiness and Well-Being* (New York: Free Press, 2011), 49; M. Seligman, "Active and Constructive Responding," YouTube video, 4:01, posted by "RefLearn," April 23, 2008, https://www.youtube.com /watch?v=MU3y2ApnG7Y.

16. S. L. Gable and H. T. Reis, "Good News! Capitalizing on Positive Events in an Interpersonal Context," *Advances in Experimental Social Psychology* 42 (2010): 195–257.

17. K. Patterson et al., *Influencer: The Power to Change Anything* (New York: McGraw Hill, 2008).

18. "The Power and Vestigiality of Positive Emotion—What's Your Happiness Ratio?" *Happier Human* (blog), http://happierhuman.com/positivity-ratio/.

19. *Merriam-Webster* online, s.v. "grace," accessed May 22, 2018, https://www.merriam -webster.com/dictionary/grace.

20. K. Weir, "Forgiveness Can Improve Mental and Physical Health," *American Psychological Association* 48, no. 1 (January 2017): 30, http://www.apa.org/monitor/2017/01/ce-corner .aspx.

21. E. Worthington, "Helping People Reach Forgiveness – Everett Worthington," YouTube video, 33:30, posted by "Dallas Theological Seminary," April 6, 2018, https://www .youtube.com/watch?v=Um2hLZLHens; see also "REACH Forgiveness of Others," Everett Worthington website, accessed April 26, 2018, http://www.evworthington-forgiveness .com/reach-forgiveness-of-others/.

CHAPTER 7: OVERCOMING TRAUMA AND GRIEF

1. K. Lansing et al., "High-Resolution Brain SPECT Imaging and Eye Movement Desensitization and Reprocessing in Police Officers with PTSD," *Journal of Neuropsychiatry and Clinical Neurosciences* 17, no. 4 (Fall 2005): 526–32, doi: 10.1176/jnp.17.4.526.

2. C. A. Raji et al., "Functional Neuroimaging with Default Mode Network Regions Distinguishes PTSD from TBI in a Military Veteran Population," *Brain Imaging and Behavior* 9, no. 3 (September 2015): 527–34, doi: 10.1007/s11682-015-9385-5; D. G. Amen et al., "Functional Neuroimaging Distinguishes Posttraumatic Stress Disorder from Traumatic Brain Injury in Focused and Large Community Datasets," *PLOS ONE* 10, no. 7 (July 1, 2015): e0129659, doi: 10.1371/journal.pone.0129659.

3. J. Guina et al., "Benzodiazepines for PTSD: A Systematic Review and Meta-Analysis," *Journal of Psychiatric Practice* 21, no. 4 (July 2015): 281–303, doi: 10.1097/PRA .0000000000000091.

4. J. I. Bisson et al., "Psychological Treatments for Chronic Post-Traumatic Stress Disorder: Systematic Review and Meta-Analysis," *British Journal of Psychiatry* 190 (February 2007): 97–104, doi: 10.1192/bjp.bp.106.021402.

5. R. M. Solomon and T. A. Rando, "Utilization of EMDR in the Treatment of Grief and Mourning," *Journal of EMDR Practice and Research* 1, no. 2 (2007): 109–17.

6. P. Gauvreau and S. P. Bouchard, "Preliminary Evidence for the Efficacy of EMDR in Treating Generalized Anxiety Disorder," *Journal of EMDR Practice and Research* 2, no. 1 (March 2008): 26–40, doi: 10.1891/1933-3196.2.1.26.

7. F. Horst et al., "Cognitive Behavioral Therapy vs. Eye Movement Desensitization and Reprocessing for Treating Panic Disorder: A Randomized Controlled Trial," *Frontiers in Psychology* 8 (2017): 1409, doi: 10.3389/fpsyg.2017.01409.

8. H. Bae et al., "Eye Movement Desensitization and Reprocessing for Adolescent Depression," *Psychiatry Investigation* 5, no. 1 (March 2008): 60–65, doi: 10.4306 /pi.2008.5.1.60.

9. F. Friedberg, "Eye Movement Desensitization in Fibromyalgia: A Pilot Study," *Complementary Therapies in Nursing and Midwifery* 10, no. 4 (2004): 245–49, doi: 10.1016 /j.ctnm.2004.06.006.

10. A. Rostaminejad et al., "Efficacy of Eye Movement Desensitization and Reprocessing on the Phantom Limb Pain of Patients with Amputations within a 24-Month Follow-Up," *International Journal of Rehabilitation Research* 40, no. 3 (September 2017): 209–14, doi: 10.1097/MRR.0000000000000227.

11. J. Zweben and J. Yeary, "EMDR in the Treatment of Addiction," *Journal of Chemical Dependency Treatment* 8, no. 2 (2006): 115–27; R. Pilz et al., "The Role of Eye Movement Desensitization and Reprocessing (EMDR) in Substance Use Disorders: A Systematic Review," *Fortschritte der Neurologie-Psychiatrie* 85, no. 10 (October 2017): 584–91, doi: 10.1055/s-0043-118338.

12. S. Foster and J. Lendl, "Eye Movement Desensitization and Reprocessing: Initial Applications for Enhancing Performance in Athletes," *Journal of Applied Sport Psychology* 7, supplement (1995): 63.

13. G. Maslovaric et al., "The Effectiveness of Eye Movement Desensitization and Reprocessing Integrative Group Protocol with Adolescent Survivors of the Central Italy Earthquake," *Frontiers in Psychology* 8 (October 23, 2017): 1826, doi: 10.3389/fpsyg.2017.01826.

14. D. G. Amen, *Healing the Hardware of the Soul* (New York: Free Press, 2002), 193.

15. C. Sachser et al., "Trauma-Focused Cognitive-Behavioral Therapy with Children and Adolescents: Practice, Evidence Base, and Future Directions," *Zeitschrift fur Kinder—und Jugendpsychiatrie und Psychotherapie* 44, no. 6 (November 2016): 479–90, doi: 10.1024 /1422-4917/a000436.

16. E. Deblinger et al., "Applying Trauma-Focused Cognitive-Behavioral Therapy in Group Format," *Child Maltreatment* 21, no. 1 (February 2016): 59–73, doi: 10.1177 /1077559515620668.

17. T. K. Jensen et al., "A Follow-Up Study from a Multisite, Randomized Controlled Trial for Traumatized Children Receiving TF-CBT," *Journal of Abnormal Child Psychology* 45, no. 8 (November 2017): 1587–97, doi: 10.1007/s10802-017-0270-0.

18. N. Gwozdziewycz and L. Mehl-Madrona, "Meta-Analysis of the Use of Narrative Exposure Therapy for the Effects of Trauma among Refugee Populations," *Permanente Journal* 17, no. 1 (Winter 2013): 70–76, doi: 10.7812/TPP/12-058.

19. D. M. Sloan et al, "A Brief Exposure-Based Treatment vs Cognitive Processing Therapy for Posttraumatic Stress Disorder: A Randomized Noninferiority Clinical Trial," *JAMA Psychiatry* 75, no. 3 (2018): 233–39, doi: 10.1001/jamapsychiatry.2017.4249.

20. A. S. Leiner et al., "Avoidant Coping and Treatment Outcome in Rape-Related Posttraumatic Stress Disorder," *Journal of Consulting and Clinical Psychology* 80, no. 2 (April 2012): 317–21, doi: 10.1037/a0026814.

21. A. J. Shallcross et al., "Let It Be: Accepting Negative Emotional Experiences Predicts Decreased Negative Affect and Depressive Symptoms," *Behaviour Research and Therapy* 48, no. 9 (September 2010): 921–29, doi: 10.1016/j.brat.2010.05.025.

22. L. Marques et al., "A Comparison of Emotional Approach Coping (EAC) between Individuals with Anxiety Disorders and Nonanxious Controls," *CNS Neuroscience and Therapeutics* 15, no. 2 (Summer 2009): 100–106, doi: 10.1111/j.1755-5949.2009.00080.x.

23. J. Lillis et al., "Binge Eating and Weight Control: The Role of Experiential Avoidance," *Behavior Modification* 35, no. 3 (May 2011): 252–64, doi: 10.1177/0145445510397178.

24. R. Chou and P. Shekelle, "Will This Patient Develop Persistent Disabling Low Back Pain?" *JAMA* 303, no. 13 (April 7, 2010): 1295–302, doi: 10.1001/jama.2010.344.

25. H. W. Sullivan et al., "The Effect of Approach and Avoidance Referents on Academic Outcomes: A Test of Competing Predictions," *Motivation and Emotions* 30, no. 2 (June 2006): 156–63, doi: 10.1007/s11031-006-9027-8.

26. J. al-Din Rumi, "The Guest House," in *The Essential Rumi*, trans. Coleman Barks (New York: HarperCollins, 2005), 109.

27. R. G. Tedeschi and L. G. Calhoun, "The Posttraumatic Growth Inventory: Measuring the Positive Legacy of Trauma," *Journal of Traumatic Stress* 9, no. 3 (July 1996): 455–71.

28. M. J. Nijdam et al., "Turning Wounds into Wisdom: Posttraumatic Growth over the Course of Two Types of Trauma-Focused Psychotherapy in Patients with PTSD," *Journal of Affective Disorders* 227 (November 11, 2017): 424–31, doi: 10.1016/j.jad.2017.11.031.

29. S. W. Jeon et al., "Eye Movement Desensitization and Reprocessing to Facilitate Posttraumatic Growth: A Prospective Clinical Pilot Study on Ferry Disaster Survivors," *Clinical Psychopharmacology and Neuroscience* 15, no. 4 (November 30, 2017): 320–27, doi: 10.9758/cpn.2017.15.4.320.

30. K. Stoller, *Oxytocin: The Hormone of Healing and Hope* (Lagunitas, CA: Dream Treader Press, 2012), 1–3.

31. M. Sack et al., "Intranasal Oxytocin Reduces Provoked Symptoms in Female Patients with Posttraumatic Stress Disorder Despite Exerting Sympathomimetic and Positive Chronotropic Effects in a Randomized Controlled Trial," *BMC Medicine* 15 (February 17, 2017): 40.

32. J. L. Frijling, "Preventing PTSD with Oxytocin: Effects of Oxytocin Administration on Fear Neurocircuitry and PTSD Symptom Development in Recently Trauma-Exposed Individuals," *European Journal of Psychotraumatology* 8, no. 1 (April 11, 2017): 1302652, doi: 10.1080/20008198.2017.1302652.

33. S. Palgi et al., "Oxytocin Improves Compassion toward Women among Patients with PTSD," *Psychoneuroendocrinology* 64 (2016): 143–49, doi: 10.1016/j.psyneuen.2015.11.008.

34. M. Kalantari et al., "Efficacy of Writing for Recovery on Traumatic Grief Symptoms of Afghani Refugee Bereaved Adolescents: A Randomized Control Trial," *Omega* 65, no. 2 (2012): 139–50, doi: 10.2190/OM.65.2.d.

35. K. van der Houwen et al., "The Efficacy of a Brief Internet-Based Self-Help Intervention for the Bereaved," *Behaviour Research and Therapy* 48, no. 5 (May 2010): 359–67, doi: 10.1016/j.brat.2009.12.009.

36. L. M. Range et al., "Does Writing about the Bereavement Lessen Grief Following Sudden, Unintentional Death?" *Death Studies* 24, no. 2 (March 2000): 115–34, doi: 10.1080 /074811800200603.

37. D. P. Hall Jr., "A Widow's Grief: The Language of the Heart" *JAMA* 268, no. 7 (August 19, 1992): 871–72; P. Taggart et al., "Anger, Emotion, and Arrhythmias: From Brain to Heart," *Frontiers in Physiology* 2 (2011): 67, doi: 10.3389/fphys.2011.00067.

38. D. Thompson, "Grief May Trigger Heart Rhythm Trouble," WebMD website, April 6, 2016, https://www.webmd.com/heart/news/20160406/death-of-loved-one-may-trigger-heart -rhythm-trouble#1.

39. J. W. James and R. Friedman, *The Grief Recovery Handbook 20th Anniversary Expanded Edition* (New York: HarperCollins, 2009), 19–20.

CHAPTER 8: CREATE IMMEDIATE AND LASTING JOY

1. "WS1988 Gm1: Scully's Call of Gibson Memorable At-Bat," YouTube video, 9:44, posted by "MLB," September 21, 2016, https://www.youtube.com/watch?v=N4nwMDZYXTI.

2. "Lessons from Leaders of the Past: Viktor Frankl," Charles Koch Institute website, accessed May 3, 2018, https://www.charleskochinstitute.org/blog/lessons-leaders -past-viktor-frankl/.

3. P. A. Boyle et al., "Effect of a Purpose in Life on Risk of Incident Alzheimer Disease and Mild Cognitive Impairment in Community-Dwelling Older Persons," *Archives of General Psychiatry* 67, no. 3 (March 2010): 304–10, doi: 10.1001/archgenpsychiatry.2009.208.

4. A. Steptoe, "Subjective Wellbeing, Health, and Ageing," *Lancet* 385, no. 9968 (February 14, 2015): 640–48, doi: 10.1016/S0140-6736(13)61489-0.

5. C. Cohen et al., "Purpose in Life and Its Relationship to All-Cause Mortality and Cardiovascular Events," *Psychosomatic Medicine* 78, no. 2 (February–March 2016): 122–33, doi: 10.1097/PSY.0000000000000274.

6. A. D. Turner et al., "Is Purpose in Life Associated with Less Sleep Disturbance in Older Adults?" *Sleep Science and Practice* 1, no. 14 (December 2017): doi: 10.1186/s41606-017 -0015-6.

7. A. L. Burrow and N. Rainone, "How Many Likes Did I Get?: Purpose Moderates Links between Positive Social Media Feedback and Self-Esteem" *Journal of Experimental Social Psychology* 69 (2016): 232–36, doi: 10.1016/j.jesp.2016.09.005.

8. A. Hart, *Thrilled to Death: How the Endless Pursuit of Pleasure Is Leaving Us Numb* (Nashville: Thomas Nelson, 2007).

9. J. B. Weaver III et al., "Health-Risk Correlates of Video-Game Playing Among Adults," *American Journal of Preventive Medicine* 37, no. 4 (October 2009): 299–305, doi: 10.1016 /j.amepre.2009.06.014.

10. N. Eyal, *Hooked: How to Build Habit-Forming Products* (New York: Portfolio/Penguin, 2014), 165.

11. "Parents, Beware: Smartphone Addiction Causes 'Imbalance' in Teenage Brains," Sputnik International website, March 12, 2017, https://sputniknews.com/society /201712031059656185-smartphone-addiction-causes-imbalance-brain/.

12. Hart, *Thrilled to Death*.

13. A. Aron et al., "Reward, Motivation, and Emotion Systems Associated with Early-Stage Intense Romantic Love," *Journal of Neurophysiology* 94, no. 1 (July 2005): 327–37, doi: 10.1152/jn.00838.2004.

14. H. E. Fisher et al., "Intense, Passionate, Romantic Love: A Natural Addiction? How the Fields That Investigate Romance and Substance Abuse Can Inform Each Other," *Frontiers in Psychology* 7 (2016): 687, doi: 10.3389/fpsyg.2016.00687.

15. M. L. Halko et al., "Entrepreneurial and Parental Love—Are They the Same?" *Human Brain Mapping* (March 13, 2017): 2923–38, doi: 10.1002/hbm.23562.

16. I. C. Duarte et al., "Tribal Love: The Neural Correlates of Passionate Engagement in

Football Fans," *Social Cognitive and Affective Neuroscience* 12, no. 5 (May 1, 2017): 718–28, doi: 10.1093/scan/nsx003.

17. D. G. Amen et al., "Reversing Brain Damage in Former NFL Players: Implications for Traumatic Brain Injury and Substance Abuse Rehabilitation," *Journal of Psychoactive Drugs* 43, no. 1 (January–March 2011): 1–5, doi: 10.1080/02791072.2011.566489.

18. G. H. Sahlgren, "Work Longer, Live Healthier," IEA Discussion Paper 46, May 2013, http://iea.org.uk/sites/default/files/publications/files/Work%20Longer,%20Live _Healthier.pdf.

19. A. O. Mechan et al., "Monoamine Reuptake Inhibition and Mood-Enhancing Potential of a Specified Oregano Extract," *British Journal of Nutrition* 105, no. 8 (April 2011): 1150–63, doi: 10.1017/S0007114510004940.

20. Some material in this section is taken from an interview with Dr. Jeff Zeig, "How Do You Find Meaning in Your Life?" on the *Brain Warrior's Way* podcast, published September 29, 2017, https://www.youtube.com/watch?v=O63vsRl2_fo.

21. V. Frankl, *Man's Search for Meaning* (Boston: Beacon Press, 1959), xv–xvi.

22. Interview with Dr. Zeig.

23. S. R. Covey, foreword to A. Patakos, *Prisoners of Our Thoughts: Viktor Frankl's Principles for Discovering Meaning in Life and Work* (San Francisco: Berrett-Koehler Publishers, 2008), viii.

24. Interview with Dr. Zeig.

25. Frankl, *Man's Search for Meaning*, 66.

26. Frankl, *Man's Search for Meaning*, 37.

27. Interview with Dr. Zeig.

28. V. Frankl, *The Doctor and the Soul: From Psychotherapy to Logotherapy* (New York: Vintage Books, 1986 edition), xix.

29. Frankl, *Man's Search for Meaning*, 112–13.

30. A. Leipzig, "How to Know Your Life Purpose in Five Minutes," Tedx Talk, February 1, 2013, https://www.youtube.com/watch?v=vVsXO9brK7M&app=desktop.

31. "54 Supplements and Drugs/Agonists to Increase Dopamine," SelfHacked website, updated March 21, 2018, https://selfhacked.com/blog/ways-to-increase-and-decrease -dopamine/.

32. Interview with Dr. Zeig.

33. E. Kübler-Ross, *Death: The Final Stage of Growth* (New York: Simon and Schuster, 1975), 164.

CHAPTER 9: THE FEEL BETTER FAST DIET

1. L. M. Pelsser et al., "Effects of a Restricted Elimination Diet on the Behaviour of Children with Attention-Deficit Hyperactivity Disorder (INCA Study): A Randomised Controlled Trial," *Lancet* 377, no. 9764 (February 5, 2011): 494–503, doi: 10.1016/S0140-6736 (10)62227-1; L. M. Pelsser et al., "Diet and ADHD, Reviewing the Evidence: A Systematic Review of Meta-Analyses of Double-Blind Placebo-Controlled Trials Evaluating the Efficacy of Diet Interventions on the Behavior of Children with ADHD," *PLOS ONE* 12, no. 1 (January 25, 2017): e0169277, doi: 10.1371/journal.pone.0169277.

2. "Preventive Health Care," Centers for Disease Control and Prevention website, accessed April 10, 2018, https://www.cdc.gov/healthcommunication/toolstemplates /entertainmented/tips/PreventiveHealth.html.

3. W. C. Willett et al., "Prevention of Chronic Disease by Means of Diet and Lifestyle Changes," in *Disease Control Priorities in Developing Countries*, 2nd edition, ed. D. T. Jamison et al. (Washington, DC: World Bank, 2006).

4. S. Khalid et al., "Is There an Association between Diet and Depression in Children and Adolescents? A Systematic Review," *British Journal of Nutrition* 116, no. 12 (December 2016): 2097–108, doi: 10.1017/S0007114516004359; R. S. Opie et al., "Dietary

Recommendations for the Prevention of Depression," *Nutritional Neuroscience* 20, no. 3 (April 2017): 161–71, doi: 10.1179/1476830515Y.0000000043; F. N. Jacka and M. Berk, "Depression, Diet and Exercise," *Medical Journal of Australia* 199, supplement 6 (September 16, 2013): S21–23.

5. F. N. Jacka et al., "The Association between Habitual Diet Quality and the Common Mental Disorders in Community-Dwelling Adults: The Hordaland Health Study," *Psychosomatic Medicine* 73, no. 6 (July–August 2011): 483–90, doi: 10.1097/PSY.0b013e318222831a.

6. A. L. Howard et al., "ADHD Is Associated with a 'Western' Dietary Pattern in Adolescents," *Journal of Attention Disorders* 15, no. 5 (July 2011): 403–11, doi: 10.1177/1087054710365990; A. Ríos-Hernández et al., "The Mediterranean Diet and ADHD in Children and Adolescents," *Pediatrics* 139, no. 2 (February 2017): e20162027, doi: 10.1542/peds.2016-2027.

7. W. B. Grant, "Using Multicountry Ecological and Observational Studies to Determine Dietary Risk Factors for Alzheimer's Disease," *Journal of the American College of Nutrition* 35, no. 5 (July 2016): 476–89, doi: 10.1080/07315724.2016.1161566; M. D. Parrott and C. E. Greenwood, "Dietary Influences on Cognitive Function with Aging: From High-Fat Diets to Healthful Eating," *Annals of the New York Academy of Sciences* 1114 (October 2007): 389–97, doi: 10.1196/annals.1396.028.

8. N. K. McGrath-Hanna et al., "Diet and Mental Health in the Arctic: Is Diet an Important Risk Factor for Mental Health in Circumpolar Peoples?—A Review," *International Journal of Circumpolar Health* 62, no. 3 (September 2003): 228–41.

9. N. Parletta et al., "A Mediterranean-Style Dietary Intervention Supplemented with Fish Oil Improves Diet Quality and Mental Health in People with Depression: A Randomized Controlled Trial (HELFIMED)," *Nutritional Neuroscience* (December 7, 2017): 1–14, doi: 10.1080/1028415X.2017.1411320.

10. L. M. Pelsser et al., "Effects of a Restricted Elimination Diet on the Behaviour of Children with Attention-Deficit Hyperactivity Disorder (INCA Study): A Randomised Controlled Trial," *Lancet* 377, no. 9764 (February 5, 2011): 494–503, doi: 10.1016/S0140-6736 (10)62227-1.

11. R. J. Hardman et al., "Adherence to a Mediterranean-Style Diet and Effects on Cognition in Adults: A Qualitative Evaluation and Systematic Review of Longitudinal and Prospective Trials," *Frontiers in Nutrition* 3 (July 22, 2016): 22, doi: 10.3389/fnut.2016.00022.

12. J. R. Hibbeln et al., "Vegetarian Diets and Depressive Symptoms among Men," *Journal of Affective Disorders* 225 (January 1, 2018): 13–17, doi: 10.1016/j.jad.2017.07.051.

13. J. J. DiNicolantonio et al., "Sugar Addiction: Is It Real? A Narrative Review," *British Journal of Sports Medicine* online (August 23, 2017): doi: 10.1136/bjsports-2017-097971.

14. M. Rao et al., "Do Healthier Foods and Diet Patterns Cost More Than Less Healthy Options? A Systematic Review and Meta-Analysis," *BMJ Open* 3, no. 12 (December 5, 2013): e004277, doi: 10.1136/bmjopen-2013-004277.

15. A. Christ et al., "Western Diet Triggers NLRP3-Dependent Innate Immune Reprogramming," *Cell* 172, nos. 1–2 (January 11, 2018): 162–75, doi: 10.1016/j.cell.2017.12.013.

16. A. O'Connor, "The Key to Weight Loss Is Diet Quality, Not Quantity, a New Study Finds," *New York Times*, February 20, 2018, https://www.nytimes.com/2018/02/20/well/eat /counting-calories-weight-loss-diet-dieting-low-carb-low-fat.html?emc=edit_ty _20180223&nl=opinion-today&nlid=20436447&te=1.

17. A. Adan, "Cognitive Performance and Dehydration," *Journal of the American College of Nutrition* 31, no. 2 (April 2012): 71–78: https://www.ncbi.nlm.nih.gov/pubmed/22855911.

18. R. O. Roberts et al., "Relative Intake of Macronutrients Impacts Risk of Mild Cognitive Impairment or Dementia," *Journal of Alzheimer's Disease* 32, no. 2 (January 1, 2012): 329–39, doi: 10.3233/JAD-2012-120862.

19. M. Dehghan et al., "Associations of Fats and Carbohydrate Intake with Cardiovascular Disease and Mortality in 18 Countries from Five Continents (PURE): A Prospective Cohort Study," *Lancet* 390, no. 10107 (November 4, 2017): 2050–62, doi: 10.1016/S0140 -6736(17)32252-3.

20. Y. Gu et al., "Nutrient Intake and Plasma β-amyloid," *Neurology* 78, no. 23 (June 5, 2012): 1832–40, doi: 10.1212/WNL.0b013e318258f7c2.

21. M. C. Houston, "Saturated Fats and Coronary Heart Disease," *Annals of Nutritional Disorders and Therapy* 4, no. 1 (2017): 1038.

22. B. A. Golomb and A. K. Bui, "A Fat to Forget: Trans Fat Consumption and Memory," *PLOS ONE* 10, no. 6 (June 17, 2015): e0128129, doi: 10.1371/journal.pone.0128129.

23. J. E. Gangwisch et al., "High Glycemic Index Diet as a Risk Factor for Depression: Analyses from the Women's Health Initiative," *American Journal of Clinical Nutrition* 102, no. 2 (August 2015): 454–63, doi: 10.3945/ajcn.114.103846.

24. R. Mujcic and A. J. Oswald, "Evolution of Well-Being and Happiness After Increases in Consumption of Fruits and Vegetables," *American Journal of Public Health* 106, no. 8 (August 2016): 1504–10, doi: 10.2105/AJPH.2016.303260; University of Warwick, "Fruit and Veggies Give You the Feel-Good Factor," *ScienceDaily*, July 10, 2016, https://www.sciencedaily.com/releases/2016/07/160710094239.htm.

25. E. Schmidt, "This Is Your Brain on Sugar: UCLA Study Shows High-Fructose Diet Sabotages Learning, Memory," UCLA Newsroom website, May 15, 2012, http://newsroom.ucla.edu/releases/this-is-your-brain-on-sugar-ucla-233992.

26. G. Addolorato et al., "Anxiety but Not Depression Decreases in Coeliac Patients after One-Year Gluten-Free Diet: A Longitudinal Study," *Scandinavian Journal of Gastroenterology* 36, no. 5 (May 2001): 502–6.

27. P. Usai et al., "Frontal Cortical Perfusion Abnormalities Related to Gluten Intake and Associated Autoimmune Disease in Adult Coeliac Disease: 99mTc-ECD Brain SPECT Study," *Digestive Liver Disease* 36, no. 8 (August 2004): 513–18, doi: 10.1016/j.dld.2004.03.010.

28. "15 Health Problems Linked to Monsanto's Roundup," EcoWatch website, accessed April 11, 2018, http://ecowatch.com/2015/01/23/health-problems-linked-to-monsanto-roundup/.

29. R. D. Abbott et al., "Midlife Milk Consumption and Substantia Nigra Neuron Density at Death," *Neurology* 86, no. 6 (February 9, 2016): 512–19, doi: 10.1212/WNL.0000000000002254; A. Kyrozis et al., "Dietary and Lifestyle Variables in Relation to Incidence of Parkinson's Disease in Greece," *European Journal of Epidemiology* 28, no. 1 (January 2013): 67–77, doi: 10.1007/s10654-012-9760-0.

30. A. Farooq et al., "A Prospective Study of the Physiological and Neurobehavioral Effects of Ramadan Fasting in Preteen and Teenage Boys," *Journal of the Academy of Nutrition and Dietetics* 115, no. 6 (June 2015): 889–97, doi: 10.1016/j.jand.2015.02.012.

31. N. M. Hussin et al., "Efficacy of Fasting and Calorie Restriction (FCR) on Mood and Depression among Ageing Men," *Journal of Nutrition, Health and Aging* 17, no. 8 (2013): 674–80, doi: 10.1007/s12603-013-0344-9.

32. T. Moro et al., "Effects of Eight Weeks of Time-Restricted Feeding (16/8) on Basal Metabolism, Maximal Strength, Body Composition, Inflammation, and Cardiovascular Risk Factors in Resistance-Trained Males," *Journal of Translational Medicine* 14, no. 1 (October 13, 2016): 290, doi: 10.1186/s12967-016-1044-0.

33. M. A. Faris et al., "Intermittent Fasting during Ramadan Attenuates Proinflammatory Cytokines and Immune Cells in Healthy Subjects," *Nutrition Research* 32, no. 12 (December 2012): 947–55, doi: 10.1016/j.nutres.2012.06.021.

34. A. R. Vasconcelos et al., "Intermittent Fasting Attenuates Lipopolysaccharide-Induced Neuroinflammation and Memory Impairment," *Journal of Neuroinflammation* 11 (May 6, 2014): 85, doi: 10.1186/1742-2094-11-85.

35. B. Spencer, "Why You Should NEVER Eat After 7 p.m.," DailyMail.com, August 31, 2016, http://www.dailymail.co.uk/health/article-3767231/Why-NEVER-eat-7pm-Late-night-meals-increases-risk-heart-attack-stroke.html.

36. A. Madjd et al., "Beneficial Effect of High Energy Intake at Lunch Rather Than Dinner on Weight Loss in Healthy Obese Women in a Weight-Loss Program: A Randomized

Clinical Trial," *American Journal of Clinical Nutrition* 104, no. 4 (October 1, 2016): 982–89, doi: 10.3945/ajcn.116.134163.

37. Authority Nutrition, "The 9 Healthiest Beans and Legumes You Can Eat," Healthline website, accessed April 12, 2018, www.healthline.com/nutrition/healthiest-beans-legumes.

38. Health Fitness Revolution, "Top 10 Healthiest Mushrooms and Their Benefits," Health Fitness Revolution website, September 5, 2016, www.healthfitnessrevolution.com/top-10-healthiest-mushrooms-and-their-benefits/.

39. D. M. Lovinger, "Serotonin's Role in Alcohol's Effects on the Brain," *Alcohol Health and Research World* 21, no. 2 (1997): 114–20, https://www.ncbi.nlm.nih.gov/pubmed/15704346.

40. R. P. Sharma and R. A. Coulombe Jr., "Effects of Repeated Doses of Aspartame on Serotonin and Its Metabolite in Various Regions of the Mouse Brain," *Food and Chemical Toxicology* 25, no. 8 (August 1987): 565–68, https://www.ncbi.nlm.nih.gov/pubmed/2442082.

41. "Foods That Fight Winter Depression," WebMD archives, accessed April 12, 2018, www.webmd.com/depression/features/foods-that-fight-winter-depression#1.

42. S. Nishizawa et al., "Differences between Males and Females in Rates of Serotonin Synthesis in Human Brain," *Proceedings of the National Academy of Sciences of the United States of America* 94, no. 10 (May 13, 1997): 5308–13, doi: 10.1073/pnas.94.10.5308.

43. J. Ding et al., "Alcohol Intake and Cerebral Abnormalities on Magnetic Resonance Imaging in a Community-Based Population of Middle-Aged Adults: The Atherosclerosis Risk in Communities (ARIC) Study," *Stroke* 35, no. 1 (January 2004): 16–21, doi: 10.1161/01.STR.0000105929.88691.8E.

44. J. Conner, "Alcohol Consumption as a Cause of Cancer," *Addiction* 112, no. 2 (February 2017): 222–28, doi: 10.1111/add.13477.

45. M. Schwarzinger et al., "Contribution of Alcohol Use Disorders to the Burden of Dementia in France 2008–13: A Nationwide Retrospective Cohort Study," *Lancet* 3, no. 3 (March 2018): e124–e132, doi: 10.1016/S2468-2667(18)30022-7.

46. S. K. Kulkarni et al., "Antidepressant Activity of Curcumin: Involvement of Serotonin and Dopamine System," *Psychopharmacology* 201, no. 3 (December 2008): 435–42, doi: 10.1007/s00213-008-1300-y.

47. T. Yamada et al., "Effects of Theanine, r-glutamylethylamide, on Neurotransmitter Release and Its Relationship with Glutamic Acid Neurotransmission," *Nutritional Neuroscience* 8, no. 4 (August 2005): 219–26, doi: 10.1080/10284150500170799.

48. "15 Brain Foods to Boost Focus and Memory," Dr. Axe website, accessed April 12, 2018, https://draxe.com/15-brain-foods-to-boost-focus-and-memory/.

49. D. Derbyshire, "A Bowl of Blueberries Keeps the Brain Active in the Afternoon," DailyMail.com, September 14, 2009, www.dailymail.co.uk/health/article-1212579/A-bowl-blueberries-day-keeps-brain-active-afternoon.html.

50. S. K. Park et al., "A Combination of Green Tea Extract and L-theanine Improves Memory and Attention in Subjects with Mild Cognitive Impairment: A Double-Blind Placebo-Controlled Study," *Journal of Medicinal Food* 14, no. 4 (April 2011): 334–43, doi: 10.1089/jmf.2009.1374.

51. S. Barker et al., "Improved Performance on Clerical Tasks Associated with Administration of Peppermint Odor," *Perceptual and Motor Skills* 97, no. 3 part 1 (December 2003): 1007–10, doi: 10.2466/pms.2003.97.3.1007.

52. P. R. Zoladz and B. Raudenbush, "Cognitive Enhancement through Stimulation of the Chemical Senses," *North American Journal of Psychology* 7, no. 1 (January 2005): 125–140; H. M. Chen and H. W. Chen, "The Effect of Applying Cinnamon Aromatherapy for Children with Attention Deficit Hyperactivity Disorder," *Journal of Chinese Medicine* 19, nos. 1–2 (2008): 27–34; "Study Finds That Peppermint and Cinnamon Lower Drivers' Frustration and Increase Alertness," Wheeling Jesuit University website, accessed April 12, 2018, http://www.wju.edu/about/adm_news_story.asp?iNewsID=1882&strBack=/about/adm_news_archive.asp.

53. D. L. Walcutt, "Chocolate and Mood Disorders," Psych Central website, accessed April 12, 2018, http://psychcentral.com/blog/archives/2009/04/27/chocolate-and-mood -disorders/; A. A. Sunni and R. Latif, "Effects of Chocolate Intake on Perceived Stress; a Controlled Clinical Study," *International Journal of Health Sciences (Qassim)* 8, no. 4 (October 2014): 393–401.

54. G. Akkasheh et al., "Clinical and Metabolic Response to Probiotic Administration in Patients with Major Depressive Disorder: A Randomized, Double-Blind, Placebo-Controlled Trial," *Nutrition* 32, no. 3 (March 2016): 315–20, doi: 10.1016/j.nut.2015.09.003; M. R. Hilimire et al., "Fermented Foods, Neuroticism, and Social Anxiety: An Interaction Model," *Psychiatry Research* 228, no. 2 (August 15, 2015): 203–8, doi: 10.1016/j.psychres .2015.04.023.

55. A. Ghajar et al., "Crocus sativus L. versus Citalopram in the Treatment of Major Depressive Disorder with Anxious Distress: A Double-Blind, Controlled Clinical Trial," *Pharmacopsychiatry* 50, no. 4 (July 2017): 152–60, doi: 10.1055/s-0042-116159; H. A. Hausenblas et al., "A Systematic Review of Randomized Controlled Trials Examining the Effectiveness of Saffron (Crocus sativus L.) on Psychological and Behavioral Outcomes," *Journal of Integrative Medicine* 13, no. 4 (July 2015): 231–40, doi: 10.1016/S2095-4964 (15)60176-5.

56. S. K. Kulkarni et al., "Antidepressant Activity of Curcumin: Involvement of Serotonin and Dopamine System," *Psychopharmacology* 201, no. 3 (December 2008): 435–42, doi: 10.1007/s00213-008-1300-y; A. L. Lopresti et al., "Curcumin for the Treatment of Major Depression: A Randomised, Double-Blind, Placebo Controlled Study," *Journal of Affective Disorders* 167 (2014): 368–75, doi: 10.1016/j.jad.2014.06.001.

57. A. L. Lopresti and P. D. Drummond, "Efficacy of Curcumin, and a Saffron/Curcumin Combination for the Treatment of Major Depression: A Randomised, Double-Blind, Placebo-Controlled Study," *Journal of Affective Disorders* 207 (January 1, 2017): 188–96, doi: 10.1016/j.jad.2016.09.047.

58. University of Warwick, "Fruit and Veggies Give You the Feel-Good Factor," *ScienceDaily*, July 10, 2016, www.sciencedaily.com/releases/2016/07/160710094239.htm.

59. L. Stojanovska et al., "Maca Reduces Blood Pressure and Depression, in a Pilot Study in Postmenopausal Women," *Climacteric* 18, no. 1 (February 2015): 69–78, doi: 10.3109 /13697137.2014.929649.

60. F. N. Jacka et al., "Western Diet Is Associated with a Smaller Hippocampus: A Longitudinal Investigation," *BMC Medicine* 13, no. 1 (September 8, 2015): 215, doi: 10.1186/s12916-015-0461-x.

61. D. Mastroiacovo et al., "Cocoa Flavanol Consumption Improves Cognitive Function, Blood Pressure Control, and Metabolic Profile in Elderly Subjects: The Cocoa, Cognition, and Aging (CoCoA) Study—A Randomized Controlled Trial," *American Journal of Clinical Nutrition* 101, no. 3 (March 1, 2015): 538–48, doi: 10.3945/ajcn.114.092189.

62. C. Poly et al., "The Relation of Dietary Choline to Cognitive Performance and White-Matter Hyperintensity in the Framingham Offspring Cohort," *American Journal of Clinical Nutrition* 94, no. 6 (December 2011): 1584–91, doi: 10.3945/ajcn.110.008938.

63. K. Kimura et al., "L-Theanine Reduces Psychological and Physiological Stress Responses," *Biological Psychology* 74, no. 1 (January 2007): 39–45, doi: 10.1016/j.biopsycho.2006.06.006.

64. J. K. Kiecolt-Glaser et al., "Omega-3 Supplementation Lowers Inflammation and Anxiety in Medical Students: A Randomized Controlled Trial," *Brain, Behavior, and Immunity* 25, no. 8 (November 2011): 1725–34, doi: 10.1016/j.bbi.2011.07.229.

CHAPTER 10: ADVANCED AND BRAIN-TYPE NUTRACEUTICALS

1. A. Pariente et al., "The Benzodiazepine-Dementia Disorders Link: Current State of Knowledge," *CNS Drugs* 30, no. 1 (January 2016): 1–7, doi: 10.1007/s40263-015 -0305-4; H. Taipale et al., "Use of Benzodiazepines and Related Drugs Is Associated with a Risk of Stroke among Persons with Alzheimer's Disease," *International Clinical Psychopharmacology* 32, no. 3 (May 2017): 135–41, doi: 10.1097/YIC.0000000000000161.

2. D. G. Amen et al., "Reversing Brain Damage in Former NFL Players: Implications for Traumatic Brain Injury and Substance Abuse Rehabilitation," *Journal of Psychoactive Drugs* 43, no. 1 (January–March 2011): 1–5, doi: 10.1080/02791072.2011.566489; D. G. Amen et al., "Effects of Brain-Directed Nutrients on Cerebral Blood Flow and Neuropsychological Testing: A Randomized, Double-Blind, Placebo-Controlled, Crossover Trial," *Advances in Mind-Body Medicine* 27, no. 2 (Spring 2013): 24–33.

3. Y. Steinbuch, "90 Percent of Americans Eat Garbage," *New York Post*, November 17, 2017, https://nypost.com/2017/11/17/90-of-americans-eat-like-garbage/?utm_campaign =iosapp&utm_source=mail_app; "Only 1 in 10 Adults Get Enough Fruits or Vegetables," CDC website, November 16, 2017, https://www.cdc.gov/media/releases/2017/p1116 -fruit-vegetable-consumption.html.

4. R. H. Fletcher and K. M. Fairfield, "Vitamins for Chronic Disease Prevention in Adults: Clinical Applications," *JAMA* 287, no. 23 (June 19, 2002): 3127–29.

5. C. W. Popper, "Single-Micronutrient and Broad-Spectrum Micronutrient Approaches for Treating Mood Disorders in Youth and Adults," *Child and Adolescent Psychiatric Clinics of North America* 23, no. 3 (July 2014): 591–672, doi: 10.1016/j.chc.2014.04.001.

6. J. J. Rucklidge et al., "Vitamin-Mineral Treatment of Attention-Deficit Hyperactivity Disorder in Adults: Double-Blind Randomised Placebo-Controlled Trial," *British Journal of Psychiatry* 204 (2014): 306–15, doi: 10.1192/bjp.bp.113.132126.

7. J. J. Rucklidge and B. J. Kaplan, "Broad-Spectrum Micronutrient Formulas for the Treatment of Psychiatric Symptoms: A Systematic Review," *Expert Review of Neurotherapeutics* 13, no. 1 (January 2013): 49–73, doi: 10.1586/ern.12.143.

8. S. J. Schoenthaler and I. D. Bier, "The Effect of Vitamin-Mineral Supplementation on Juvenile Delinquency among American Schoolchildren: A Randomized, Double-Blind Placebo-Controlled Trial," *Journal of Alternative and Complementary Medicine* 6, no. 1 (February 2000): 7–17, doi: 10.1089/act.2000.6.7.

9. J. J. Rucklidge et al., "Shaken but Unstirred? Effects of Micronutrients on Stress and Trauma after an Earthquake: RCT Evidence Comparing Formulas and Doses," *Human Psychopharmacology* 27, no. 5 (September 2012): 440–54, doi: 10.1002/hup.2246.

10. B. J. Kaplan et al., "A Randomised Trial of Nutrient Supplements to Minimise Psychological Stress after a Natural Disaster," *Psychiatry Research* 228, no. 3 (August 30, 2015): 373–79, doi: 10.1016/j.psychres.2015.05.080.

11. D. O. Kennedy et al., "Effects of High-Dose B Vitamin Complex with Vitamin C and Minerals on Subjective Mood and Performance in Healthy Males," *Psychopharmacology* 211, no. 1 (July 2010): 55–68, doi: 10.1007/s00213-010-1870-3.

12. C. Haskell et al., "Cognitive and Mood Effects in Healthy Children during 12 Weeks' Supplementation with Multi-Vitamin/Minerals," *British Journal of Nutrition* 100, no. 5 (November 2008): 1086–96, doi: 10.1017/S0007114508959213.

13. "Smoking, High Blood Pressure and Being Overweight Top Three Preventable Causes of Death in the U.S.," Harvard T.H. Chan School of Public Health website, April 27, 2009, https://www.hsph.harvard.edu/news/press-releases/smoking-high-blood-pressure -overweight-preventable-causes-death-us/.

14. T. A. Mori and L. J. Beilin, "Omega-3 Fatty Acids and Inflammation," *Current Atherosclerosis Reports* 6, no. 6 (November 2004): 461–67; D. Moertl et al., "Dose-Dependent Effects of Omega-3-Polyunsaturated Fatty Acids on Systolic Left Ventricular Function, Endothelial Function, and Markers of Inflammation in Chronic Heart Failure of Nonischemic Origin: A Double-Blind, Placebo-Controlled, 3-Arm Study," *American Heart Journal* 161, no. 5 (May 2011): 915.e1-9, doi: 10.1016/j.ahj.2011.02.011; J. G. Devassy et al., "Omega-3 Polyunsaturated Fatty Acids and Oxylipins in Neuroinflammation and Management of Alzheimer Disease," *Advances in Nutrition* 7, no. 5 (September 15, 2016): 905–16, doi: 10.3945/an.116.012187.

15. C. von Schacky, "The Omega-3 Index as a Risk Factor for Cardiovascular Diseases," *Prostaglandins and Other Lipid Mediators* 96, nos. 1–4 (November 2011): 94–98, doi: 10.1016/j.prostaglandins.2011.06.008; S. P. Whelton et al., "Meta-Analysis of

Observational Studies on Fish Intake and Coronary Heart Disease," *American Journal of Cardiology* 93, no. 9 (May 1, 2004): 1119–23, doi: 10.1016/j.amjcard.2004.01.038.

16. E. Messamore et al., "Polyunsaturated Fatty Acids and Recurrent Mood Disorders: Phenomenology, Mechanisms, and Clinical Application," *Progress in Lipid Research* 66 (April 2017): 1–13, doi: 10.1016/j.plipres.2017.01.001; J. Sarris et al., "Omega-3 for Bipolar Disorder: Meta-Analyses of Use in Mania and Bipolar Depression," *Journal of Clinical Psychiatry* 73, no. 1 (January 2012): 81–86, doi: 10.4088/JCP.10r06710; R. J. Mocking et al., "Meta-Analysis and Meta-Regression of Omega-3 Polyunsaturated Fatty Acid Supplementation for Major Depressive Disorder," *Translational Psychiatry* 6 (March 15, 2016): e756, doi:10.1038/tp.2016.2.

17. J. R. Hibbeln and R. V. Gow, "The Potential for Military Diets to Reduce Depression, Suicide, and Impulsive Aggression: A Review of Current Evidence for Omega-3 and Omega-6 Fatty Acids," *Military Medicine* 179, Supplement 11 (November 2014): 117–28, doi: 10.7205/MILMED-D-14-00153; M. Huan et al., "Suicide Attempt and n-3 Fatty Acid Levels in Red Blood Cells: A Case Control Study in China," *Biological Psychiatry* 56, no. 7 (October 1, 2004): 490–96, doi: 10.1016/j.biopsych.2004.06.028; M. E. Sublette et al., "Omega-3 Polyunsaturated Essential Fatty Acid Status as a Predictor of Future Suicide Risk," *American Journal of Psychiatry* 163, no. 6 (June 2006): 1100–1102, doi: 10.1176/ajp .2006.163.6.1100; M. D. Lewis et al., "Suicide Deaths of Active-Duty US Military and Omega-3 Fatty-Acid Status: A Case-Control Comparison," *Journal of Clinical Psychiatry* 72, no. 12 (December 2011): 1585–90, doi: 10.4088/JCP.11m06879.

18. C. M. Milte et al., "Increased Erythrocyte Eicosapentaenoic Acid and Docosahexaenoic Acid Are Associated With Improved Attention and Behavior in Children With ADHD in a Randomized Controlled Three-Way Crossover Trial," *Journal of Attention Disorders* 19, no. 11 (November 2015): 954–64, doi: 10.1177/1087054713510562; M. H. Bloch and A. Qawasmi, "Omega-3 Fatty Acid Supplementation for the Treatment of Children with Attention-Deficit/Hyperactivity Disorder Symptomatology: Systematic Review and Meta-Analysis," *Journal of the American Academy of Child and Adolescent Psychiatry* 50, no. 10 (October 2011): 991–1000, doi: 10.1016/j.jaac.2011.06.008.

19. Y. Zhang et al., "Intakes of Fish and Polyunsaturated Fatty Acids and Mild-to-Severe Cognitive Impairment Risks: A Dose-Response Meta-Analysis of 21 Cohort Studies," *American Journal of Clinical Nutrition* 103, no. 2 (February 2016): 330–40, doi: 10.3945/ajcn .115.124081; T. A. D'Ascoli et al., "Association between Serum Long-Chain Omega-3 Polyunsaturated Fatty Acids and Cognitive Performance in Elderly Men and Women: The Kuopio Ischaemic Heart Disease Risk Factor Study," *European Journal of Clinical Nutrition* 70, no. 8 (August 2016): 970–75, doi: 10.1038/ejcn.2016.59; K. Lukaschek et al., "Cognitive Impairment Is Associated with a Low Omega-3 Index in the Elderly: Results from the KORA-Age Study," *Dementia and Geriatric Cognitive Disorders* 42, nos. 3–4 (2016): 236–45, doi: 10.1159/000448805.

20. C. Couet et al., "Effect of Dietary Fish Oil on Body Fat Mass and Basal Fat Oxidation in Healthy Adults," *International Journal of Obesity and Related Metabolic Disorders* 21, no. 8 (August 1997): 637–43; J. D. Buckley and P. R. Howe, "Anti-Obesity Effects of Long-Chain Omega-3 Polyunsaturated Fatty Acids," *Obesity Reviews* 10, no. 6 (November 2009): 648–59, doi: 10.1111/j.1467-789X.2009.00584.x.

21. D. G. Amen et al., "Quantitative Erythrocyte Omega-3 EPA Plus DHA Are Related to Higher Regional Cerebral Blood Flow on Brain SPECT," *Journal of Alzheimer's Disease* 58, no. 4 (2017): 1189–99, doi: 10.3233/JAD-170281.

22. C. W. Skovlund et al., "Association of Hormonal Contraception with Suicide Attempts and Suicides," *American Journal of Psychiatry* 175, no. 4 (April 1, 2018): 336–42, doi: 10.1176 /appi.ajp.2017.17060616.

23. G. Small et al., "Memory and Brain Amyloid and Tau Effects of a Bioavailable Form of Curcumin in Non-Demented Adults: A Double-Blind, Placebo-Controlled 18-Month Trial," *American Journal of Geriatric Psychiatry* 26, no. 3 (March 2018): 266–77, doi: 10.1016/j.jagp .2017.10.010.

24. D. G. Amen and B. Carmichael, "High Resolution Brain SPECT Imaging in ADHD," *Annals of Clinical Psychiatry* 9, no. 2 (June 1997): 81–86.

25. R. F. Santos, "Cognitive Performance, SPECT, and Blood Viscosity in Elderly Non-Demented People Using Ginkgo Biloba," *Pharmacopsychiatry* 36, no. 4 (July 2003): 127–33, doi: 10.1055/s-2003-41197.

26. H. Y. Kim, et al., "Phosphatidylserine in the Brain: Metabolism and Function," *Progress in Lipid Research* 56 (October 2014): 1–18, doi: 10.1016/j.plipres.2014.06.002.

27. A. E. Capello and C. R. Markus, "Effect of Sub Chronic Tryptophan Supplementation on Stress-Induced Cortisol and Appetite in Subjects Differing in 5-HTTLPR Genotype and Trait Neuroticism," *Psychoneuroendocrinology* 45 (July 2014): 96–107, doi: 10.1016/j.psyneuen.2014.03.005.

28. A. Nantel-Vivier et al., "Serotonergic Contribution to Boys' Behavioral Regulation," *PLOS ONE* 6, no. 6 (2011):e20304, doi: 10.1371/journal.pone.0020304.

29. M. H. Mohajeri et al., "Chronic Treatment with a Tryptophan-Rich Protein Hydrolysate Improves Emotional Processing, Mental Energy Levels and Reaction Time in Middle-Aged Women," *British Journal of Nutrition* 113, no. 2 (January 28, 2015): 350–65, doi: 10.1017/S0007114514003754.

30. S. E. Murphy et al., "Tryptophan Supplementation Induces a Positive Bias in the Processing of Emotional Material in Healthy Female Volunteers," *Psychopharmacology* 187, no. 1 (July 2006): 121–30, doi: 10.1007/s00213-006-0401-8.

31. P. Jangid et al., "Comparative Study of Efficacy of L-5-Hydroxytryptophan and Fluoxetine in Patients Presenting with First Depressive Episode," *Asian Journal of Psychiatry* 6, no. 1 (February 2013): 29–34, doi: 10.1016/j.ajp.2012.05.011; J. Angst et al., "The Treatment of Depression with L-5-Hydroxytryptophan versus Imipramine. Results of Two Open and One Double-Blind Study," *Archiv fur Psychiatrie und Nervenkrankheiten* 224, no. 2 (October 11, 1977):175–86.

32. "5-HTP," Examine.com, accessed April 16, 2018, https://examine.com/supplements/5-htp/.

33. "Saffron," Examine.com, accessed April 16, 2018, https://examine.com/supplements/saffron/; A. L. Lopresti and P. D. Drummond, "Saffron (Crocus sativus) for Depression: A Systematic Review of Clinical Studies and Examination of Underlying Antidepressant Mechanisms of Action," *Human Psychopharmacology* 29, no. 6 (November 2014): 517–27, doi: 10.1002/hup.2434.

34. M. Tsolaki et al., "Efficacy and Safety of Crocus sativus L. in Patients with Mild Cognitive Impairment," *Journal of Alzheimer's Disease* 54, no. 1 (July 27, 2016): 129–33, doi: 10.3233/JAD-160304.

35. L. Kashani et al., "Saffron for Treatment of Fluoxetine-Induced Sexual Dysfunction in Women: Randomized Double-Blind Placebo-Controlled Study," *Human Psychopharmacology* 28, no. 1 (January 2013): 54–60, doi: 10.1002/hup.2282.

36. M. Agha-Hosseini et al., "Crocus sativus L. (Saffron) in the Treatment of Premenstrual Syndrome: A Double-Blind, Randomised and Placebo-Controlled Trial," *BJOG* 115, no. 4 (March 2008): 515–19, doi: 10.1111/j.1471-0528.2007.01652.x.

37. M. N. Shahi et al., "The Impact of Saffron on Symptoms of Withdrawal Syndrome in Patients Undergoing Maintenance Treatment for Opioid Addiction in Sabzevar Parish in 2017," *Advances in Medicine* 2017 (2017): Article ID 1079132, doi: 10.1155/2017/1079132.

38. T. Bottiglieri, "S-Adenosyl-L-Methionine (SAMe): From the Bench to the Bedside—Molecular Basis of a Pleiotrophic Molecule," *American Journal of Clinical Nutrition* 76, no. 5 (November 2002): 1151S–7S, doi: 10.1093/ajcn/76/5.1151S.

39. A. Sharma et al., "S-Adenosylmethionine (SAMe) for Neuropsychiatric Disorders: A Clinician-Oriented Review of Research," *Journal of Clinical Psychiatry* 78, no. 6 (June 2017): e656–e667, doi: 10.4088/JCP.16r11113.

40. F. Di Pierro et al., "Role of Betaine in Improving the Antidepressant Effect of

S-adenosyl-methionine in Patients with Mild-to-Moderate Depression," *Journal of Multidisciplinary Healthcare* 8 (2015): 39–45, doi: 10.2147/JMDH.S77766; F. Di Pierro and R. Settembre, "Preliminary Results of a Randomized Controlled Trial Carried Out with a Fixed Combination of S-adenosyl-L-methionine and Betaine versus Amitriptyline in Patients with Mild Depression," *International Journal of General Medicine* 8 (February 4, 2015): 73–78, doi: 10.2147/IJGM.S79518.

CHAPTER 11: THINK DIFFERENT

1. D. G. Amen et al., "Multi-Site Six Month Outcome Study of Complex Psychiatric Patients Evaluated with Addition of Brain SPECT Imaging," *Advances in Mind-Body Medicine* 27, no. 2 (Spring 2013): 6–16.

2. J. F. Thornton et al., "Improved Outcomes Using Brain SPECT-Guided Treatment versus Treatment-as-Usual in Community Psychiatric Outpatients: A Retrospective Case-Control Study," *Journal of Neuropsychiatry and Clinical Neurosciences* 26, no. 1 (Winter 2014): 51–56, doi: 10.1176/appi.neuropsych.12100238.

3. D. G. Amen et al., "Specific Ways Brain SPECT Imaging Enhances Clinical Psychiatric Practice," *Journal of Psychoactive Drugs* 44, no. 2 (April-June 2012): 96–106, doi: 10.1080/02791072.2012.684615.

4. D. G. Amen, *Change Your Brain, Change Your Life*, rev. ed., (New York: Harmony Books, 2015), 15.

5. "What a Psychiatrist Learned from 87,000 Brain Scans," Facebook video, November 13, 2017, https://www.facebook.com/Illumeably/videos/283984572006650.

CHAPTER 12: LOVE IS YOUR SECRET WEAPON

1. A. Moosavi and A. M. Ardekani, "Role of Epigenetics in Biology and Human Diseases," *Iranian Biomedical Journal* 20, no. 5 (November 2016): 246–58.

2. K. Northstone et al., "Prepubertal Start of Father's Smoking and Increased Body Fat in His Sons: Further Characterisation of Paternal Transgenerational Responses," *European Journal of Human Genetics* 22, no. 12 (December 2014): 1382–86, doi: 10.1038/ejhg.2014.31.

3. C. S. Lewis, *The Four Loves* (New York: Harcourt, Brace, 1960), 1.

4. C. M. Karns et al., "The Cultivation of Pure Altruism via Gratitude: A Functional MRI Study of Change with Gratitude Practice," *Frontiers in Human Neuroscience* 11 (December 2017): article 599, doi: 10.3389/fnhum.2017.00599.

5. Michael Wines, "In Memoir, Barbara Bush Recalls Private Trials of a Political Life," *New York Times*, September 8, 1994, http://www.nytimes.com/1994/09/08/us/in-memoir-barbara-bush-recalls-private-trials-of-a-political-life.html; "Barbara Bush Says She Fought Depression in '76," *Washington Post*, May 20, 1990, https://www.washingtonpost.com/archive/politics/1990/05/20/barbara-bush-says-she-fought-depression-in-76/0ac40655-923e-448d-bfcc-aa3ea5cb88c8/?utm_term=.1bb20fdb6707.

6. K. E. Buchanan and A. Bardi, "Acts of Kindness and Acts of Novelty Affect Life Satisfaction," *Journal of Social Psychology* 150, no. 3 (May–June 2010): 235–37, doi: 10.1080/00224540903365554.

7. L. B. Aknin et al, "Happiness Runs in a Circular Motion: Evidence for a Positive Feedback Loop between Prosocial Spending and Happiness," *Journal of Happiness Studies* 13, no. 2 (April 2012): 347–55, doi: 10.1007/s10902-011-9267-5.

8. S. Q. Park et al., "A Neural Link between Generosity and Happiness," *Nature Communications* 8 (2017): 159674, doi: 10.1038/ncomms15964; S. G. Post, "Altruism, Happiness, and Health: It's Good to Be Good," *International Journal of Behavioral Medicine* 12, no. 2 (2005): 66–77, doi: 10.1207/s15327558ijbm1202_4; L. B. Aknin et al., "Giving Leads to Happiness in Young Children," *PLOS ONE* 7, no. 6 (2012): e39211, doi: 10.1371/journal.pone.0039211.

APPENDIX A

1. R. Boussi-Gross et al., "Hyperbaric Oxygen Therapy Can Improve Post Concussion Syndrome Years after Mild Traumatic Brain Injury—Randomized Prospective Trial," *PLOS ONE* 8, no. 11 (November 15, 2013): e79995, doi: 10.1371/journal.pone.0079995; S. Tal et al., "Hyperbaric Oxygen May Induce Angiogenesis in Patients Suffering from Prolonged Post-Concussion Syndrome Due to Traumatic Brain Injury," *Restorative Neurology and Neuroscience* 33, no. 6 (2015): 943–51, doi: 10.3233/RNN-150585; P. G. Harch et al., "A Phase I Study of Low-Pressure Hyperbaric Oxygen Therapy for Blast-Induced Post-Concussion Syndrome and Post-Traumatic Stress Disorder," *Journal of Neurotrauma* 29, no. 1 (January 1, 2012): 168–85, doi: 10.1089/neu.2011.1895.

2. S. Efrati et al., "Hyperbaric Oxygen Induces Late Neuroplasticity in Post Stroke Patients—Randomized, Prospective Trial," *PLOS ONE* 8, no. 1 (January 2013): e53716, doi: 10.1371/journal.pone.0053716.

3. S. Efrati et al., "Hyperbaric Oxygen Therapy Can Diminish Fibromyalgia Syndrome—Prospective Clinical Trial," *PLOS ONE* 10, no. 5 (May 26, 2015): e0127012, doi: 10.1371/journal.pone.0127012.

4. C. Y. Huang et al., "Hyperbaric Oxygen Therapy as an Effective Adjunctive Treatment for Chronic Lyme Disease," *Journal of the Chinese Medical Association* 77, no. 5 (May 2014): 269–71, doi: 10.1016/j.jcma.2014.02.001.

5. I. I. H. Chiang et al., "Adjunctive Hyperbaric Oxygen Therapy in Severe Burns: Experience in Taiwan Formosa Water Park Dust Explosion Disaster," *Burns* 43, no. 4 (June 2017): 852–57, doi: 10.1016/j.burns.2016.10.016.

6. M. Löndahl et al., "Relationship between Ulcer Healing after Hyperbaric Oxygen Therapy and Transcutaneous Oximetry, Toe Blood Pressure and Ankle-Brachial Index in Patients with Diabetes and Chronic Foot Ulcers," *Diabetologia* 54, no. 1 (January 2011): 65–68, doi: 10.1007/s00125-010-1946-y.

7. A. M. Eskes et al., "Hyperbaric Oxygen Therapy: Solution for Difficult to Heal Acute Wounds? Systematic Review," *World Journal of Surgery* 35, no. 3 (March 2011): 535–42, doi: 10.1007/s00268-010-0923-4; J. J. Shaw et al., "Not Just Full of Hot Air: Hyperbaric Oxygen Therapy Increases Survival in Cases of Necrotizing Soft Tissue Infections," *Surgical Infections* 15, no. 3 (June 2014): 328–35, doi: 10.1089/sur.2012.135.

8. M. T. Asl et al., "Brain Perfusion Imaging with Voxel-Based Analysis in Secondary Progressive Multiple Sclerosis Patients with a Moderate to Severe Stage of Disease: A Boon for the Workforce," *BMC Neurology* 16 (May 26, 2016): 79, doi: 10.1186/s12883-016-0605-4.

9. P. S. Dulai et al., "Systematic Review: The Safety and Efficacy of Hyperbaric Oxygen Therapy for Inflammatory Bowel Disease," *Alimentary Pharmacology and Therapeutics* 39, no. 11 (June 2014): 1266–75, doi: 10.1111/apt.12753.

10. D. N. Teguh et al., "Early Hyperbaric Oxygen Therapy for Reducing Radiotherapy Side Effects: Early Results of a Randomized Trial in Oropharyngeal and Nasopharyngeal Cancer," *International Journal of Radiation Oncology, Biology, Physics* 75, no. 3 (November 1, 2009): 711–16, doi: 10.1016/j.ijrobp.2008.11.056; N. A. Schellart et al., "Hyperbaric Oxygen Treatment Improved Neurophysiologic Performance in Brain Tumor Patients after Neurosurgery and Radiotherapy: A Preliminary Report," *Cancer* 177, no. 15 (August 1, 2011): 3434–44, doi: 10.1002/cncr.25874.

11. D. A. Rossignol et al., "The Effects of Hyperbaric Oxygen Therapy on Oxidative Stress, Inflammation, and Symptoms in Children with Autism: An Open-Label Pilot Study," *BMC Pediatrics* 7 (November 16, 2007): 36, doi: 10.1186/1471-2431-7-36; D. A. Rossignol et al., "Hyperbaric Treatment for Children with Autism: A Multicenter, Randomized, Double-Blind, Controlled Trial," *BMC Pediatrics* 9 (March 13, 2009): 21, doi: 10.1186/1471-2431-9-21.

12. A. Mukherjee et al., "Intensive Rehabilitation Combined with HBO$_2$ Therapy in Children with Cerebral Palsy: A Controlled Longitudinal Study," *Undersea and Hyperbaric Medicine* 41, no. 2 (March–April 2014): 77–85.

13. T. Perera et al., "The Clinical TMS Society Consensus Review and Treatment Recommendations for TMS Therapy for Major Depressive Disorder," *Brain Stimulation* 9, no. 3 (May–June 2016): 336–46, doi: 10.1016/j.brs.2016.03.010.

14. D. White and S. Tavakoli, "Repetitive Transcranial Magnetic Stimulation for Treatment of Major Depressive Disorder with Comorbid Generalized Anxiety Disorder," *Annals of Clinical Psychiatry* 27, no. 3 (August 2015): 192–96.

15. M. Ceccanti et al., "Deep TMS on Alcoholics: Effects on Cortisolemia and Dopamine Pathway Modulation. A Pilot Study," *Canadian Journal of Physiology and Pharmacology* 93, no. 4 (April 2015): 283–90, doi: 10.1139/cjpp-2014-0188.

16. L. Dinur-Klein et al., "Smoking Cessation Induced by Deep Repetitive Transcranial Magnetic Stimulation of the Prefrontal and Insular Cortices: A Prospective, Randomized Controlled Trial," *Biological Psychiatry* 76, no. 9 (November 1, 2014): 742–49, doi: 10.1016/j.biopsych.2014.05.020.

17. P. S. Boggio et al., "Noninvasive Brain Stimulation with High-Frequency and Low-Intensity Repetitive Transcranial Magnetic Stimulation Treatment for Posttraumatic Stress Disorder," *Journal of Clinical Psychiatry* 71, no. 8 (August 2010): 992–99, doi: 10.4088/JCP.08m04638blu.

18. A. P. Trevizol et al., "Transcranial Magnetic Stimulation for Obsessive-Compulsive Disorder: An Updated Systematic Review and Meta-analysis," *The Journal of ECT* 32, no. 4 (December 2016): 262–66, doi: 10.1097/YCT.0000000000000335.

19. H. L. Drumond Marra et al., "Transcranial Magnetic Stimulation to Address Mild Cognitive Impairment in the Elderly: A Randomized Controlled Study," *Behavioural Neurology* 2015 (2015): 287843, doi: 10.1155/2015/287843; W. M. McDonald, "Neuromodulation Treatments for Geriatric Mood and Cognitive Disorders," *American Journal of Geriatric Psychiatry* 24, no. 12 (December 2016): 1130–41, doi: 10.1016/j.jagp.2016.08.014; J. M. Rabey and E. Dobronevsky, "Repetitive Transcranial Magnetic Stimulation (rTMS) Combined with Cognitive Training Is a Safe and Effective Modality for the Treatment of Alzheimer's Disease: Clinical Experience," *Journal of Neural Transmission (Vienna)* 123, no. 12 (December 2016): 1449–55, doi: 10.1007/s00702-016-1606-6.

20. M. Yilmaz et al., "Effectiveness of Transcranial Magnetic Stimulation Application in Treatment of Tinnitus," *Journal of Craniofacial Surgery* 25, no. 4 (July 2014): 1315–18, doi: 10.1097/SCS.0000000000000782.

21. T. V. Kulishova and O. V. Shinkorenko, "The Effectiveness of Early Rehabilitation of the Patients Presenting with Ischemic Stroke," *Voprosy Kurortologii Fizioterapii, i Lechebnoi Fizicheskoi Kultury* 6 (November–December 2014): 9–12.

22. H. L. Drumond Marra et al., "Transcranial Magnetic Stimulation to Address Mild Cognitive Impairment in the Elderly: A Randomized Controlled Study," *Behavioural Neurology* 2015 (2015): 287843, doi: 10.1155/2015/287843.

23. C. Andrade, "Ketamine for Depression, 1: Clinical Summary of Issues Related to Efficacy, Adverse Effects, and Mechanism of Action," *Journal of Clinical Psychiatry* 78, no. 4 (April 2017): e415–e419, doi: 10.4088/JCP.17f11567; M. F. Grunebaum et al., "Ketamine for Rapid Reduction of Suicidal Thoughts in Major Depression: A Midazolam-Controlled Randomized Clinical Trial," *American Journal of Psychiatry* 175, no. 4 (April 1, 2018): 327–35, doi: 10.1176/appi.ajp.2017.17060647.

24. J. Guez et al., "Influence of Electroencephalography Neurofeedback Training on Episodic Memory: A Randomized, Sham-Controlled, Double-Blind Study," *Memory* 23, no. 5 (2015): 683–94, doi: 10.1080/09658211.2014.921713; S. Xiong et al., "Working Memory Training Using EEG Neurofeedback in Normal Young Adults," *Bio-Medical Materials and Engineering* 24, no. 6 (2014): 3637–44, doi: 10.3233/BME-141191; J. R. Wang and S. Hsieh, "Neurofeedback Training Improves Attention and Working Memory Performance," *Clinical Neurophysiology* 124, no. 12 (December 2013): 2406–20, doi: 10.1016/j.clinph.2013.05.020.

25. S. E. Kober et al., "Specific Effects of EEG Based Neurofeedback Training on Memory Functions in Post-Stroke Victims," *Journal of Neuroengineering and Rehabilitation* 12 (December 1, 2015): 107, doi: 10.1186/s12984-015-0105-6.

26. V. Meisel et al., "Neurofeedback and Standard Pharmacological Intervention in ADHD: A Randomized Controlled Trial with Six-Month Follow-Up," *Biological Psychology* 94, no. 1 (September 2013): 12–21, doi: 10.1016/j.biopsycho.2013.04.015.

27. J. Kopřivová et al., "Prediction of Treatment Response and the Effect of Independent Component Neurofeedback in Obsessive-Compulsive Disorder: A Randomized, Sham-Controlled, Double-Blind Study," *Neuropsychobiology* 67, no. 4 (2013): 210–23, doi: 10.1159/000347087.

28. E. J. Cheon et al., "The Efficacy of Neurofeedback in Patients with Major Depressive Disorder: An Open Labeled Prospective Study," *Applied Psychophysiology and Biofeedback* 41, no. 1 (September 2015): 103–10, doi: 10.1007/s10484-015-9315-8.

29. T. Surmeli et al., "Quantitative EEG Neurometric Analysis-Guided Neurofeedback Treatment in Postconcussion Syndrome (PCS): Forty Cases. How Is Neurometric Analysis Important for the Treatment of PCS and as a Biomarker?" *Clinical EEG and Neuroscience* 48, no. 3 (June 27, 2016): 217–30, doi: 10.1177/1550059416654849.

30. R. Rostami and F. Dehghani-Arani, "Neurofeedback Training as a New Method in Treatment of Crystal Methamphetamine Dependent Patients: A Preliminary Study," *Applied Psychophysiology and Biofeedback* 40, no. 3 (September 2015): 151–61, doi: 10.1007/s10484-015-9281-1.

31. P. Kubik et al., "Neurofeedback Therapy Influence on Clinical Status and Some EEG Parameters in Children with Localized Epilepsy," *Przeglad Lekarski* 73, no. 3 (2016): 157–60.

32. M. P. Jensen et al., "Use of Neurofeedback to Enhance Response to Hypnotic Analgesia in Individuals with Multiple Sclerosis," *International Journal of Clinical and Experimental Hypnosis* 64, no. 1 (2016): 1–23, doi: 10.1080/00207144.2015.1099400.

33. A. Azarpaikan et al., "Neurofeedback and Physical Balance in Parkinson's Patients," *Gait Posture* 40, no. 1 (2014): 177–81, doi: 10.1016/j.gaitpost.2014.03.179.

34. M. Y. Cheng et al., "Sensorimotor Rhythm Neurofeedback Enhances Golf Putting Performance," *Journal of Sport & Exercise Psychology* 37, no. 6 (December 2015): 626–36, doi: 10.1123/jsep.2015-0166.

35. J. Gruzelier et al., "Acting Performance and Flow State Enhanced with Sensory-Motor Rhythm Neurofeedback Comparing Ecologically Valid Immersive VR and Training Screen Scenarios," *Neuroscience Letters* 480, no. 2 (August 16, 2010): 112–16, doi: 10.1016/j.neulet.2010.06.019.

36. N. Rahmati et al., "The Effectiveness of Neurofeedback on Enhancing Cognitive Process Involved in Entrepreneurship Abilities among Primary School Students in District No. 3 Tehran," *Basic and Clinical Neuroscience* 5, no. 4 (October 2014): 277–84.

37. T. L. Huang and C. Charyton, "A Comprehensive Review of the Psychological Effects of Brainwave Entrainment," *Alternative Therapies in Health and Medicine* 14, no. 5 (September–October 2008): 38–50.

38. J. C. Mazziotta et al., "Tomographic Mapping of Human Cerebral Metabolism: Subcortical Responses to Auditory and Visual Stimulation," *Neurology* 34, no. 6 (June 1984): 825–28, doi: 10.1212/WNL.34.6.825.

39. P. T. Fox and M. E. Raichle, "Stimulus Rate Determines Regional Brain Blood Flow in Striate Cortex," *Annals of Neurology* 17, no. 3 (March 1985): 303–5.

40. H. Y. Tang et al., "A Pilot Study of Audio-Visual Stimulation as a Self-Care Treatment for Insomnia in Adults with Insomnia and Chronic Pain," *Applied Psychophysiology and Biofeedback* 39, nos. 3–4 (December 2014): 219–25, doi: 10.1007/s10484-014-9263-8; V. Abeln et al., "Brainwave Entrainment for Better Sleep and Post-Sleep State of Young Elite Soccer Players—A Pilot Study," *European Journal of Sport Science* 14, no. 5 (2014): 393–402, doi: 10.1080/17461391.2013.819384.

41. Ibid.; C. Gagnon and F. Boersma, "The Use of Repetitive Audio-Visual Entrainment in the Management of Chronic Pain," *Medical Hypnoanalysis Journal* 7, no. 3 (1992): 462–68.

42. Huang and Charyton, "A Comprehensive Review of the Psychological Effects of Brainwave Entrainment," 38–50.

43. D. Anderson, "The Treatment of Migraine with Variable Frequency Photo-Stimulation," *Headache* 29 (March 1989): 154–55.

44. K. Berg and D. Siever, "A Controlled Comparison of Audio-Visual Entrainment for Treating Seasonal Affective Disorder," *Journal of Neurotherapy* 13, no. 3 (2009): 166–75, doi: 10.1080/10874200903107314; D. S. Cantor and E. Stevens, "QEEG Correlates of Auditory-Visual Entrainment Treatment Efficacy of Refractory Depression," *Journal of Neurotherapy* 13, no. 2 (April 2009): 100–108, doi: 10.1080/10874200902887130.

45. D. Siever, "Audio-Visual Entrainment: History, Physiology, and Clinical Studies," The Association for Applied Psychophysiology and Biofeedback website, accessed May 7, 2018, https://www.aapb.org/files/news/Entrainment.pdf.

APPENDIX B

1. Centers for Disease Control and Prevention, "CDC Report: Mental Illness Surveillance among Adults in the United States," CDC website, last edited December 2, 2011, https://www.cdc.gov/mentalhealthsurveillance/fact_sheet.html.

2. Kaiser Permanente, "Only One-Third of Patients Diagnosed with Depression Start Treatment: Likelihood of Beginning Treatment Is Especially Low among Ethnic and Racial Minorities and the Elderly," *ScienceDaily*, February 8, 2018, www.sciencedaily.com/releases /2018/02/180208141239.htm.

3. C. Battaglia et al., "Participation in a 9-Month Selected Physical Exercise Program Enhances Psychological Well-Being in a Prison Population," *Criminal Behaviour and Mental Health* 25, no. 5 (December 2015): 343–54, doi: 10.1002/cbm.1922.

4. A. M. Abdou et al., "Relaxation and Immunity Enhancement Effects of Gamma-Aminobutyric Acid (GABA) Administration in Humans," *Biofactors* 26, no. 3 (2006): 201–8; A. Yoto et al., "Oral Intake of γ-aminobutyric Acid Affects Mood and Activities of Central Nervous System during Stressed Condition Induced by Mental Tasks," *Amino Acids* 43, no. 3 (September 2012): 1331–37, doi: 10.1007/s00726-011-1206-6.

5. K. Kimura et al., "L-Theanine Reduces Psychological and Physiological Stress Responses," *Biological Psychology* 74, no. 1 (January 2007): 39–45, doi: 10.1016/j.biopsycho.2006.06.006.

6. J. Knapen et al., "Exercise Therapy Improves Both Mental and Physical Health in Patients with Major Depression," *Disability and Rehabilitation* 37, no. 16 (2015): 1490–95, doi: 10.3109/09638288.2014.972579; C. Battaglia et al., "Participation in a 9-Month Selected Physical Exercise Program Enhances Psychological Well-Being in a Prison Population," *Criminal Behaviour and Mental Health* 25, no. 5 (December 2015): 343–54, doi: 10.1002/cbm.1922.

7. M. Hosseinzadeh et al., "Empirically Derived Dietary Patterns in Relation to Psychological Disorders," *Public Health Nutrition* 19, no. 2 (February 2016): 204–17, doi: 10.1017 /S136898001500172X.

8. K. Niu et al., "A Tomato-Rich Diet Is Related to Depressive Symptoms among an Elderly Population Aged 70 Years and Over: A Population-Based, Cross-Sectional Analysis," *Journal of Affective Disorders* 144, nos. 1–2 (January 10, 2013): 165–70, doi: 10.1016 /j.jad.2012.04.040.

9. G. Grosso et al., "Role of Omega-3 Fatty Acids in the Treatment of Depressive Disorders: A Comprehensive Meta-Analysis of Randomized Clinical Trials," *PLOS ONE* 9, no. 5 (May 7, 2014): e96905, doi: 10.1371/journal.pone.0096905; B. Hallahan et al., "Efficacy of Omega-3 Highly Unsaturated Fatty Acids in the Treatment of Depression," *British Journal of Psychiatry* 209, no. 3 (September 2016): 192–201, doi: 10.1192/bjp.bp.114.160242; J. G. Martins, "EPA but Not DHA Appears to Be Responsible for the Efficacy of Omega-3 Long Chain Polyunsaturated Fatty Acid Supplementation in Depression: Evidence from a Meta-Analysis of Randomized Controlled Trials," *Journal of the American College of Nutrition* 28, no. 5 (October 2009): 525–42.

10. D. J. Carpenter, "St. John's Wort and S-Adenosyl Methionine as 'Natural' Alternatives to Conventional Antidepressants in the Era of the Suicidality Boxed Warning: What Is the Evidence for Clinically Relevant Benefit?" *Alternative Medicine*

Review 16, no. 1 (March 2011): 17–39; G. I. Papkostas et al., "S-Adenosyl Methionine (SAMe) Augmentation of Serotonin Reuptake Inhibitors for Antidepressant Nonresponders with Major Depressive Disorder: A Double-Blind, Randomized Clinical Trial," *American Journal of Psychiatry* 167, no. 8 (August 2010): 942–8, doi: 10.1176/appi.ajp.2009.09081198; J. Sarris et al., "S-Adenosyl Methionine (SAMe) versus Escitalopram and Placebo in Major Depression RCT: Efficacy and Effects of Histamine and Carnitine as Moderators of Response," *Journal of Affective Disorders* 164 (August 2014): 76–81, doi: 10.1016/j.jad.2014.03.041.

11. J. Sarris et al., "Is S-Adenosyl Methionine (SAMe) for Depression Only Effective in Males? A Re-Analysis of Data from a Randomized Clinical Trial," *Pharmacopsychiatry* 48, nos. 4–5 (July 2015): 141–44, doi: 10.1055/s-0035-1549928.

12. A. L. Lopresti and P. D. Drummond, "Efficacy of Curcumin, and a Saffron/Curcumin Combination for the Treatment of Major Depression: A Randomised, Double-Blind, Placebo-Controlled Study," *Journal of Affective Disorders* 207 (January 1, 2017): 188–96, doi: 10.1016/j.jad.2016.09.047.

13. Z. Sepehrmanesh et al., "Vitamin D Supplementation Affects the Beck Depression Inventory, Insulin Resistance, and Biomarkers of Oxidative Stress in Patients with Major Depressive Disorder: A Randomized, Controlled Clinical Trial," *Journal of Nutrition* 146, no. 2 (February 2016): 243–48, doi: 10.3945/jn.115.218883; H. Mozaffari-Khosravi et al., "The Effect of 2 Different Single Injections of High Dose of Vitamin D on Improving the Depression in Depressed Patients with Vitamin D Deficiency: A Randomized Clinical Trial," *Journal of Clinical Psychopharmacology* 33, no. 3 (June 2013): 378–85, doi: 10.1097/JCP.0b013e31828f619a.

14. R. T. Ackermann and J. W. Williams, "Rational Treatment Choices for Non-Major Depressions in Primary Care: An Evidence-Based Review," *Journal of General Internal Medicine* 17, no. 4 (April 2002) 293–301.

15. A. S. Yeung et al., "A Pilot Study of Acupuncture Augmentation Therapy in Antidepressant Partial and Non-Responders with Major Depressive Disorder," *Journal of Affective Disorders* 130, nos. 1–2 (April 2011): 285–89, doi: 10.1016/j.jad.2010.07.025; J. Wu et al., "Acupuncture for Depression: A Review of Clinical Applications," *Canadian Journal of Psychiatry* 57, no. 7 (July 2012): 397–405, doi: 10.1177/070674371205700702.

16. G. I. Papakostas et al., "L-Methylfolate as Adjunctive Therapy for SSRI-Resistant Major Depression: Results of Two Randomized, Double-Blind, Parallel-Sequential Trials," *American Journal of Psychiatry* 169, no. 12 (December 2012): 1267–74, doi: 10.1176/appi.ajp.2012.11071114.

17. A. S. de Sá Filho et al., "Potential Therapeutic Effects of Physical Exercise for Bipolar Disorder," *CNS & Neurological Disorders Drug Targets* 14, no. 10 (2015): 1255–59.

18. R. K. McNamara et al., "Adolescents with or at Ultra-High Risk for Bipolar Disorder Exhibit Erythrocyte Docosahexaenoic Acid and Eicosapentaenoic Acid Deficits: A Candidate Prodromal Risk Biomarker," *Early Intervention in Psychiatry* 10, no. 3 (June 2016): 203–11, doi: 10.1111/eip.12282; J. Sarris et al., "Omega-3 for Bipolar Disorder: Meta-Analyses of Use in Mania and Bipolar Depression," *Journal of Clinical Psychiatry* 73, no. 1 (January 2012): 81–86, doi: 10.4088/JCP.10r06710.

19. A. P. Silva et al., "Measurement of the Effect of Physical Exercise on the Concentration of Individuals with ADHD," *PLOS ONE* 10, no. 3 (March 24, 2015): e0122119, doi: 10.1371/journal.pone.012119; B. W. Tan et al., "A Meta-Analytic Review of the Efficacy of Physical Exercise Interventions on Cognition in Individuals with Autism Spectrum Disorder and ADHD," *Journal of Autism and Developmental Disorders* 46, no. 9 (September 2016): 3126–43, doi: 10.1007/s10803-016-2854-x; B. Hoza et al., "A Randomized Trial Examining the Effects of Aerobic Physical Activity on Attention-Deficit/Hyperactivity Disorder Symptoms in Young Children," *Journal of Abnormal Child Psychology* 43, no. 4 (May 2015): 655–67, doi: 10.1007/s10802-014-9929-y.

20. E. Hawkey and J. T. Nigg, "Omega3 Fatty Acid and ADHD: Blood Level Analysis and Meta-Analytic Extension of Supplementation Trials," *Clinical Psychology Review* 34, no. 6 (August 2014): 496–505, doi: 10.1016/j.cpr.2014.05.005; C. M. Milte et al., "Increased

Erythrocyte Eicosapentaenoic Acid and Docosahexaenoic Acid Are Associated with Improved Attention and Behavior in Children with ADHD in a Randomized Controlled Three-Way Crossover Trial," *Journal of Attention Disorders* 19, no. 11 (November 2015): 954–64, doi: 10.1177/1087054713510562; K. Widenhorn-Müller et al., "Effect of Supplementation with Long-Chain Ω3 Polyunsaturated Fatty Acids on Behavior and Cognition in Children with Attention Deficit/Hyperactivity Disorder (ADHD): A Randomized Placebo-Controlled Intervention Trial," *Prostaglandins, Leukotrienes, and Essential Fatty Acids* 91, nos. 1–2 (July–August 2014): 49–60, doi: 10.1016/j.plefa .2014.04.004; H. Perera et al., "Combined Ω3 and Ω6 Supplementation in Children with Attention-Deficit Hyperactivity Disorder (ADHD) Refractory to Methylphenidate Treatment: A Double-Blind, Placebo-Controlled Study," *Journal of Child Neurology* 27, no. 6 (June 2012): 747–53, doi: 10.1177/0883073811435243; D. J. Bos et al., "Reduced Symptoms of Inattention after Dietary Omega3 Fatty Acid Supplementation in Boys with and without Attention Deficit/Hyperactivity Disorder," *Neuropsychopharmacology* 40, no. 10 (September 2015): 2298–306, doi: 10.1038/npp.2015.73.

21. P. Toren et al., "Zinc Deficiency in Attention-Deficit Hyperactivity Disorder," *Biological Psychiatry* 40, no. 12 (December 15, 1996): 1308–10; O. Oner et al., "Effects of Zinc and Ferritin Levels on Parent and Teacher Reported Symptom Scores in Attention Deficit Hyperactivity Disorder," *Child Psychiatry and Human Development* 41, no. 4 (August 2010): 441–47, doi: 10.1007/s10578-010-0178-1; O. Yorbik et al., "Potential Effects of Zinc on Information Processing in Boys with Attention Deficit Hyperactivity Disorder," *Progress in Neuro-Psychopharmacology & Biological Psychiatry* 32, no. 3 (April 1, 2008): 662–67, doi: 10.1016/j.pnpbp.2007.11.009; S. Akhondzadeh et al., "Zinc Sulfate as an Adjunct to Methylphenidate for the Treatment of Attention Deficit Hyperactivity Disorder in Children: A Double Blind and Randomized Trial," *BMC Psychiatry* 4 (April 8, 2004): 9, doi: 10.1186/1471-244X-4-9.

22. M. Mousain-Bosc et al., "Improvement of Neurobehavioral Disorders in Children Supplemented with Magnesium-Vitamin B6. I. Attention Deficit Hyperactivity Disorders," *Magnesium Research* 19, no. 1 (March 2006): 46–52; M. Huss et al., "Supplementation of Polyunsaturated Fatty Acids, Magnesium and Zinc in Children Seeking Medical Advice for Attention-Deficit/Hyperactivity Problems—An Observational Cohort Study," *Lipids in Health and Disease* 9 (September 24, 2010): 105, doi: 10.1186/1476-511X-9-105.

23. J. S. Halterman et al., "Iron Deficiency and Cognitive Achievement among School-Aged Children and Adolescents in the United States," *Pediatrics* 107, no. 6 (June 2001): 1381–86.

24. S. Hirayama et al., "The Effect of Phosphatidylserine Administration on Memory and Symptoms of Attention-Deficit Hyperactivity Disorder: A Randomised, Double-Blind, Placebo-Controlled Clinical Trial," *Journal of Human Nutrition & Dietetics* 27, Supplement 2 (April 2014): 284–91, doi: 10.1111/jhn.12090; I. Manor et al., "The Effect of Phosphatidylserine Containing Omega3 Fatty-Acids on Attention-Deficit Hyperactivity Disorder Symptoms in Children: A Double-Blind Placebo-Controlled Trial, Followed by an Open-Label Extension," *European Psychiatry* 27, no. 5 (July 2012): 335–42, doi: 10.1016 /j.eurpsy.2011.05.004.

25. L. Chen et al., "Eye Movement Desensitization and Reprocessing versus Cognitive-Behavioral Therapy for Adult Posttraumatic Stress Disorder: Systematic Review and Meta-Analysis," *Journal of Nervous and Mental Disease* 203, no. 6 (June 2015): 443–51, doi: 10.1097/NMD.0000000000000306.

26. D. J. Kearney et al., "Loving-Kindness Meditation for Posttraumatic Stress Disorder: A Pilot Study," *Journal of Traumatic Stress* 26, no. 4 (August 2013): 426–34, doi: 10.1002 /jts.21832; D. J. Kearney et al., "Loving-Kindness Meditation and the Broaden-and-Build Theory of Positive Emotions among Veterans with Posttraumatic Stress Disorder," *Medical Care* 52, Supplement 5 (December 2014): S32–S38, doi: 10.1097/MLR .0000000000000221.

27. Mayo Clinic Staff, "Exercise and Stress: Get Moving to Manage Stress," Mayo Clinic website, accessed April 29, 2018, http://www.mayoclinic.org/healthy-lifestyle/stress -management/in-depth/exercise-and-stress/art-20044469.

28. J. N. Belding et al., "Social Buffering by God: Prayer and Measures of Stress," *Journal of Religion and Health* 49, no. 2 (June 2010): 179–87, doi: 10.1055/s-0042-116159.

29. K. Bluth et al., "A Pilot Study of a Mindfulness Intervention for Adolescents and the Potential Role of Self-Compassion in Reducing Stress," *Explore (NY)* 11, no. 4 (July–August 2015): 292–95, doi: 10.1016/j.explore.2015.04.005; W. Turakitwanakan et al., "Effects of Mindfulness Meditation on Serum Cortisol of Medical Students," *Journal of the Medical Association of Thailand* 96, Supplement 1 (January 2013): S90–95.

30. A. Ghajar et al., "Crocus sativus L. versus Citalopram in the Treatment of Major Depressive Disorder with Anxious Distress: A Double-Blind, Controlled Clinical Trial," *Pharmacopsychiatry* 50, no. 4 (July 2017): 152–60, doi: 10.1055/s-0042-116159; H. Fukui et al., "Psychological and Neuroendocrinological Effects of Odor of Saffron (Crocus sativus)," *Phytomedicine* 18, nos. 8–9 (June 15, 2011): 726–30, doi: 10.1016/j.phymed .2010.11.013.

31. R. A. Emmons and M. E. McCullough, "Counting Blessings versus Burdens: An Experimental Investigation of Gratitude and Subjective Well-Being in Daily Life," *Journal of Personality and Social Psychology* 84, no. 2 (February 2003): 377–89.

32. M. Ingall, "Chocolate Can Do Good Things for Your Heart, Skin and Brain," December 22, 2006, *Health*, posted on CNN website, http://www.cnn.com/2006/HEALTH/12/20/health .chocolate/.

33. Deutches Aertzeblatt International, "The Healing Powers of Music: Mozart and Strauss for Treating Hypertension," June 20, 2016, *ScienceDaily*, https://www.sciencedaily.com /releases/2016/06/160620112512.htm.

34. E. Brodwin, "Psychologists Discover the Simplest Way to Boost Your Mood," *Business Insider*, April 3, 2015, http://www.businessinsider.com/how-to-boost-your-mood-2015-4.

35. K. Kimura et al., "L-Theanine Reduces Psychological and Physiological Stress Responses," *Biological Psychology* 74, no. 1 (January 2007): 39–45, doi: 10.1016/j .biopsycho.2006.06.006.

36. M. Rudd et al., "Awe Expands People's Perception of Time, Alters Decision Making, and Enhances Well-Being," *Psychological Science* 23, no. 10 (October 1, 2012): 1130–36, doi: 10.1177/0956797612438731.

37. Y. Miyazaki et al., "Preventive Medical Effects of Nature Therapy," *Nihon Eiseigaku Zasshi* 66, no. 4 (September 2011): 651–56.

38. G. N. Bratman et al., "Nature Experience Reduces Rumination and Subgenual Prefrontal Cortex Activation," *Proceedings of the National Academy of Sciences of the United States of America* 112, no. 28 (July 14, 2015): 8567–72, doi: 10.1073/pnas.1510459112.

39. S. Slon, "7 Health Benefits of Going Barefoot Outside," MindBodyGreen website, March 29, 2012, http://www.mindbodygreen.com/0-4369/7-Health-Benefits-of-Going-Barefoot -Outside.html.

40. L. Taruffi and S. Koelsch, "The Paradox of Music-Evoked Sadness: An Online Survey," *PLOS ONE* 9, no. 10 (October 20, 2014): e110490, doi: 10.1371/journal.pone.0110490.

41. Y. H. Liu et al., "Effects of Music Listening on Stress, Anxiety, and Sleep Quality for Sleep-Disturbed Pregnant Women," *Women & Health* 56, no. 3 (2016): 296–311, doi: 10.1080/03630242.2015.1088116.

42. T. Bradberry, "How Complaining Rewires Your Brain for Negativity," *HuffPost* (blog), December 26, 2016, http://www.huffingtonpost.com/dr-travis-bradberry/how -complaining-rewires-y_b_13634470.html.

43. "Can You Catch Depression? Being Surrounded by Gloomy People Can Make You Prone to Illness," DailyMail.com, April 19, 2013, http://www.dailymail.co.uk/health/article -2311523/Can-CATCH-depression-Being-surrounded-gloomy-people-make-prone -illness-say-scientists.html.

44. R. T. Howell et al., "Momentary Happiness: The Role of Psychological Need Satisfaction," *Journal of Happiness Studies* 12, no. 1 (March 2011): 1–15.

45. C. Gregoire, "Older People Are Happier Than You. Why?" *Huffington Post*, posted on CNN website, April 24, 2015, http://www.cnn.com/2015/04/24/health/old-people-happy/.

46. M. Mela et al., "The Influence of a Learning to Forgive Programme on Negative Affect among Mentally Disordered Offenders," *Criminal Behaviour and Mental Health* 27, no. 2 (April 2017): 162–75, doi: 10.1002/cbm.1991.

47. L. Bolier et al., "Positive Psychology Interventions: A Meta Analysis of Randomized Controlled Studies," *BMC Public Health* 13 (February 8, 2013): 119, doi: 10.1186/1471-2458-13-119.

48. P. Bentley, "What Really Makes Us Happy? How Spending Time with Your Friends Is Better for You Than Being with Family," DailyMail.com, June 30, 2013, http://www.dailymail.co.uk/news/article-2351870/What-really-makes-happy-How-spending-time-friends-better-family.html.

49. D. G. Blanchflower and A. J. Oswald, "Money, Sex and Happiness: An Empirical Study," *Scandinavian Journal of Economics* 106, no. 3 (2004): 393–415, doi: 10.3386/w10499.

50. M. Purcell, "The Health Benefits of Journaling," PsychCentral website, accessed April 30, 2018, http://psychcentral.com/lib/the-health-benefits-of-journaling/.

APPENDIX C

1. "Cancers Associated with Overweight and Obesity Make Up 40 Percent of Cancers Diagnosed in the United States," Centers for Disease Control and Prevention website, October 3, 2017, https://www.cdc.gov/media/releases/2017/p1003-vs-cancer-obesity.html.

2. G. Kolata, "Under New Guidelines, Millions More Americans Will Need to Lower Blood Pressure," *New York Times*, November 13, 2017, https://www.nytimes.com/2017/11/13/health/blood-pressure-treatment-guidelines.html?_r=0; S. Scutti, "Nearly Half of Americans Now Have High Blood Pressure, Based on New Guidelines," CNN website, November 14, 2017, https://www.cnn.com/2017/11/13/health/new-blood-pressure-guidelines/index.html.

3. P. K. Elias et al., "Serum Cholesterol and Cognitive Performance in the Framingham Heart Study," *Psychosomatic Medicine* 67, no. 1 (January–February 2005): 24–30, doi: 10.1097/01.psy.0000151745.67285.c2.

4. M. M. Mielke et al., "High Total Cholesterol Levels in Late Life Associated with a Reduced Risk of Dementia," *Neurology* 64, no. 10 (May 24, 2005): 1689–95, doi: 10.1212/01.WNL.0000161870.78572.A5; A. W. Weverling-Rijnsburger et al., "Total Cholesterol and Risk of Mortality in the Oldest Old," *Lancet* 350, no. 9085 (October 18, 1997): 1119–23.

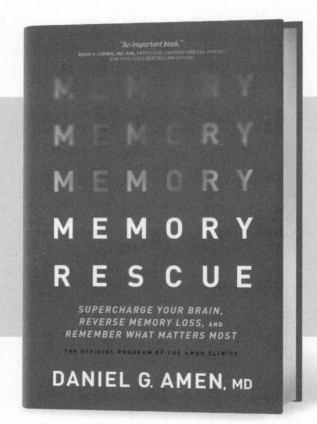

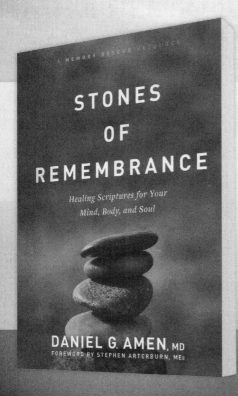

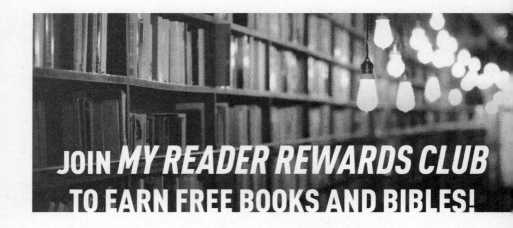
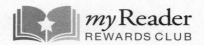